Lippincott's Illustrated Q&A Review of

Biochemistry

Michael A. Lieberman
Distinguished Teaching Professor
Department of Molecular Genetics,
Biochemistry, and Microbiology
University of Cincinnati College of Medicine
Cincinnati, Ohio

Rick Ricer
Professor Emeritus
Department of Family Medicine
University of Cincinnati College of Medicine
Cincinnati, Ohio

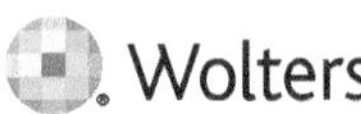
Wolters Kluwer | Lippincott Williams & Wilkins
Health

Philadelphia • Baltimore • New York • London
Buenos Aires • Hong Kong • Sydney • Tokyo

Acquisitions Editor: Charles W. Mitchell
Managing Editor: Kelley A. Squazzo
Marketing Manager: Jennifer Kuklinski
Designer: Doug Smock
Compositor: SPI Technologies

First Edition

351 West Camden Street
Baltimore, MD 21201

530 Walnut Street
Philadelphia, PA 19106

Printed in the United States of America.

Library of Congress Cataloging-in-Publication Data

Lieberman, Michael, 1950–
Lippincott's illustrated Q & A review of biochemistry / Michael A. Lieberman, Rick Ricer.—1st ed.
p. ; cm.
Includes index.
ISBN 978-1-60547-302-4
1. Clinical biochemistry—Examinations, questions, etc. 2. Biochemistry—Examinations, questions, etc. I. Ricer, Rick E. II. Title. III. Title: Lippincott's illustrated Q and A review of biochemistry. IV. Title: Illustrated Q & A review of biochemistry.
[DNLM: 1. Biochemistry—Examination Questions. QU 18.2 L695L2010]
RB112.5.L54 2010
616.07076—dc22 2009023149

To purchase additional copies of this book, call our customer service department at (800) 638–3030 or fax orders to (301) 223–2320. International customers should call (301) 223–2300.

Visit Lippincott Williams & Wilkins on the Internet: http://www.LWW.com. Lippincott Williams & Wilkins customer service representatives are available from 8:30 am to 6:00 pm, EST.

9 8 7

Preface and Acknowledgments

The molecular basis of disease is best understood through a thorough comprehension of biochemistry and molecular biology. Diseases alter the normal flow of metabolites through biochemical pathways, and treatment of disease is aimed toward restoring this normal flow. Why should an inability to metabolize phenylalanine lead to neuronal damage? Why is an inability to transmit the insulin signal so detrimental to long-term survival? Why is obesity linked to heart disease and diabetes? Understanding biochemistry provides insights into understanding the human body, which is the basis of medicine. Understanding biochemistry allows the student to recognize how a basic pathway has malfunctioned, to think through the pathophysiology results and treatment possibilities, to rationally differentiate pharmacotherapeutic treatment, and to understand and predict the unwanted side effects of pharmaceuticals. All of these skills are critical to the practice of medicine. The questions in this book are geared toward allowing the student to learn and apply biochemical principles to disease states.

This book has been designed to present questions that take the student through the various aspects of biochemistry, starting with the basic chemical building blocks of the discipline through human genetics and the biochemistry of cancer. The questions have been written such that students completing their second year of medical school should be able to answer them, although first year students can also use the book as they review biochemistry. Many of the questions were written in National Board format and require two levels of thought. The first is to determine a diagnosis from the information presented in the question, and the second is to understand the biochemistry behind the diagnosis. However, understanding biochemistry also requires an understanding of the vocabulary of the subject, and many of the online questions will test a student's understanding of the vocabulary.

All questions are written such that one best answer is required, and the explanations accompanying the questions are designed to reinforce the biochemistry underlying the question. As biochemistry is a cumulative subject, concepts learned in earlier chapters are required to aid in answering questions in later chapters. Working through the 630 questions associated with the book and online materials will enable a student to better master the relationship between biochemistry and medicine.

In a book of this nature, it is possible that certain questions will have mixed interpretations (twenty-five years of teaching medical students has definitely brought that point home to the authors). Any errors in the book are the sole responsibility of the authors, and they would like to be informed of such errors, or alternative interpretations, by the readers. Through this feedback, future printings of the book will reflect the correction of these errors.

The authors would like to thank the staff at LWW for their assistance in the preparation of this manuscript, particularly Ms Kelley Squazzo, for her patience with the authors as they struggled, at times, to write the perfect questions. We would also like to thank the reviewers of the manuscript for their excellent comments for improving the questions found in the text. Finally, the authors would also like to thank the many classes of medical students whom they have taught for their feedback on the questions we have used to evaluate them as they progressed through their first year of medical school. This feedback has proved to be invaluable to the authors as they continually assess and modify their evaluation methods every year.

Contents

Chapter 1

Biochemical Compounds

This chapter is designed to have the student think about the basic building blocks of biochemical compounds, such as amino acids, which lead to proteins; nitrogenous bases, which lead to nucleosides, nucleotides, and nucleic acids; and fatty acids, which lead to phospholipids. The student will also consider the biochemical function of intracellular compartmentation in eukaryotes, such as the nucleus, endoplasmic reticulum, Golgi apparatus, lysosome, mitochondria, peroxisome, and membranes. As this is a building block chapter, the references to disease are sparse but will increase in later chapters of this book.

QUESTIONS

Select the single best answer.

1 The procedure of Southern blotting involves treatment of the solid support (nitrocellulose) containing the DNA with NaOH to denature the double helix. Treatment of a Northern blot with NaOH, however, will lead to the hydrolysis of the nucleic acid on the filter paper. This is due to which major chemical feature of the nucleic acids involved in a Northern blot?

(A) The presence of thymine
(B) The presence of uracil
(C) The presence of a 2′-hydroxyl group
(D) The presence of a 3′-hydroxyl group
(E) The presence of a 3′–5′ phosphodiester linkage

2 A 6-month-old infant, with a history of chronic diarrhea and multiple pneumonias, is seen again by the pediatrician for a possible episode of pneumonia. The chest X-ray shows a pneumonia, but also reveals an abnormally small thymus. Blood work shows a distinct lack of circulating lymphocytes. The most likely inherited enzymatic defect in this child leads to an inability to alter a purine nucleotide at which position of the ring structure?

(A) 1
(B) 3
(C) 6
(D) 7
(E) 8

3 An African native who is going to college in the United States experiences digestive problems (bloating, diarrhea, and flatulence) whenever she eats foods containing milk products. She is most likely deficient in splitting which type of chemical bond?

(A) A sugar bond
(B) An ester linkage
(C) A phosphodiester bond
(D) An amide bond
(E) A glycosidic bond

4 Consider the amino acid shown below. The configuration about which atom (labeled A through E) will determine whether the amino acid is in the D or L configuration?

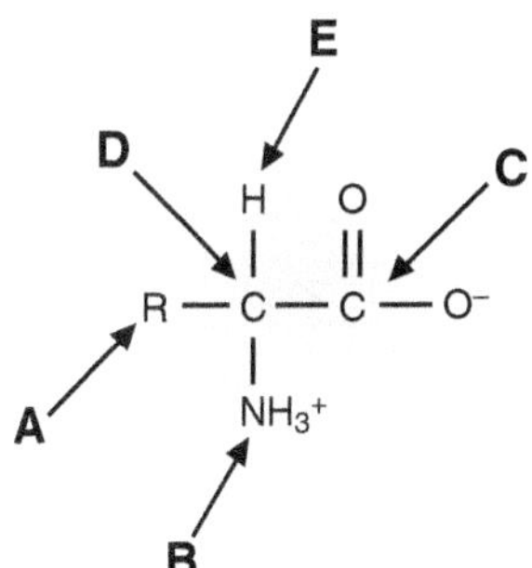

5 Your patient has a mechanical heart valve and is chronically anemic due to damage to red blood cells as they pass through this valve. One of the signals that target damaged red blood cells for removal from the circulation is the presence of phosphatidylserine in the outer leaflet of the red cell membrane. Phosphatidylserine is an integral part of cell membranes and is normally found in the inner leaflet of the red cell membrane. This flip-flop of phosphatidylserine between membrane

leaflets exposes which part of the phosphatidylserine to the environment?
(A) The head group
(B) Fatty acids
(C) Sphingosine
(D) Glycerol
(E) Ceramide

6 Which of the following is the type of bond that allows nucleotides to form long polymers?

A $R-C(=O)-N(H)-R'$

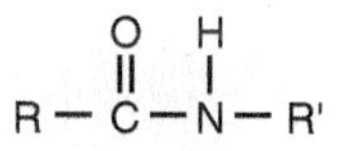

B $R-C(=O)-O-R'$

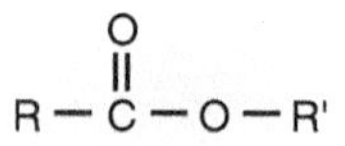

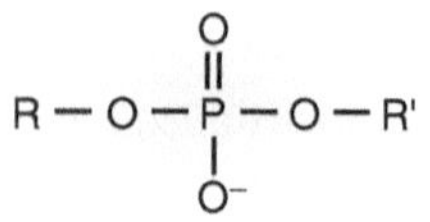

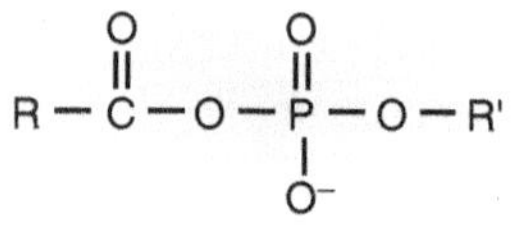

C $R-O-P(=O)(O^-)-O-R'$

D $R-C(=O)-O-P(=O)(O^-)-O-R'$

E $R-O-R'$

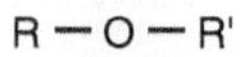

7 A couple has had five children, all of who exhibit short stature, eyelid droop, and some degree of muscle weakness and hearing loss (some severe, some mild). The mother also has such problems, although at a mild level. The father has no symptoms. The mutation that afflicts the children most likely resides in DNA found in which intracellular organelle?
(A) Mitochondria
(B) Peroxisome
(C) Lysosome
(D) Endoplasmic reticulum
(E) Nucleus

8 Lysosomal enzymes have a pH optimum between 4 and 6. The intralysosomal contents are kept at this pH by which of the following mechanisms?
(A) The active pumping of protons out of the organelle
(B) The free diffusion of protons out of the organelle
(C) The active pumping of protons into the organelle
(D) The free diffusion of protons into the organelle
(E) The synthesis of carboxylic acids within the lysosome

9 A type 1 diabetic is brought to the emergency department due to lethargy and rapid breathing. Blood measurements indicated elevated levels of glucose and ketone bodies. Blood pH was 7.1. The patient was exhibiting enhanced breathing to exhale which one of the following gases in order to correct the abnormal blood pH?
(A) Oxygen
(B) Nitrogen
(C) Nitrous oxide
(D) Carbon dioxide
(E) Superoxide

10 The protein albumin is a major buffer of the pH in the blood, which is normally kept between 7.2 and 7.4. Which of the following is an amino acid side chain of albumin that participates in this buffering range?
(A) Histidine
(B) Aspartate
(C) Glutamate
(D) Lysine
(E) Arginine

11 Consider the following structure:

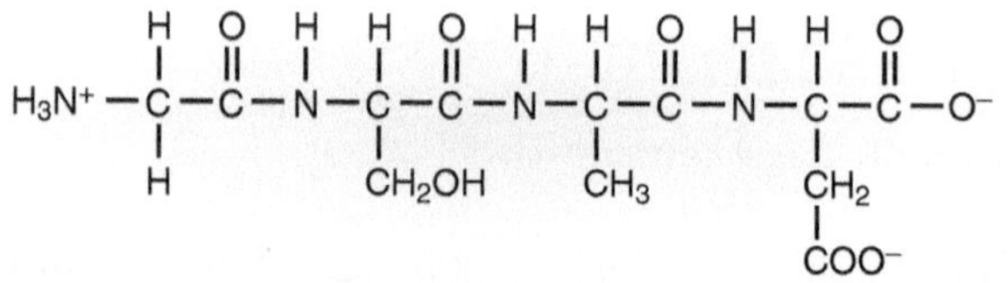

$$H_3N^+-CH_2-C(=O)-NH-CH(CH_2OH)-C(=O)-NH-CH(CH_3)-C(=O)-NH-CH(CH_2COO^-)-C(=O)-O^-$$

This structure is best described as which of the following?
(A) An amino acid
(B) A tripeptide
(C) A tetrapeptide
(D) A lipid
(E) A carbohydrate

12 A drug contains one ionizable group, a weak base with a pK_a of 9.0. The drug enters cells via free diffusion through the membrane in its uncharged form. This will occur most readily at which of the following pH values?
(A) 3.5
(B) 5.5
(C) 7.0
(D) 7.6
(E) 9.2

13 Consider the five functional groups shown below.

(i) $R-NH_2$

(ii) $R-C(=O)-OH$

(iii) $R-OH$

(iv) $R-CH_3$

(v) $R-CH=CH_2$

A hydrogen bond would form between which pair of groups?
(A) iii and iv
(B) iii and v
(C) ii and iv
(D) ii and iii
(E) i and v

14 Water is the universal solvent for biological systems. Compared to ethanol, for example, water has a relatively high boiling point and high freezing point. This is due primarily to which one of the following properties of water?
(A) Its hydrophobic effect
(B) Ionic interactions between water molecules
(C) The pH
(D) Hydrogen bonds between water molecules
(E) Van der Waals interactions

15 Membrane formation occurs, in part, due to low lipid solubility in water due to primarily which of the following?
(A) Hydrogen bond formation between lipids and water
(B) Covalent bond formation between lipids and water
(C) A decrease in water entropy
(D) An increase in water entropy
(E) Ionic bond formation between lipids and water

16 A 47-year-old woman visits the emergency department due to severe pain in the metatarsophalangeal (MTP) joint of her right great toe. Upon examination, the toe is bright red, swollen, warm, and very sensitive to the touch. Analysis of joint fluid shows crystals. The patient is given indomethacin to reduce the severity of the symptoms. The crystals that are accumulating in this patient are most likely derived from which type of molecule?
(A) Purines
(B) Pyrimidines
(C) Nicotinamides
(D) Amino acids
(E) Fatty acids

17 A single-stranded DNA molecule contains 20%A, 25%T, 30%G, and 25%C. When the complement of this strand is synthesized, the T content of the resulting *duplex* will be which one of the following?
(A) 20%
(B) 22.5%
(C) 25%
(D) 27.5%
(E) 30%

18 The activated form of the drug omeprazole (used to treat peptic ulcer disease) prevents acid secretion by forming a covalent bond with the H^+, K^+-ATPase, thereby inhibiting the enzyme's transport capabilities. Analysis of the drug-treated protein demonstrated that an internal cysteine residue was involved in the covalent interaction with the drug. Further analysis indicated that the bond was not susceptible to acid or base catalyzed hydrolysis. Based on this information, one would expect the drug to contain which of the following functional groups that would be critical for its inhibitory action?
(A) A carboxylic acid
(B) A free primary amino group
(C) An imidazole group
(D) A reactive sulfhydryl group
(E) A phosphate group

19 Your diabetic patient has a hemoglobin A1c (HbA1c) of 8.8. HbA1c differs from unmodified hemoglobin by which one of the following?
(A) Amino acid sequence
(B) Serine acylation
(C) Valine glycosylation
(D) Intracellular location
(E) Rate of degradation

20 Liver catabolism of xenobiotic compounds, such as acetaminophen (Tylenol), is geared toward increasing the solubility of such compounds for safe excretion from the body. This can occur via the addition of which compound below in a covalent linkage with the xenobiotic?
(A) Phenylalanine
(B) Palmitate
(C) Linoleate
(D) Glucuronate
(E) Cholesterol

ANSWERS

1 **The answer is C: The presence of a 2′-hydroxyl group.** RNA is susceptible to alkaline hydrolysis, whereas DNA is not. The major difference between the two polynucleotides is the presence of a 2′-hydroxyl group on the sugar ribose in RNA, versus its absence in deoxyribose, a component of DNA. Under alkaline conditions, the hydroxyl group can act as a nucleophile and attack the phosphodiester linkage between adjacent nucleotides, breaking the linkage and leading to the transient formation of a cyclic nucleotide. As this can occur at every phosphodiester linkage in RNA, hydrolysis of the RNA will occur due to these reactions. As DNA lacks the 2′-hydroxyl group, this reaction cannot occur, and DNA is very stable under alkaline conditions. The fact that DNA contains thymine, and RNA uracil (both true statements) does not address the base stability of DNA as compared to RNA. Both DNA and RNA contain 3′-hydroxyl groups, which are usually in 3′–5′ phosphodiester bonds in the DNA backbone. The procedure of Southern blotting is used in the diagnosis of various disorders, including some instances of hemoglobinopathies and diseases induced by triplet-repeat expansions of DNA (such as myotonic dystrophy).

2 **The answer is C: 6.** The child is exhibiting the symptoms of adenosine deaminase deficiency, an inherited immunodeficiency syndrome that is a cause of severe combined immunodeficiency. The disease is caused by the lack of adenosine deaminase (a gene found on chromosome 20), which converts adenosine to inosine (part of the salvage and degradative pathway of adenosine, see the figure below). This disorder leads to an accumulation of deoxyadenosine and S-adenosylhomocysteine, which are toxic to immature lymphocytes in the thymus. As indicated in the figure below, the amino group at position 6 is deaminated and is replaced by a double-bond oxygen, to produce the base hypoxanthine, and the nucleoside inosine. The same type of reaction occurs in tRNA anticodons, in which a 5′ position adenine is converted to hypoxanthine, to produce the nucleoside inosine. Inosine is a wobble base pair former, having the ability to base pair with adenine, uracil, or cytosine.

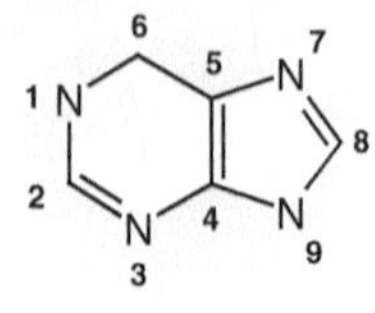

Numbering of the purine ring

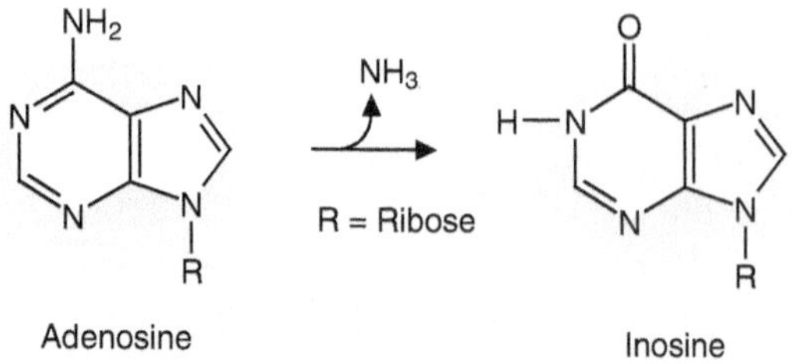

NH_2 | NH_3 | R = Ribose | O

Adenosine | Inosine

Adenosine deaminase reaction

3 **The answer is E: A glycosidic bond.** The patient is exhibiting the classic signs of lactose intolerance, in which intestinal lactase levels are low, and the major dietary component of milk products (lactose) cannot be digested. Lactase will split the β-1,4 linkage between galactose and glucose in lactose. The lactose thus passes unmetabolized to the bacteria inhabiting the gut, and their metabolism of the disaccharide leads to the observed symptoms. Combining two sugars in a dehydration reaction creates a glycosidic bond. Adding a sugar to the nitrogen of a nitrogenous base also creates an *N*-glycosidic bond. A sugar bond is not an applicable term in biochemistry. Ester linkages contain an oxygen linked to a carbonyl group. A phosphodiester bond is a phosphate in two ester linkages with two different compounds (such as the 3′–5′ link in the sugar phosphate backbone of DNA and RNA). An amide bond is the joining of an amino group with a carboxylic acid with the loss of water. These types of bonds are shown below.

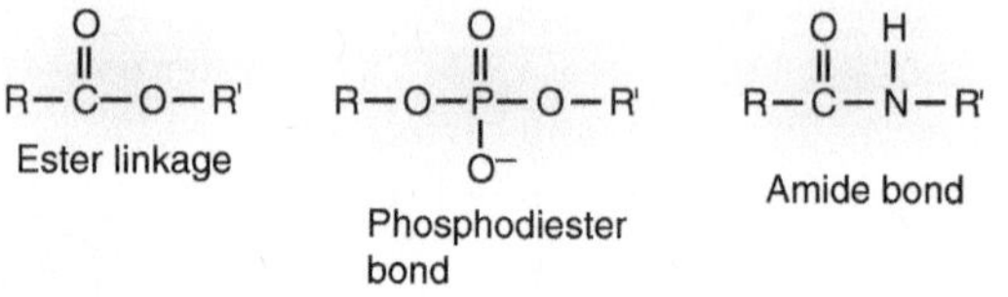

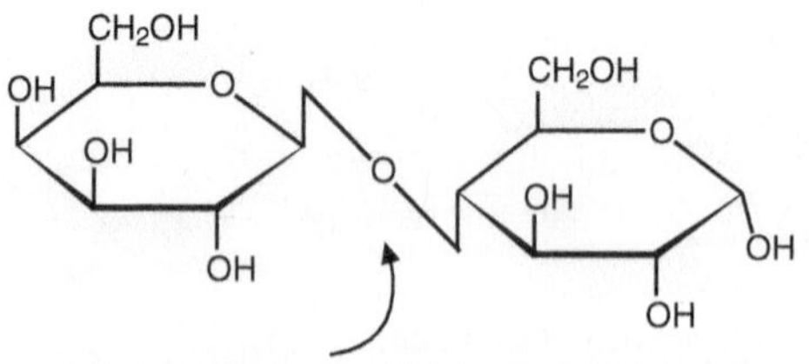

R–C(=O)–O–R′ Ester linkage | R–O–P(=O)(O⁻)–O–R′ Phosphodiester bond | R–C(=O)–N(H)–R′ Amide bond

A β-glycosidic bond, which is cleaved by lactase

4 **The answer is D.** The central (or α) carbon of amino acids has four different substituents (as long as R is not H, in which case the amino acid is glycine). Due to having four different substituents, this is considered an asymmetric carbon, and the orientation of the substituents around this carbon can be in either the D or L configuration. None of the other choices refer to an asymmetric carbon atom. Many biochemical compounds (including drugs) are only active as either the D or L isomer. Fenfluramine, an appetite suppressant, in only active in its D form; in its L form it induces drowsiness.

5 **The answer is A: The head group.** Phospholipids contain a very hydrophobic backbone and a "head group" that is primarily hydrophilic. The hydrophobic portion of the phospholipid remains embedded in the membrane while the hydrophilic head group faces the aqueous environment of the cell. As seen in the figure below, the glycerol portion (or ceramide portion, which contains sphingosine) of the phospholipid, as well as the fatty acids, remains embedded in the membrane while only the head group (R) faces the aqueous environment. Thus, when a phospholipid flip-flops across the membrane, the head group will always end up facing the aqueous environment.

Aqueous phase

Interior of membrane bilayer

6 **The answer is C.** A phosphodiester bond links nucleotides in nucleic acids. Answer A is an amide bond (the type found linking amino acids together in proteins). Answer B is an ester linkage (the type found in triacylglycerol, in which fatty acids are attached to a glycerol backbone). Answer D is a phosphoanhydride bond (similar to that found at the 1 position of 1,3 bisphosphoglycerate), and answer E is an ether linkage (found in ether lipids, for example).

7 **The answer is A: Mitochondria.** The mother and children are experiencing the effects of a mitochondrial disorder. Eukaryotic cells actually have two genomes; one in the nucleus, and another in the mitochondria. The mitochondrial genome codes for a small number of proteins which are found in the mitochondria. In order to make these proteins the mitochondria also synthesize their own tRNA molecules. As only the mother transmits mitochondria to her children, mitochondrial diseases display a unique inheritance pattern. None of the other organelles listed, other than the nucleus, contain DNA, and these symptoms and inheritance pattern are not consistent with a mutation in nuclear DNA. The mitochondrial genome is 15,569 base pairs in size, encoding 37 genes. These genes include two different molecules of rRNA, 22 different tRNA molecules, and 13 polypeptides (seven subunits of NADH dehydrogenase, or complex I, three subunits of cytochrome *c* oxidase, or complex IV, two subunits of the proton translocating ATP synthase, and cytochrome *b*). There are multiple mitochondrial disorders associated with muscular dystrophy, including Kearns–Sayer syndrome (this case), Leigh syndrome (non-X-linked), Pearson syndrome, mitochondrial DNA depletion syndrome, and mitochondrial encephalomyopathy.

8 **The answer is C: The active pumping of protons into the organelle.** Lysosomal membranes contain an enzyme which actively pumps protons into the organelle, thereby maintaining a low intraorganelle pH. This enzyme is the proton-translocating ATPase, as ATP hydrolysis provides the energy to pump protons against their concentration gradient. The removal of protons from the lysosome would raise pH, not lower it (thereby rendering answers A and B incorrect). Free diffusion of protons would not allow uptake of protons against a concentration gradient, as diffusion is the flow from a higher concentration to a lower concentration. Since the cytoplasmic pH is in the range of 7.2, if protons were freely diffusible across the lysosomal membrane, the protons would leave the lysosomes and enter the cytoplasm. The lysosomes do not synthesize large amounts of carboxylic acids (a weak acid) in order to lower the pH inside the organelle.

9 **The answer is D: Carbon dioxide.** The patient is in the midst of diabetic ketoacidosis, in which the production, but nonuse, of ketone bodies (which are acids) results in a significant lowering of blood pH. This patient will be creating a respiratory alkalosis to attempt to compensate for a metabolic acidosis. Under conditions of an acidosis, the proton concentration of the blood needs to be reduced. Due to the presence of carbonic anhydrase in the red blood cell, as carbon dioxide is exhaled, protons are removed from solution. As the concentration of carbon dioxide is reduced, bicarbonate (HCO_3^-) reacts with a proton (H^+) to form carbonic acid, which then dissociates to form water (H_2O) and carbon dioxide (CO_2). These reactions are summarized in the figure below. Thus, as carbon dioxide is exhaled, the proton concentration decreases, and the acidosis is reduced. The exhalation of oxygen or nitrogen will not affect the proton levels in the blood, nor will the loss of nitrous oxide or superoxide.

$$CO_2 + H_2O \rightleftharpoons H_2CO_3 \rightleftharpoons H^+ + HCO_3^-$$

As the concentration of carbon dioxide decreases, the equilibrium is shifted to the left, thereby also decreasing the proton concentration, resulting in a rise in pH.

10 **The answer is A: Histidine.** Of the amino acid choices listed only histidine has a side chain which could conceivably buffer in the range of 7.2 to 7.4. The imidazole group of histidine has a pK_a of 6.0, but this can be altered by the local environment of the protein. Aspartic acid and glutamic acid have side chain carboxylic acids,

each of which has a pK_a about 4.0 and would not be able to contribute to buffering at neutral pH. Both lysine and arginine have basic side chains, with pK_a values about 9.5, and those too will not be able to buffer near neutral pH.

11 **The answer is C: A tetrapeptide.** The structure consists of four amino acids linked by three peptide bonds, generating a tetrapeptide (the amino acids are glycine, serine, alanine, and aspartic acid). The structure contains no lipid or carbohydrate.

12 **The answer is E: 9.2.** With a pK_a of 9.0, the weak base needs to lose a proton to enter cells in its uncharged form (this base is most likely $-NH_3^+$ below pH 9.0, and $-NH_2$ above pH 9.0). Thus, the higher the pH, the greater the proportion of drug which is in its unionized form. At pH values less than 9.0, greater than 50% of the drug will be ionized, which will slow its entry into cells. At pH 9.2, less than 50% of the drug is ionized, and as the unionized form enters the cell, it will reduce the concentration of unionized drug in the circulation, thereby forcing a re-equilibration and generating more unionized drug. At the next highest pH value listed, 7.6, less than 8% of the drug is unionized, and the rate of transport would be much less than at pH 9.2.

13 **The answer is D: ii and iii.** Hydrogen bonds are formed when two electronegative atoms share a hydrogen. The atom which has a greater affinity for the hydrogen is known as the hydrogen bond donor, and the atom with the lesser affinity the hydrogen bond acceptor. Hydrogens linked to carbons never participate in hydrogen bonding, as the electrons in the bond are evenly shared by the hydrogen and the carbon. In the case of hydrogens bound to nitrogen, or oxygen, the electronegative atom has a higher affinity for the electrons, thereby allowing hydrogen to "bond" to another electronegative atom. Of the structures shown, structure i could be a hydrogen bond acceptor or donor, and the carbonyl group of structure ii could be a hydrogen bond acceptor. The hydroxyl group in structure iii can either be a donor or the oxygen can be an acceptor. Compounds iv and v will not participate in hydrogen bonding due to containing exclusively C–H bonds. Thus, of the choices listed, only compounds ii and iii would form a hydrogen bond, as indicated below.

R—O(*)—H ······ O(*)=C—R'
R—O ······ HO—C

* = Hydrogen bond acceptor

14 **The answer is D: Hydrogen bonds between water molecules.** Water exhibits its unique properties due to the extensive hydrogen bonding that can occur between water molecules, and due to the extremely high concentration of water (at 18 g/mol, 1 L of water contains 55 moles of water, for a concentration approximating 55 M). Water forms hydrogen bonds in a latticelike structure (see the figure below), which makes it difficult for water to leave and become gaseous (thus the high boiling point). As water movement is reduced due to low temperature, the lattice becomes a solid (ice), explaining the relatively high freezing point of water. The hydrophobic effect of water comes into play when a hydrophobic substance enters water; it does not apply to water itself. The concentration of water molecules, with a charge, is very small (at pH 7.0, there is 1×10^{-7} M H^+ and OH^- ions, out of a 55 M solution), so ionic interactions between water molecules are minimal and do not contribute to its high boiling and freezing points. The pH of the water refers to the concentration of protons, which will not affect the hydrogen bonding capacity of the water molecules. Van der Waals interactions do not play a role in the physical properties of water.

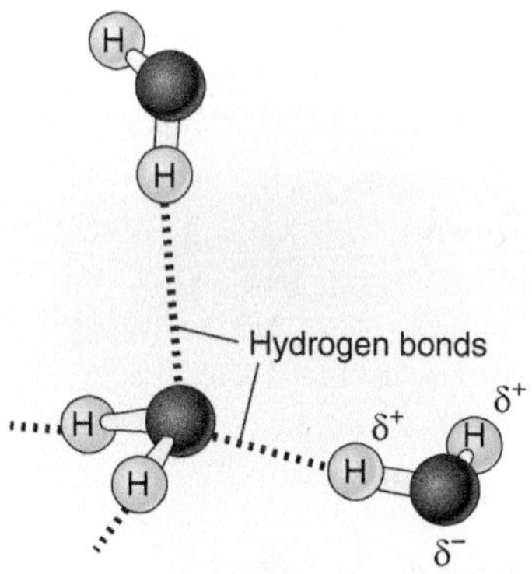

15 **The answer is D: An increase in water entropy.** Lipids are hydrophobic molecules which do not form hydrogen bonds with water. Due to this, water molecules will form a "cage" around the lipid molecules, surrounding them. Cage forming decreases water entropy, which is unfavorable, and this leads to the hydrophobic effect, in which the lipid molecules all come together such that only one large cage needs to be formed about the lipid molecules, rather than many small cages about each individual lipid molecule. The lipids do not form covalent or ionic bonds with water, and, as mentioned above, lipids in water leads to a decrease in water entropy (which is unfavorable), rather than an increase in the entropy of water (which would be a favorable event). The figure below shows a "cage" of water surrounding ten lipid molecules.

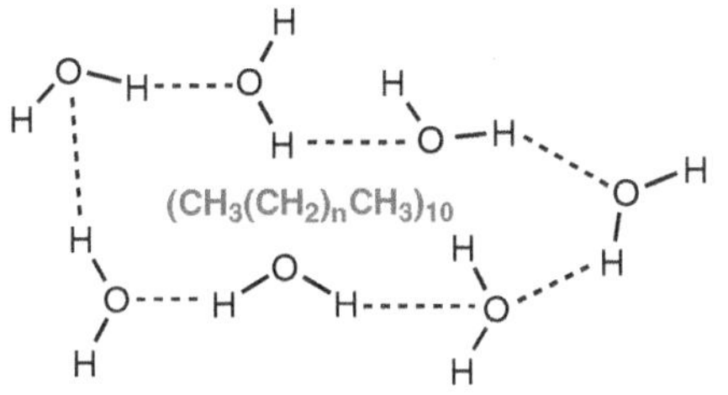

H
O—H·····O
H
H······O—H
O—H
(CH$_3$(CH$_2$)$_n$CH$_3$)$_{10}$
H H H
O···· H O H······O
H H

16 **The answer is A: Purines.** The patient is suffering from a gout attack due to the buildup of uric acid in the blood, and precipitation of uric acid in "cold" areas of the body, such as the great toe. Uric acid has the basic ring structure of the purines and is the degradative product of adenine and guanine. As shown in the figure below, the ring structure of uric acid is not at all similar to pyrimidines, nicotinamides (derived from the vitamin niacin), amino acids, or fatty acids.

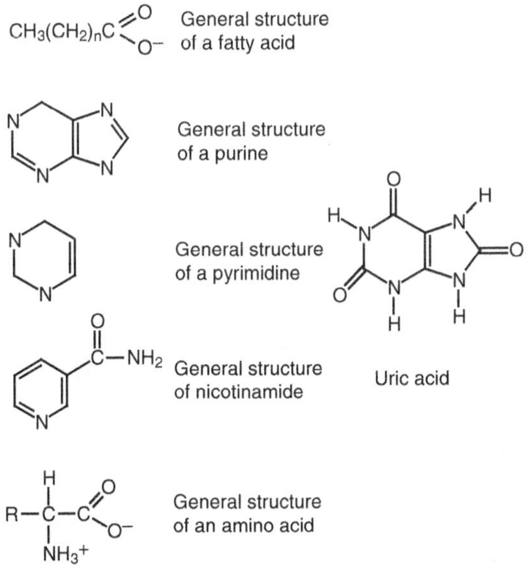

$CH_3(CH_2)_nCOO^-$ General structure of a fatty acid

General structure of a purine

General structure of a pyrimidine

Uric acid

General structure of nicotinamide

General structure of an amino acid

17 **The answer is B: 22.5%.** The given strand of DNA contains 25%T; the complementary strand will contain 20%T (this must be equivalent to the content of A in the given strand, since A and T base pair, and [A] = [T] in duplex DNA). For the entire duplex then, the T content is the average of 25% and 20%, or 22.5% for the duplex. The [A] in the duplex will also be 22.5% (again, since [A] = [T]), and the concentrations of [G] and [C] will each be 27.5% for the duplex.

18 **The answer is D: A reactive sulfhydryl group.** A free sulfhydryl group in the drug would be able to form a disulfide bond with the protein (-CH_2–S–S–CH_2), which is an oxidation reduction reaction. This would render the disulfide resistant to acid or base-catalyzed hydrolysis. Forming a bond with the other groups listed would lead to relatively easy hydrolysis reactions, rendering the inhibitory bond unstable. Since the inhibition is stable, the best choice is a sulfhydryl group. The drug is a proton pump inhibitor and reduces acid secretion by the chief cells in the stomach, thereby alleviating symptoms of acid reflux in the patient.

19 **The answer is C: Valine glycosylation.** HbA1c is glycosylated hemoglobin, reflecting the level of blood glucose over the lifetime of the erythrocyte (120 days). The higher the concentration of HbA1c, the more poorly controlled blood glucose levels are (normal is about 5.5% HbA1c). The glycosylation primarily occurs on the N-terminal valine residues of the β chains (which contain a free amino group). The amino acid sequences of hemoglobin and HbA1c are the same, there is no fatty acid addition (acylation) to the hemoglobin, the red cell contains no intracellular organelles for compartmentation to be an issue, and the rate of degradation of non-modified hemoglobin and HbA1c are the same.

20 **The answer is D: Glucuronate.** In order to make a xenobiotic more soluble, a hydrophilic group needs to be added to the xenobiotic. Of the possible answer choices, only glucuronic acid (glucose with a carboxylic acid at position 6 instead of an alcohol group) is a hydrophilic molecule. Glucuronic acid is added to the xenobiotic at position 1, using the activated intermediate UDPglucuronate. Once added to the xenobiotic, the highly soluble glucuronate confers enhanced solubility to the adduct. Phenylalanine contains a hydrophobic side chain, and palmitate, linoleate, and cholesterol are all very hydrophobic molecules. Their addition to a xenobiotic would decrease, rather than increase, its solubility.

Chapter 2

Protein Structure and Function

In this chapter, questions will cover various aspects of protein structure and function, including enzyme kinetics, the transport of molecules across cell membranes, various mechanisms of catalysis, the binding of oxygen to hemoglobin, and various diseases that result from altered protein folding. There will be a mixture of clinical and nonclinical questions seen in this chapter.

QUESTIONS

Select the single best answer.

1 A kinetic analysis of the effect of a drug on an enzyme's activity was performed, and the results shown below were obtained. The drug would be best classified as which one of the following?

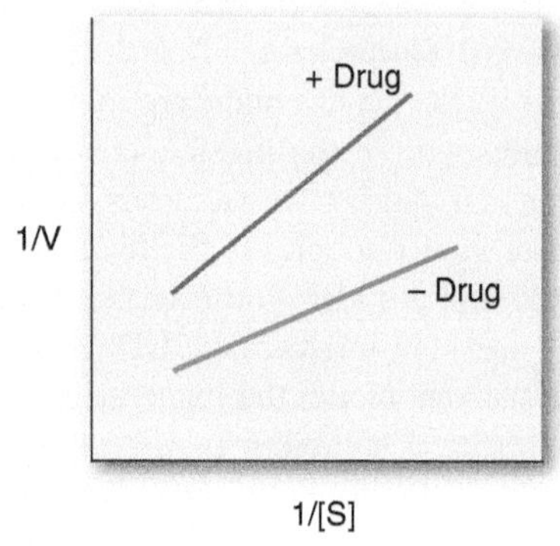

(A) A competitive inhibitor
(B) A noncompetitive inhibitor
(C) An uncompetitive inhibitor
(D) A competitive activator of the enzyme
(E) A noncompetitive activator of the enzyme

2 A critical histidine side chain in an enzyme's active site displays a pK_a value of 8.2. Which of the following best describes the local environment in which this histidine residue resides?

(A) A surface-associated domain
(B) A very hydrophobic environment
(C) A very polar environment
(D) Buried deep within the core of this globular protein
(E) Surrounded by phenylalanine, valine, and leucine residues

3 A major driving force for protein folding is the hydrophobic effect, in which hydrophobic amino acid side chains tend to cluster together, usually in the core of globular proteins. This occurs primarily due to which of the following?

(A) Increasing hydrogen bond formation
(B) Increasing the entropy of water
(C) Increasing disulfide bond formation
(D) Minimizing van der Waals interactions
(E) Reducing steric hindrance between amino acid side chains

4 A 7-year-old African American male is admitted to the hospital with severe abdominal pain. A blood workup indicated anemia, and an abnormal blood smear (see below). The molecular event triggering this disease is which of the following?

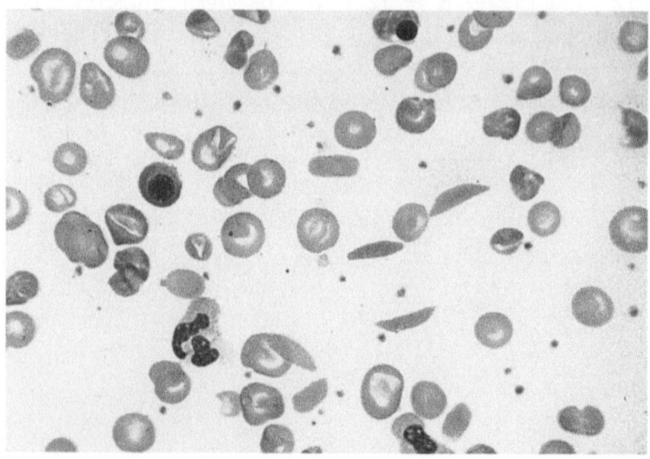

(A) A loss of quaternary structure of the hemoglobin molecule
(B) An increase in oxygen binding to hemoglobin
(C) A gain of ionic interactions, stabilizing the "T" form of hemoglobin
(D) An increase in hydrophobic interactions between deoxyhemoglobin molecules
(E) An alteration in hemoglobin secondary structure leading to loss of the "α" helix

5 A 56-year-old pathologist was taken to his family doctor by his son for he was showing mood changes, minor loss of memory, and decreased motor skills. During the patient history, it became clear that over the course of his career he had, on occasion, cut himself using the instruments he had been using on the cadavers he had been working on. A potential explanation for his symptoms is abnormal aggregation of which of the following proteins?

(A) Hemoglobin in the red blood cells
(B) Fibrillin in the extracellular compartments of the brain
(C) A truncated neuronal protein
(D) A misfolded form of a normal protein
(E) A truncated extracellular protein

6 A teenager, new to your practice, comes in for a routine physical exam. His family had just moved to the city, and the boy had rarely seen a doctor before. Upon examination, you notice a high, arched palate, disproportionately long arms and fingers, a sunken chest, and mild scoliosis. The patient has been complaining of lack of breath while doing routine chores, and upon listening to his heart, you detect an aortic regurgitation murmur. Careful examination of the eyes is indicated by the figure below. Based on your physical exam and history, you are suspicious of an inborn error of metabolism in which of the following proteins?

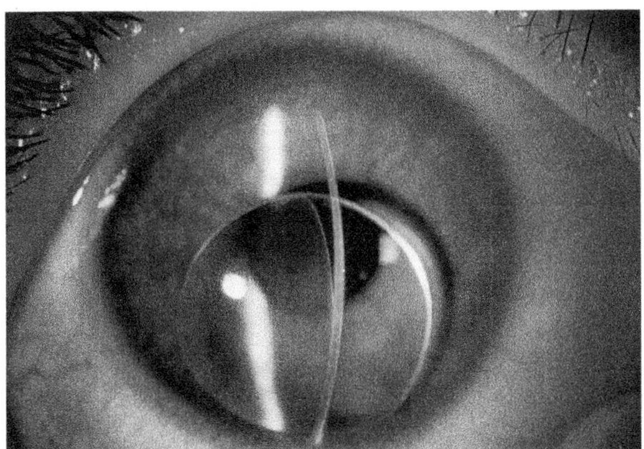

(A) Collagen
(B) Fibrillin
(C) Elastin
(D) Dystrophin
(E) β-catenin

7 While working an overnight shift in the emergency department you are called to see an 8-year-old boy who appears to have a fracture in his arm. Upon taking a history, you learn that this child has been to the ER multiple times for fractures, and the incidents that lead to the fracture would be described as mild trauma at best. X-rays indicate a number of healed fractures that the boy and his parents were unaware of (see example of arm X-ray below). Physical exam shows sky blue sclera. The parents then inform you that the child is taking bisphosphonates for his condition. The mechanism whereby the frequency of fractures is being reduced in this patient is which of the following?

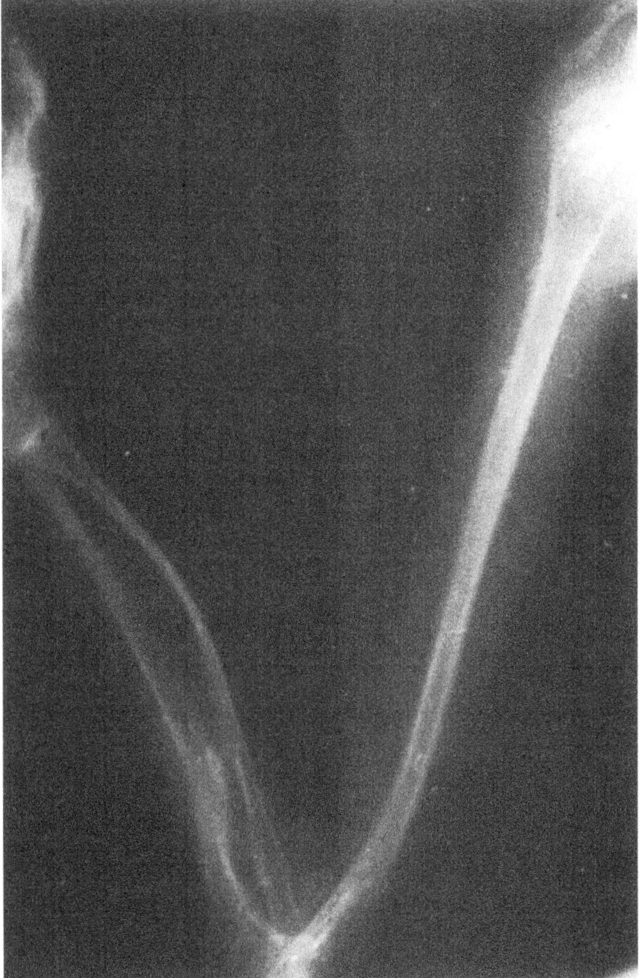

(A) Increased synthesis of collagen
(B) Increased resorption of collagen
(C) Decreased synthesis of collagen
(D) Decreased resorption of collagen
(E) Increased synthesis of fibrillin

8 You are visited by a 40-year-old female patient complaining of weight loss, numbness in the hands and

feet, fatigue, and difficulty swallowing. Physical exam notes an enlarged tongue, enlarged liver, a rubbery feeling around the joints, and bruising around the eyes. A bone marrow biopsy shows an abnormal staining of denatured protein (see below). These denatured proteins are most likely to be which of the following?

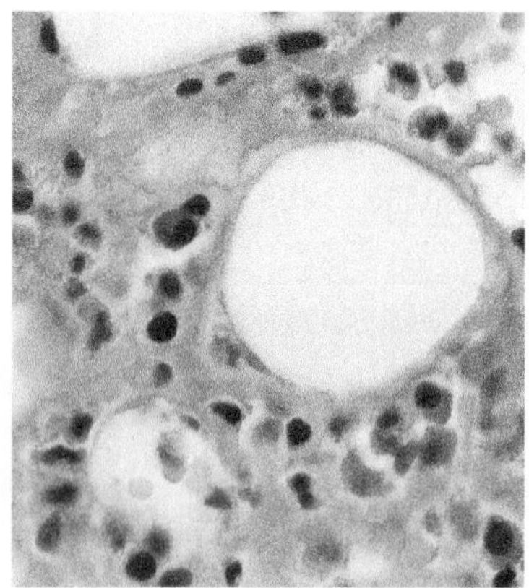

(A) Antibody light chains
(B) Collagen
(C) Fibrillin
(D) Albumin
(E) Transaminases

9 A family of four from New Jersey has embarked on a vacation in the Rocky Mountains. All four required a 24 to 48 h acclimation to the high altitude, as all were breathing at a rapid pace until the acclimation took effect. In addition to increasing the number of red blood cells in circulation, what other compensatory mechanism occurred within the red blood cell during this acclimation period?
(A) Increased synthesis of lactic acid
(B) Decreased synthesis of lactic acid
(C) Increased synthesis of 2,3-bisphosphoglycerate
(D) Decreased synthesis of 2,3-bisphosphoglycerate
(E) Decreased degradation of bilirubin, producing less carbon monoxide

10 In the 1800s, British sailors on long sea journeys developed sore and bleeding gums, sometimes to the point that their teeth would loosen and fall out. The introduction of limes to their diets helped to prevent these occurrences. The biochemical step that was lacking in these sailors was which of the following?
(A) Creating lysine cross-links in collagen
(B) Mobilization of calcium into bone
(C) Hydroxylation of proline residues in collagen
(D) Glycosylation of fibrillin
(E) Conversion of glycine to proline in collagen

11 A patient, who was recently diagnosed with cystic fibrosis, displays an increased blood clotting time. This is most likely due to which of the following?
(A) Lack of proline hydroxylation
(B) Inability to catalyze transaminations
(C) Lack of dolichol and an inability to glycosylate serum proteins
(D) Inability to carboxylate glutamic acid side chains
(E) Reduction in the synthesis of blood clotting factors due to lack of lipids for energy production

12 You order a hemoglobin electrophoresis on a patient suspected of having sickle cell disease. A blood sample was obtained and the red cells were isolated. Disruption of the red cells released the hemoglobin, which was run on a polyacrylamide gel. Following the electrophoresis, a Western blot was performed to locate the hemoglobin. The results of the Western blot are shown below. Which one of the following statements best represents the interpretation of the results?

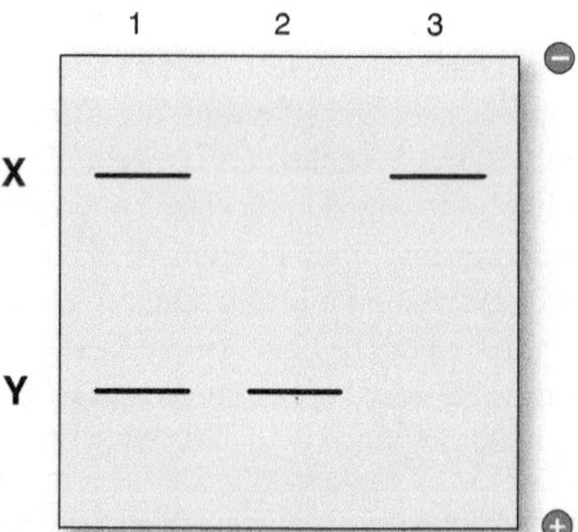

(A) The band marked as X refers to the wild-type hemoglobin protein
(B) The band in lane 2 represents an individual with sickle cell disease.
(C) A carrier of sickle cell disease is represented by the band in lane 3
(D) Lane 1 represents an individual with sickle cell disease
(E) Lane 3 represents an individual with sickle cell disease

13 Shown below is a section of a protein which forms a typical α-helix. In the form of an α-helix, a hydrogen bond would be formed between which two of the labeled atoms?

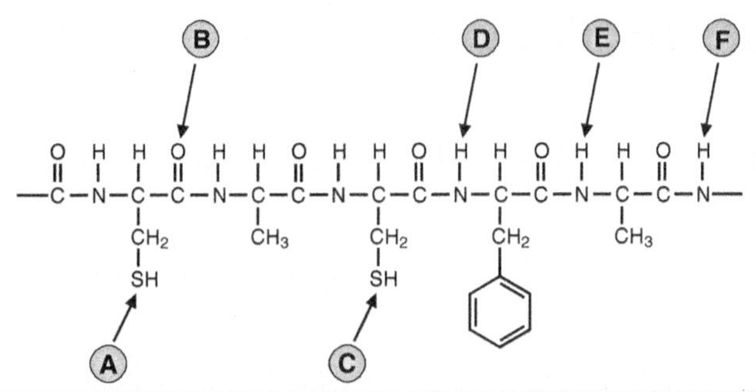

(A) A and C
(B) B and D
(C) B and E
(D) B and F
(E) D and F

14 A 37-year-old female has trouble keeping her eyes open and swallowing and is beginning to slur her speech. The patient has also noticed a weakness in her arms and legs. Treatment with edrophonium chloride results in a temporary relief of symptoms. The underlying etiology of this disorder involves auto-antibodies that do which of the following?
(A) Destroy acetylcholine
(B) Block acetylcholine receptors
(C) Inhibit acetylcholinesterase
(D) Inhibit acetylcholine synthesis
(E) Stimulate acetylcholine release into the synapse

15 You see a patient on an initial visit and are struck by the bluish coloring of the skin and mucous membranes. You ask the patient about this and you are told that it is a blood problem that the patient has had for his or her entire life. The patient's father had a similar condition, but not the mother. This condition could result from which one of the following changes within the erythrocyte?
(A) An increase of 2,3-bisphosphoglycerate in the erythrocyte
(B) An E to V mutation at position 6 of the β-chain of hemoglobin
(C) Increased oxidation of heme iron to the +3 state
(D) Enhanced oxygen binding to hemoglobin
(E) A mutated hemoglobin which no longer exhibited the Bohr effect

16 Many drugs function by acting as inhibitors of particular enzyme reactions. If an enzyme's V_{max} is 15 units/min/mg protein, with a K_m of 1.25 μM in the absence of inhibitor, but in the presence of 5 μM inhibitor the V_{max} is 6 units/min/mg protein, with the same K_m, what is the velocity of the reaction in the presence of 5 μM inhibitor at a substrate concentration of 2.50 μM?
(A) 2 units/min/mg protein
(B) 4 units/min/mg protein
(C) 6 units/min/mg protein
(D) 8 units/min/mg protein
(E) 10 units/min/mg protein

17 A 3-year-old boy is evaluated by the pediatrician as the child has trouble rising from a sitting position. Examination reveals calf hypertrophy and limb-girdle weakness. The inborn error in this patient is due to which of the following?
(A) Defective muscle mitochondria
(B) A mutation in the β-chain of hemoglobin
(C) A defect in the structure of the hepatocyte membrane
(D) A defect in the structure of the sarcolemma
(E) A defect in the transcription of muscle-specific genes

18 An 8-month-old infant exhibits jaundice and lethargy. Physical exam detects splenomegaly. Blood work displays a microcytic anemia with abnormal erythrocytes (see picture below) under all conditions. This defect is most likely due to a hereditary mutation in which of the following?

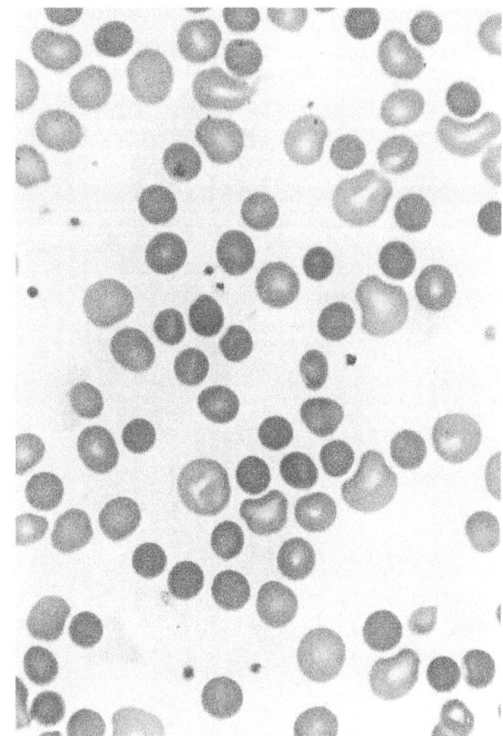

(A) Hemoglobin
(B) Glucose-6-phosphate dehydrogenase
(C) Iron transport into the erythrocyte
(D) Spectrin
(E) Methemoglobin reductase

19 A laboratory worker was working with a potent organophosphorus inhibitor of acetylcholinesterase in the lab when a drop of the inhibitor flew into his eye. This resulted in a pin-point pupil in that eye that was non-reactive and unresponsive to atropine. He eventually (over a period of weeks) recovered from this incident. The reason for the long recovery period is which of the following?

(A) Retraining of the ciliary muscles
(B) Regrowth of neurons which were damaged by the inhibitor
(C) Resynthesis of the inhibited enzyme
(D) Induction of enzymes which take the place of the inhibited enzyme
(E) Induction of proteases to reactivate the inhibited enzyme

20 A patient has midlife onset of the following symptoms: abnormal, involuntary jerking body movements, an unsteady gait, personality changes, and chewing and swallowing difficulty, which has led to a gradual weight loss. The patient's father had similar symptoms before his death at the age of 45. Cellular analysis indicated precipitated proteins in the nucleus. This disease has, at its origins, which biochemical problem?

(A) An exonic deletion
(B) A polyglutamine tract in an exon of the defective gene
(C) A nonsense mutation leading to the production of a truncated protein
(D) A splicing mutation, leading to the insertion of intronic sequences into the mature protein
(E) Production of an unstable mRNA, leading to reduced protein production

ANSWERS

1 **The answer is B: A noncompetitive inhibitor.** Analysis of the data indicates that in the presence of the inhibitor, the K_m of the enzyme is the same as in the absence of the inhibitor, but the V_{max} is significantly reduced (the extrapolated lines intersect on the x-axis). These characteristics are the hallmark of noncompetitive inhibition; the inhibitor binds to a site distinct from the substrate binding site and alters the protein's conformation such that activity is reduced, but not substrate binding. A competitive inhibitor would demonstrate an increased K_m, but an unaltered V_{max} (line intersection on the y-axis). Activation of the enzyme would either decrease the K_m or increase the V_{max}, or both. Uncompetitive inhibitors are very rare in pharmacology. Such an inhibitor alters both the K_m and V_{max} such that parallel lines are seen on double-reciprocal plots. The basic concept behind this question is critical for an understanding of how drugs alter enzyme activities (the basis for pharmacology).

2 **The answer is C: A very polar environment.** The normal pK_a for a histidine side chain is 6.0, meaning that at pH 6.0, 50% of the histidine side chains are protonated and 50% deprotonated. For the pK_a to be raised to 8.2, there must be an environment which stabilizes the protonated form of the side chain (because now one has to reach a pH of 8.2 before 50% of the histidine side chains have lost their proton). A polar environment would stabilize histidine holding on to its proton, as compared to a hydrophobic environment, which would promote side chain deprotonation at a low pH. The core of globular proteins is usually composed of hydrophobic amino acids (such as phenylalanine, valine, and leucine), and in that environment, one would expect the pK_a of the histidine side chain to be reduced. Surface-associated domains usually interact with water and are not where active sites are often found (it is too difficult to control the environment of the active site if water can freely enter the site). At a surface-associated domain, one would not expect much change in the histidine side chain pK_a. Many enzymes catalyze reactions based on the ability of amino acid side chains to accept or donate protons, which will be a function of the pK_a of the dissociable proton on the amino acid side chain.

3 **The answer is B: Increasing the entropy of water.** The tendency for hydrophobic side chains to cluster is driven by the entropy of water. Water will form a cage around hydrophobic molecules, which requires a decrease in water entropy. The decrease in entropy will be minimized, however, if water only has to form one large cage around a cluster of hydrophobic molecules, rather than a large number of small cages around separate hydrophobic molecules. Thus, the driving force for the hydrophobic side chains to cluster is to minimize their interactions with water and to allow water to maximize its entropy. It is not related to disulfide bond formation (cysteine is not a hydrophobic residue) nor to hydrogen bond formation of the side chains (hydrophobic side chains do not participate in hydrogen bonding). The clustering of hydrophobic side chains may increase van der Waals interactions (just by placing these residues in close proximity), but it will not necessarily minimize them. Steric hindrance between side chains occurs as a protein folds, as the negative van der Waals interactions will prevent side chains from interfering with each other and the overall protein structure. The polymerization of sickle-cell hemoglobin molecules is due to hydrophobic interactions between adjacent deoxygenated HbS molecules.

4 **The answer is D: An increase in hydrophobic interactions between deoxyhemoglobin molecules.** The boy is suffering from sickle cell anemia, which is due to a substitution of valine for glutamate at position 6 of the β-chain. This change, from a negatively charged amino acid side chain (glutamate) to a hydrophobic side chain (valine), allows deoxygenated hemoglobin to polymerize and form long rods within the red blood cell. Deoxygenated hemoglobin has a hydrophobic patch on its surface (created by A70, F85, and L88), which the valine in position 6 on another hemoglobin chain can associate with via hydrophobic interactions (this does not occur in normal hemoglobin as there is a charged glutamate residue at this position, which will not interact with a surface hydrophobic patch—see the figure below). The binding of hemoglobin molecules to

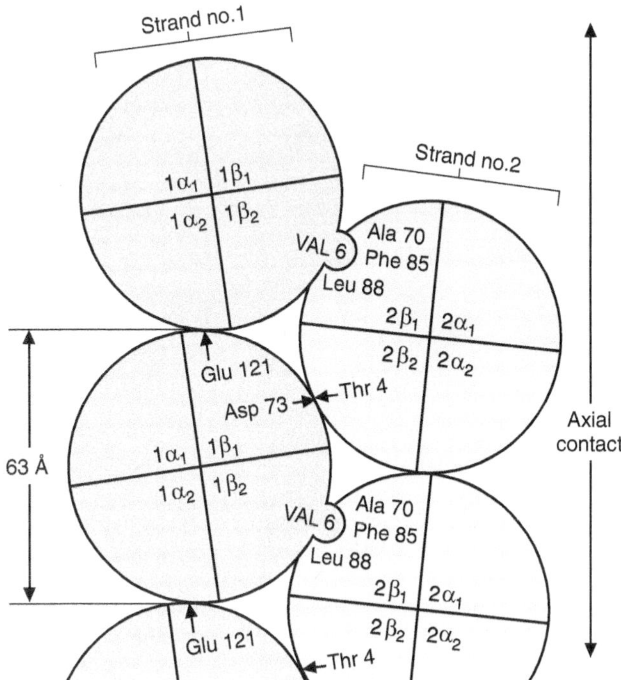

Hydrophobic interactions involved in deoxyhemoglobin S forming long polymers.

each other results in the polymerization. Oxygenated hemoglobin does not present a hydrophobic surface to other hemoglobin molecules, so polymerization is much less likely in the oxygenated state. The polymerization is not caused by a loss of quaternary structure, an increase in oxygen binding (which would actually reduce sickling), a gain of ionic interactions, or the loss of any α-helical structure in the final conformation of the protein.

5 **The answer is D: A misfolded form of a normal protein.** The pathologist is showing early clinical signs of Creutzfeldt–Jakob disease, caused by a misfolded prion protein, leading to protein aggregates in the brain. The initial seed for the aggregation was obtained from a cadaver that the pathologist was working on. Prions can exist in two states, the normal, nonaggregated form and an alternative conformation that is prone to aggregation (see differences in structure below, where PrP^c is the normal conformation, and PrP^{sc} is the abnormal structure). Once the alternative form reaches a critical concentration, aggregation ensues and shifts the equilibrium between the normal and abnormal forms to produce more abnormal form, feeding the aggregation. The prion is not a truncated neuronal protein (its primary structure can be the same in both forms of the protein), nor is it a truncated extracellular protein. This disorder is not due to alterations in hemoglobin or fibrillin. This patient will probably die within 1 year. There is no current treatment for the disease. As the disease progresses, he will probably develop blindness, involuntary movements, and severe deterioration of mental function.

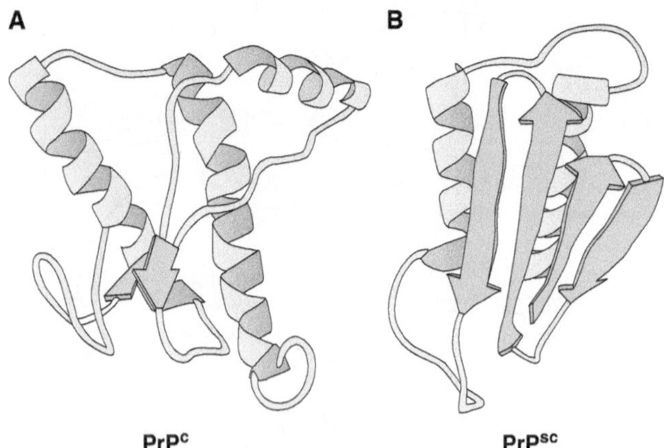

Note the difference in structure between PrP^c (normal; three major helices and two minor β-sheets) and PrP^{sc} (abnormal; four major β-sheets and two major helices). The abnormal form is much more prone to aggregate, due to the alterations in tertiary structure.

6 **The answer is B: Fibrillin.** The boy is showing the symptoms of Marfan syndrome, which is caused by mutations in fibrillin, an extracellular protein. Fibrillin helps to form, along with other proteins, microfibrils, which are present in elastic fibers (containing primarily elastin), which help to give various tissues their elastic properties. The exact mechanism whereby mutations in fibrillin lead to the symptoms of Marfan syndrome has yet to be established. Mutations in any of the other proteins listed do not give rise to Marfan's (although collagen defects give rise to osteogenesis imperfecta, and dystrophin mutations give rise to various forms of muscular dystrophy, depending on the type of mutation). Marfan's is an autosomal dominant disorder of connective tissue (not collagen). It is caused by mutations in the FBN1 gene (located on chromosome 15), which encodes fibrillin-1, a glycoprotein. The picture is of a dislocated lens, a classical finding in patients with Marfan's.

7 **The answer is D: Decreased resorption of collagen.** The patient has a form of osteogenesis imperfecta, which is due to a mutation in collagen, generating brittle bones. Mild trauma is sufficient to break the bones. Bisphosphonates decrease bone resorption by the osteoclasts, thereby strengthening the bone, even with the defective collagen molecule. Bisphosphonates do not affect the synthesis of collagen or fibrillin.

8 **The answer is A: Antibody light chains.** The patient is exhibiting the symptoms of primary amyloidosis, which is a protein folding disease in which immunoglobulin light chains are improperly processed and cannot be degraded. These proteins then form fibrils in tissues, which are insoluble. This disrupts the normal function of the tissue, and many tissues can accumulate these fibrils. Primary amyloidosis does not occur with abnormal deposits of collagen, fibrillin, albumin, or serum transaminases.

9 **The answer is C: Increased synthesis of 2,3-bisphosphoglycerate.** 2,3-bisphosphoglycerate (2,3-BPG) will bind to and stabilize the deoxygenated form of hemoglobin. Thus, if 2,3-BPG levels are increased, the binding of this molecule will aid in removing oxygen from hemoglobin in the tissues (where the concentration of oxygen is low) and therefore increase oxygen delivery to the tissues. In the lungs, where the oxygen concentration is high, the high levels of oxygen can overcome the effects of 2,3-BPG and bind to hemoglobin. Lactic acid levels do not directly affect oxygen binding (and lactate does not accumulate in the red cell), although changes in proton concentration (pH) can. Decreased pH will reduce oxygen binding to hemoglobin due to the Bohr effect. Bilirubin degradation, even though it does produce CO, does not effect oxygen binding to hemoglobin.

10 **The answer is C: Hydroxylation of proline residues in collagen.** Limes provided vitamin C, which is a required cofactor for prolyl hydroxylase, the enzyme which hydroxylates proline residues in collagen. Lysine cross-links in collagen do not require vitamin C (although lysine hydroxylation, for the purpose of glycosylation, does). Vitamin C does not affect calcium mobilization (that is vitamin D), and fibrillin is not the problem in vitamin C deficiency. Glycine residues in collagen cannot be converted to proline within the polypeptide.

11 **The answer is D: Inability to carboxylate glutamic acid side chains.** Cystic fibrosis patients have a thickening of the pancreatic duct, leading to nutrient malabsorption, as pancreatic enzymes have difficulty reaching the intestinal lumen. Lipid malabsorption syndromes frequently lead to deficiencies in fat-soluble vitamin uptake (vitamins E, D, K, and A). Vitamin K is required for the carboxylation of glutamic acid side chains on blood clotting proteins. This provides a means for these proteins to chelate calcium, and to bind to platelet surfaces. In the absence of gamma-carboxylation of glutamate, the clotting complexes cannot form, and a clotting disorder is observed. Vitamin C is required for proline hydroxylation, and as vitamin C is a water-soluble vitamin, lipid malabsorption does not affect vitamin C uptake. Transaminations require vitamin B_6, another water-soluble vitamin. Dolichol can be synthesized in the body, so its absorption is not an issue under these conditions. Endogenous fatty acids will provide energy for protein synthesis in individuals with lipid malabsorption problems.

12 **The answer is E: Lane 3 represents an individual with sickle cell disease.** The mutation in sickle cell disease is a valine for glutamate substitution at position 6 of the β-chain. This substitution removes a negative charge from the β-chain such that when the β-chain is migrated through an electric field it will not travel as far towards the positive pole as does the nonmutated protein. Thus, in the gel shown in the question, band X represents the hemoglobin S β-chain (since it does not migrate as far towards the positive pole), and band Y represents the nonmutated protein. The pattern shown in lane 1 is that of a carrier of HbS (one normal β-chain and one mutated β-chain). The pattern shown in lane 2 represents a person who does not carry a mutant allele (two normal alleles). Lane 3 represents someone with the disease (two mutant genes).

13 **The answer is C: B and E.** In a typical α-helix, there are 13 atoms between hydrogen bonds (formed between the carbonyl oxygen of one amino acid and the amide nitrogen of the amino acid four residues up in the chain). This is referred to as a 3.6/13 helix (3.6 amino acids per turn, with 13 atoms between hydrogen bonds). Other variants of the helix are 3/10 and 4.4/16. As shown below, in a linear fashion, are the hydrogen bonds formed in all three types of helices.

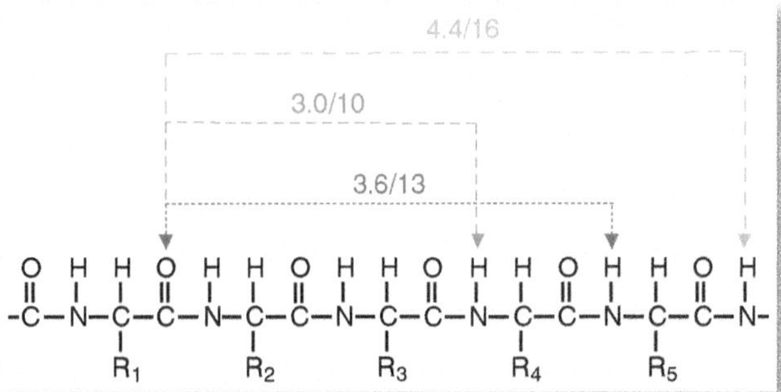

14 **The answer is B: Block acetylcholine receptors.** The patient has myasthenia gravis, in which she generates antibodies against the acetylcholine receptor. Treatment with edrophonium chloride leads to a transient increase in acetylcholine levels (through the temporary inactivation of acetylcholinesterase) such that acetylcholine can bind to receptors (via competition with the antibodies). Normal levels of acetylcholine are too low for such competition to be successful. This disorder does not generate antibodies which lead to acetylcholine destruction, inhibition of acetylcholinesterase, inhibition of acetylcholine synthesis, or release of acetylcholine at the synapse.

15 **The answer is C: Increased oxidation of heme iron to the +3 state.** The patient is exhibiting methemoglobinemia, in which an increased percentage of his hemoglobin has the iron in the +3 oxidation state (normal is +2), which is a form that cannot bind oxygen. This condition can arise by a variety of mutations within hemoglobin which lead to destabilization of the iron in the heme ring. The red blood cell contains methemoglobin reductase, which will reduce the iron back to the +2 state (using NADPH as the electron donor), and mutations within the reductase can also lead to this condition. An acquired form of methemoglobinemia can be caused by exposure to oxidizing drugs or toxins (aniline dyes, nitrates, nitrites, and lidocaine) which exceed the reduction capacity of the red blood cells. Surprisingly, the majority of patients with this syndrome show no ill effects, other than the bluish discoloration of certain tissues. Excessive 2,3-bisphosphoglycerate in the erythrocyte would lead to increased oxygen delivery to the tissues as 2,3-bisphosphoglycerate stabilizes the deoxygenated form of hemoglobin (as would a mutant hemoglobin with an enhanced ability to bind 2,3-BPG). The E to V mutation at position 6 of the β-chain of hemoglobin leads to sickle cell disease.

16 **The answer is B: 4 units/min/mg protein.** This is solved using the Michaelis–Menten equation, $v = V_{max}/(1 + [K_m/S])$. Under inhibited conditions V_{max} is 6 units/min/

mg protein, the K_m is 1.25 μM, and the substrate concentration is 2.50 μM. Plugging these numbers into the equation leads to a value of v of 4 units/min/mg protein.

17 **The answer is D: A defect in the structure of the sarcolemma.** The boy has Duchenne muscular dystrophy, which is due to mutations in the protein dystrophin, found in the muscle sarcolemma (plasma membrane). The lack of dystrophin alters the permeability properties of the plasma membrane, eventually leading to cell death. The disorder is not found in mitochondria, the liver, or in the β-chain of hemoglobin. This disease also does not alter gene transcription. As the muscles weaken, their function is compromised, leading to the complications of this form of muscular dystrophy.

18 **The answer is D: Spectrin.** The child is exhibiting the symptoms of hereditary spherocytosis, a defect in spectrin in the erythrocyte membrane. This membrane problem leads to an abnormal shape of the red blood cell, such that the spleen removes them from circulation (hence, the large spleen), leading to an anemia due to a reduction of red blood cells in circulation. This defect is not due to a loss of hemoglobin or glucose-6-phosphate dehydrogenase (a lack of glucose-6-phosphate dehydrogenase will lead to red cell damage and cell fragments on peripheral smear under oxidizing conditions, conditions not observed with this patient). A lack of iron in the erythrocyte can lead to an anemia (due to insufficient oxygen binding to hemoglobin and reduced oxygen delivery to the tissues), but it would not lead to an altered cell shape. A loss of methemoglobin reductase would lead to increased levels of methemoglobin, which cannot bind oxygen, but would also not lead to a cell shape change. The placement of spectrin in the red cell membrane is shown in the figure.

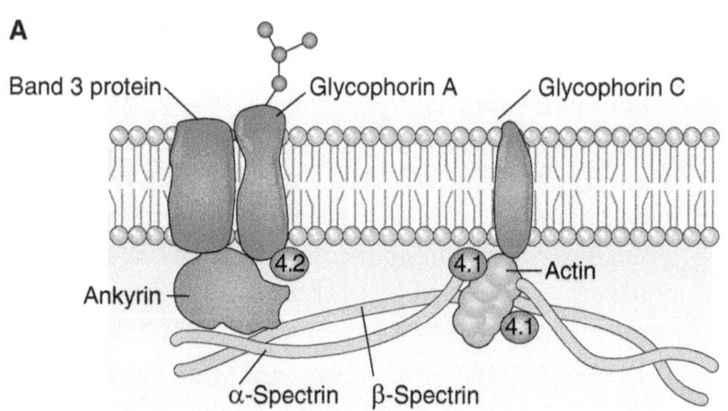

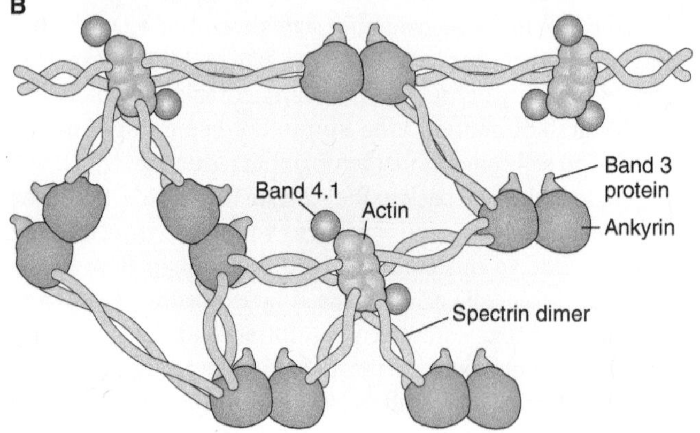

19 **The answer is C: Resynthesis of the inhibited enzyme.** Once acetylcholinesterase has been covalently modified by an inhibitor, it cannot be reactivated. The only way to regain this activity is by new synthesis of acetylcholinesterase, which would not have the covalent modification found in the inhibited enzyme. Since acetylcholine is released at nerve muscle junctions, once new acetylcholinesterase has been synthesized the released acetylcholine can be cleaved in order to allow relaxation of the muscle.

20 **The answer is B: A polyglutamine tract in an exon of the defective gene.** The patient is suffering from Huntington disease, which is transmitted in an autosomal dominant pattern in which a triplet repeat is expanded within the Huntington disease gene. This triplet repeat codes for a polyglutamine tract in the mature protein, which leads to its eventual failure and disease symptoms. Huntington's is not caused by an exonic deletion or a nonsense mutation. Splicing is normal for the gene, and the mature mRNA is stable.

Chapter 3

DNA Structure, Replication, and Repair

The questions in this chapter examine a student's ability to think through questions relating to DNA. As DNA is the human genetic material, it must be replicated faithfully; otherwise, potential deleterious mutations could result, harming the species' ability to survive in future generations. As such, repairing errors during replication and repairing errors that occur before replication (as induced by environmental agents) are crucial for the species' long-term survival. This chapter presents questions concerning a wide variety of topics relating to this theme.

QUESTIONS

Select the single best answer.

1 A clinic was studying patients with xeroderma pigmentosum and ran experiments to determine how many different complementation groups were represented in their patient sample. Fibroblast cell lines were created from five different patients and fused with each other (all possible fusions were examined, as shown in Table 3-1). The resultant heterodikaryons were then examined for their resistance to UV light, as indicated below (a "+" indicates resistance to UV damage, while a "–" indicates sensitivity to UV damage).

Table 3-1.

Cell Number	1	2	3	4	5
1	–	+	+	+	+
2	+	–	–	+	+
3	+	–	–	+	+
4	+	+	+	–	–
5	+	+	+	–	–

The number of complementation groups represented by these patients is which of the following?

(A) 1
(B) 2
(C) 3
(D) 4
(E) 5

2 Analysis of a cell line that rapidly transforms into a tumor cell line demonstrated an increased mutation rate within the cell. Further analysis indicated that there was a mutation in the DNA polymerase enzyme that synthesizes the leading strand. This inactivating mutation is likely to be in which of the following activities of this DNA polymerase?

(A) 5′–3′ exonuclease activity
(B) 3′–5′ exonuclease activity
(C) Phosphodiester bond making capability
(D) Uracil-DNA glycosylase activity
(E) Ligase activity

3 A 13-year-old exhibited developmental delay, learning disabilities, mood swings, and at times, autistic behavior when he was younger. His current physical exam shows a long face, large ears, and large, fleshy hands. His fingers exhibit hyperextensible joints. Examination of fibroblasts cultured from the boy showed abnormal DNA damage, but only in the absence of folic acid. This disorder has, at the genetic level, which one of the following?

(A) A single missense mutation
(B) A large deletion
(C) An extended triplet nucleotide repeat
(D) A nonsense mutation
(E) Gene inactivation via methylation

4 An 8-month-old child is brought to the pediatrician's office due to excessive sensitivity to the sun. Skin areas exposed to the sun for only a brief period of time were reddened with scaling. Irregular dark spots have also appeared. The pediatrician suspects a genetic disorder in which of the following processes?

(A) DNA replication
(B) Transcription
(C) Base excision repair
(D) Nucleotide excision repair
(E) Translation

5 Spontaneous deamination of certain bases in DNA occurs at a constant rate under all conditions. Such deamination can lead to mutations if not repaired. Which deamination indicated below would lead to a mutation in a resulting protein if not repaired?

(A) T to U
(B) C to U
(C) G to A
(D) A to G
(E) U to C

6 A couple sees an obstetrician due to difficulties of the woman keeping a pregnancy to term. She has had three miscarriages over the past 6 years, and the couple is searching for an answer. Karyotype analysis of the woman gave the result of 45,XX,der(14;21). A likely potential cause of the miscarriages may be which of the following?

(A) Imbalance of DNA in polyploid conceptions
(B) Imbalance of DNA in euploid conceptions
(C) Triple X conceptions
(D) Zero X conceptions
(E) Trisomy 21 conceptions

7 A 32-year-old woman exhibited a high fever, malaise, generalized lymphadenopathy, weight loss, and esophageal candidiasis. She had a history of drug abuse and needle sharing. Blood analysis indicated a CD4 lymphocyte count of less than 200. Which of the following compounds would be a drug of choice for this patient?

A

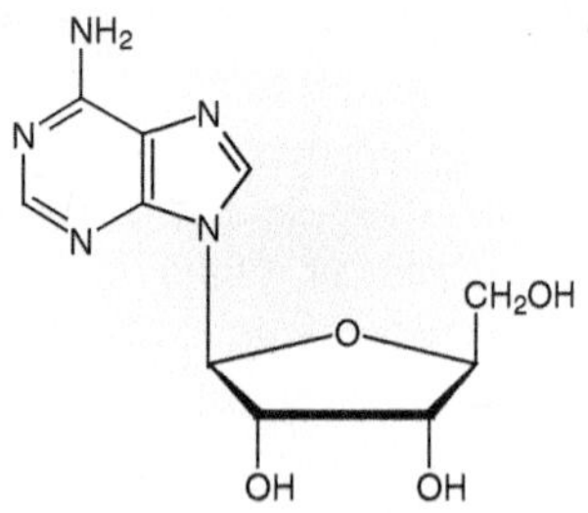

B

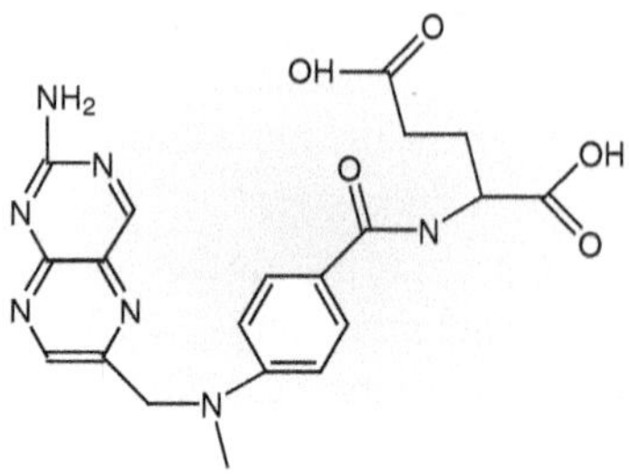

C

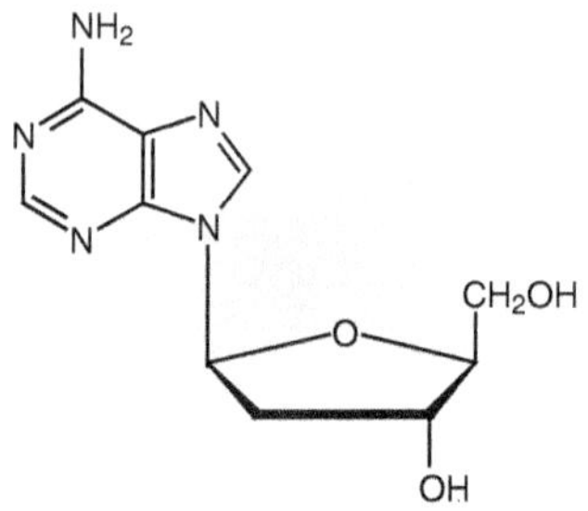

D

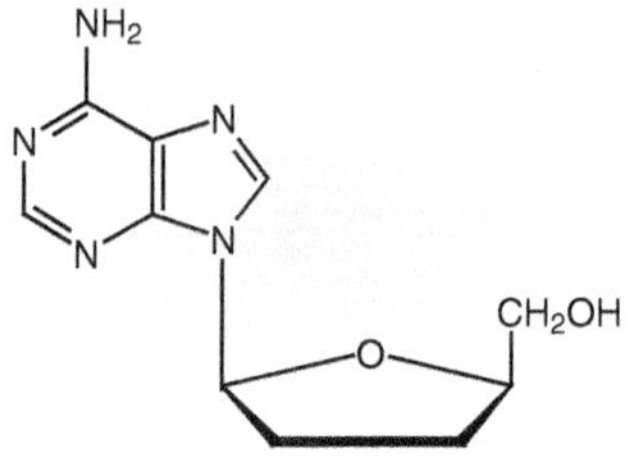

E

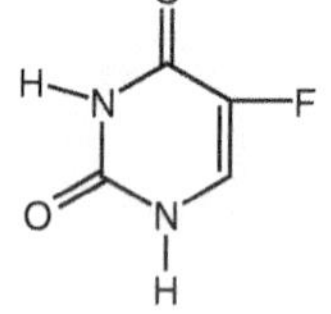

8 The high mutation rate of the human immunodeficiency virus (HIV) is due in part to a property of which of the following host cell enzymes?

(A) DNA polymerase
(B) RNA polymerase
(C) DNA primase
(D) Telomerase
(E) DNA ligase

9 Consider the DNA replication fork shown below. DNA ligase will be required to finish synthesis at which labeled points on the figure?

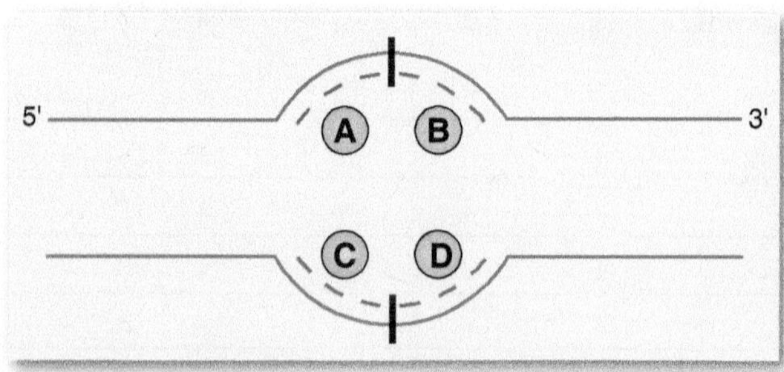

(A) A and B
(B) C and D
(C) A and C
(D) D and B
(E) B and C

10 The sequence of part of a DNA strand is the following: –ATTCGATTGCCCACGT–. When this strand is used as a template for DNA synthesis, the product will be which one of the following?
(A) TAAGCTAACGGGTGCA
(B) UAAGCUAACGGGUGCA
(C) ACGUGGGCAAUCGAAU
(D) ACGTGGGCAATCGAAT
(E) TGCACCCGTTAGCTTA

11 You have been following a newborn who first presented with hypotonia and trouble sucking. Special feeding techniques were required for the child to gain nourishment. As the child aged, there appeared to be developmental delay, and the child then gained a great interest in eating, and rapidly became obese. Developmental delay was still evident, as was hypotonia. A karyotype analysis of this patient would indicate which of the following?
(A) A monosomy
(B) A trisomy
(C) A duplication
(D) A chromosomal inversion
(E) A deletion

12 You see a 2-year-old child of Ashkenazi Jewish descent who is very small for her age. The patient exhibits a long, narrow face, small lower jaw, and prominent eyes and ears. The child is very sensitive to being outdoors in the sun, often burning easily, with butterfly-shaped patches of redness on her skin. Upon testing, the child is also slightly developmentally delayed. The defective protein in this child is which of the following?
(A) DNA polymerase
(B) DNA ligase
(C) RNA polymerase
(D) DNA helicase
(E) Reverse transcriptase

13 Concerned parents are referred to a specialty clinic by their family physician due to abnormalities in their 18-month-old child's development. The child displays delayed psychomotor development, and is mentally retarded. The child is photosensitive, and also appears to be aging prematurely, with a stooped posture and sunken eyes. The altered process in this autosomal recessive disorder is which of the following?
(A) Base excision repair
(B) DNA replication
(C) Transcription-coupled DNA repair
(D) Proofreading by DNA polymerase
(E) Sealing nicks in DNA

14 A woman visits her physician due to fever and pain upon urination. Urinary analysis shows bacteria, leukocytes, and leukocyte esterase in the urine, and the physician places the woman on a quinolone antibiotic (ciprofloxacin). The mammalian counterpart to the bacterial enzyme inhibited by this drug is which of the following?
(A) DNA polymerase α
(B) Topoisomerase
(C) Ligase
(D) Primase
(E) Helicase

15 Which answer below best predicts the effect of the following drug on the pathways indicated?

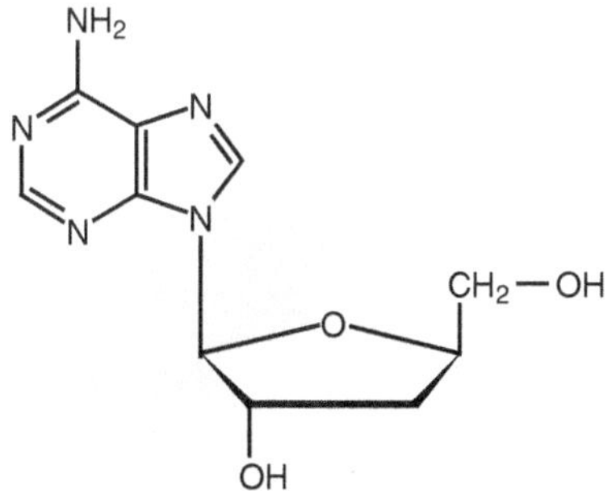

NH$_2$ — N — N — N — N — O — CH$_2$—OH — OH

	DNA Synthesis	RNA Synthesis	Protein Synthesis
(A)	Inhibit	Inhibit	No effect
(B)	Inhibit	No effect	No effect
(C)	No effect	Inhibit	No effect
(D)	No effect	No effect	No effect
(E)	No effect	No effect	Inhibit

16 A new patient visits your practice due to his concern of developing colon cancer. A large number of relatives have had premature (less than the age of 45) colon cancer, and all cases were right-sided, with the only visible polyps being found on that side. The molecular basis for this form of colon cancer is which of the following?

(A) A defect in DNA mismatch repair
(B) A defect in base excision repair
(C) A defect in the Wnt signaling pathway
(D) A defect in repairing double-strand DNA breaks
(E) A defect in telomerase

17 Over 50% of human tumors have developed an inactivating mutation in p53 activity. The lack of this activity contributes to tumor cell growth via which one of the following mechanisms?
(A) Loss of Wnt signaling
(B) Increase in DNA mutation rates
(C) Activation of MAP kinases
(D) Increase in apoptotic events
(E) Increase in transcription-coupled DNA repair

18 The isolation of nascent Okazaki fragments during DNA replication led to the surprising discovery of uracil in the fragment. The uracil is present due to which of the following?
(A) Deamination of cytosine
(B) Chemical modification of thymine
(C) An error in DNA polymerase
(D) Failure of mismatch repair
(E) The need for a primer

19 You have a patient with an elevated white blood cell count and a feeling of malaise. Molecular analysis of the white

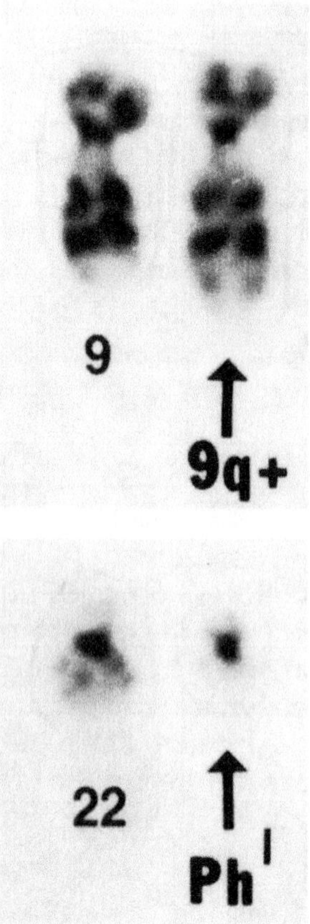

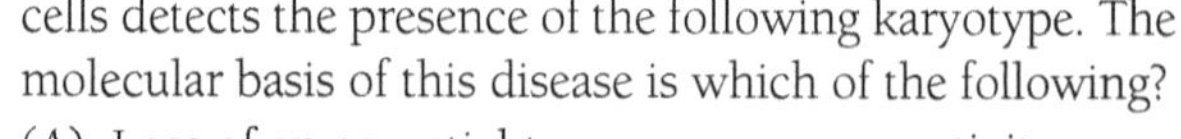
cells detects the presence of the following karyotype. The molecular basis of this disease is which of the following?
(A) Loss of an essential tumor suppressor activity
(B) Increased rate of DNA mutation due to loss of DNA repair enzymes
(C) Creation of a fusion protein not normally found in cells
(D) Loss of a critical tyrosine kinase activity
(E) Gain of a critical ser/thr kinase activity

20 A scientist is replicating human DNA in a test tube and has added intact DNA, the replisome complex, and the four deoxyribonucleoside triphosphates. To the surprise of the scientist, there was no DNA synthesized, as determined by the incorporation of radio-labeled precursors into acid-precipitable material. The scientist's failure to synthesize DNA is most likely due to a lack of which of the following in his reaction mixture?
(A) Reverse transcriptase
(B) Ribonucleoside triphosphates
(C) Templates
(D) Dideoxynucleoside triphosphates
(E) Sigma factor

ANSWERS

1 **The answer is C: 3.** Cell lines complement each other if their mutations are in different genes. For the purpose of this question, let us assume there are three genes involved, lettered x, y, and z. Cell line 1 is deficient in gene x, but since it can complement every other cell line, cell lines 2 through 5 cannot be deficient in gene x. When fused, the other cell lines (2 through 5) produce normal x protein, which complements the deficiency in cell line 1. Similarly, cell line 1 produces normal copies of the genes that are deficient in cell lines 2 through 5. This indicates that there are at least two complementation groups available. Cell line 2 complements cell lines 1, 4, and 5, but not 3. Thus, the mutation in cell line 2 (call it gene y) is also present in cell line 3 (since the two cell lines cannot complement each other), but not in cell lines 4 and 5. Thus, at this point, cell line 1 is deficient in gene x, and cell lines 2 and 3 are deficient in gene y. Cell line 4 complements cell lines 1, 2, and 3, but not 5. Thus, cell lines 4 and 5 have similar mutations, but in a gene distinct from genes x and y. Thus, cell lines 4 and 5 can be deficient in gene z. The cell lines are thus 1 (x^-), 2 and 3 (y^-) and 4 and 5 (z^-). So, as an example, when cell line 1 is fused with cell line 2, cell line 1 is x^-y^+, and cell line 2 is x^+y^-, so the fused cell ($x^-y^+/x^+/y^-$) produces both normal x and y.

2 **The answer is B: 3′–5′ exonuclease activity.** DNA polymerase rarely makes mistakes when inserting bases into a newly synthesized strand and base-pairing with the template strand. However, mistakes do occur at a frequency of about one in a million bases synthesized, but DNA polymerase has an error checking capability which enables it to remove the mispaired base before proceeding with the next base insertion. This is due to the 3′–5′ exonuclease activity of DNA polymerase by which, prior to adding the next nucleotide to the growing DNA chain, the base put into place in the previous step is examined for correct base-pairing properties. If it is incorrect, the enzyme goes "backwards" and removes the incorrect base, then replaces it with the correct base. The 5′–3′ exonuclease activity of DNA polymerase moves ahead, and is used to remove RNA primers from newly synthesized DNA. If the enzyme could no longer synthesize phosphodiester bonds (the primary responsibility of the enzyme), DNA synthesis would halt. A loss of uracil-DNA glycosylase activity is not a property of DNA polymerase, but that of a separate enzyme system which repairs spontaneous deamination of cytosine bases to uracil within DNA strands. If these were left intact, mutations would increase in DNA. A loss of ligase activity would lead to unstable DNA, as the Okazaki fragments would not be able to be sealed together to form one continuous piece of DNA, and this would most likely lead to cell death, not an increased mutation rate.

3 **The answer is C: An extended triplet nucleotide repeat.** The boy is displaying the symptoms of fragile X syndrome. Fragile X contains a triplet nucleotide repeat (CGG) on the X chromosome in the 5′ untranslated region of the FMR1 gene. The triplet repeat expansion leads to no expression of the FMR1 gene, which produces a protein required for brain development. Its function appears to be that of an mRNA shuttle, moving mRNA from the nucleus to appropriate sites in the cytoplasm for translation to occur. Depending on the level of expression of FMR1 (which is dependent on the number of repeats), the symptoms can vary from mild to severe. Less than 1% of cases of fragile X are due to missense or nonsense mutations; the vast majority are due to the expansion of the triplet repeat at the 5' end of the gene. Gene inactivation by methylation, or deletion, are not causes of fragile X syndrome. The syndrome was called fragile X because the X chromosome that carries the repeat expansion is subject to DNA strand break under certain conditions (such as lack of folic acid), which does not occur with normal X chromosomes. The area containing the repeat alters the staining pattern of the X chromosome, allowing this to be seen in a karyotype (as seen below). Fragile X is the most common inheritable cause of mental retardation. Males are more severely affected. In early childhood, developmental delay, speech and language problems, and autisticlike behavior are noticeable. After puberty, the classic physical signs develop (large testicles, long-thin face, mental retardation, large ears, and prominent jaw).

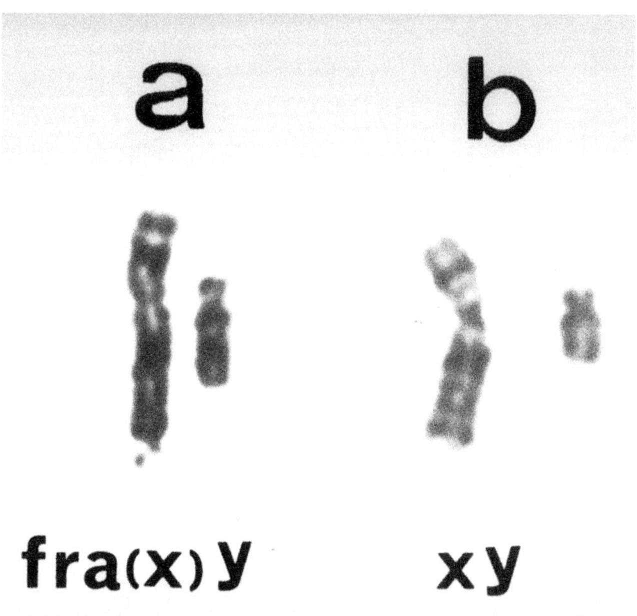

Picture of a fragile X chromosome and normal X and Y chromosomes. Note the end of the long arm (q), and the differences between the two chromosomes.

4 **The answer is D: Nucleotide excision repair.** The child is suffering from a form of xeroderma pigmentosum, a disorder in which thymine dimers (created by exposure to UV light) cannot be appropriately repaired in DNA. Nucleotide excision repair enzymes recognize bulky distortions in the helix, whereas base excision repair recognizes only specific lesions of a small, single, damaged base. The mechanism whereby thymine dimers are removed from DNA is nucleotide excision repair in which entire nucleotides are removed from the damaged DNA. In base excision repair, only a single base is removed; the sugar phosphate backbone is initially left intact (see the figure below for comparisons between these two systems for repairing DNA). This disorder is not due to alterations in transcription (synthesizing RNA from DNA), DNA replication, or translation (synthesizing proteins from mRNA). Another example of a disease resulting from a defect in nucleotide excision repair is Cockayne syndrome. Neurological diseases (such as Alzheimer's) may also have a deficiency in nucleotide excision repair.

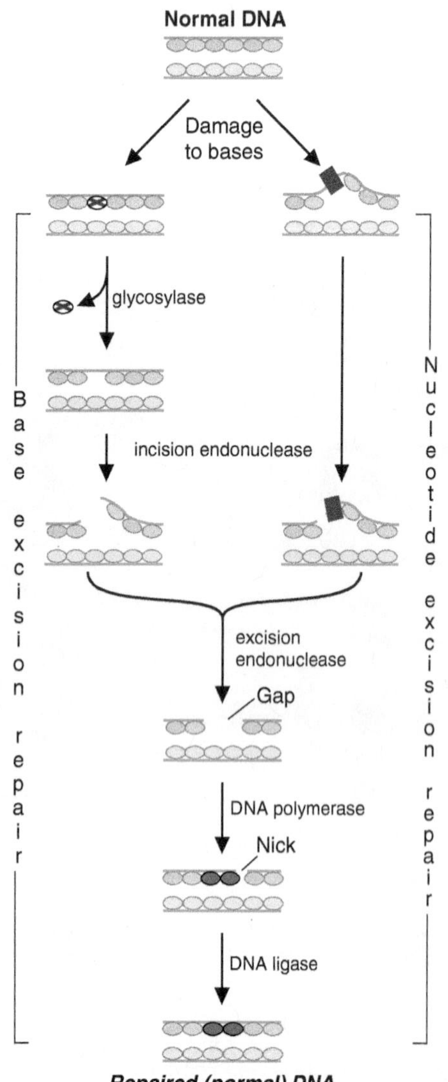

A comparison of nucleotide excision repair and base excision repair.

5 **The answer is B: C to U.** Cytosine spontaneously deaminates to form uracil while in DNA. This error is repaired by the uracil-DNA glycosylase system, which recognizes this abnormal base in DNA and initiates the process of base excision repair to correct the mistake. Neither thymine nor uracil contains an amino group to deaminate (thus, answers A and E are incorrect). When adenine deaminates, the base hypoxanthine is formed (inosine as part of a nucleoside), and guanine deamination will lead to xanthine production. The deamination of cytosine and conversion to uridine is shown below.

The deamination of cytidine to uridine (C to U within a DNA strand).

6 **The answer is B: Imbalance of DNA in euploid conceptions.** The woman has a Robertsonian translocation between chromosomes 14 and 21 (the two chromosomes are fused together at their stalks; see the figure on page 23). When she creates her eggs, there is an imbalance in the amount of DNA representing chromosomes 14 and 21 in the eggs, such that fertilization of the eggs will lead to either monosomy or trisomy with these chromosomes, most of which are incompatible with life. The figure below indicates these potential outcomes. Polyploid outcomes would be three or more times the normal number of chromosomes, which does not occur here; and the Robertsonian translocation will not affect the distribution of the X chromosome. Trisomy 21 will lead to a live birth, Down syndrome, although there is still a risk of miscarriage with trisomy 21 conceptions. The risk is lower, however, than an imbalance of DNA brought about by the segregation of the chromosomes containing the Robertsonian translocation. Euploid cells have a number of chromosomes which are exact multiples of the haploids (in humans haploid is 23, diploid is 46, and polyploid is 69 or 92 chromosomes).

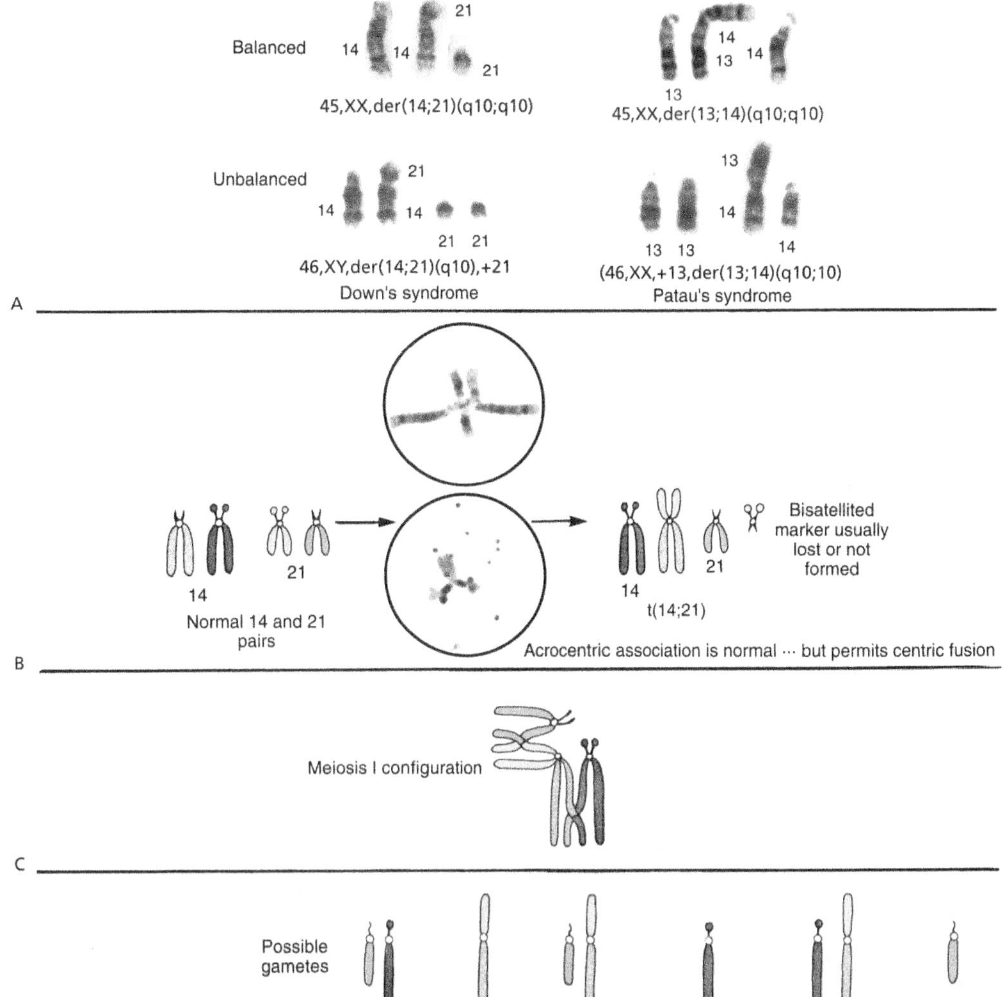

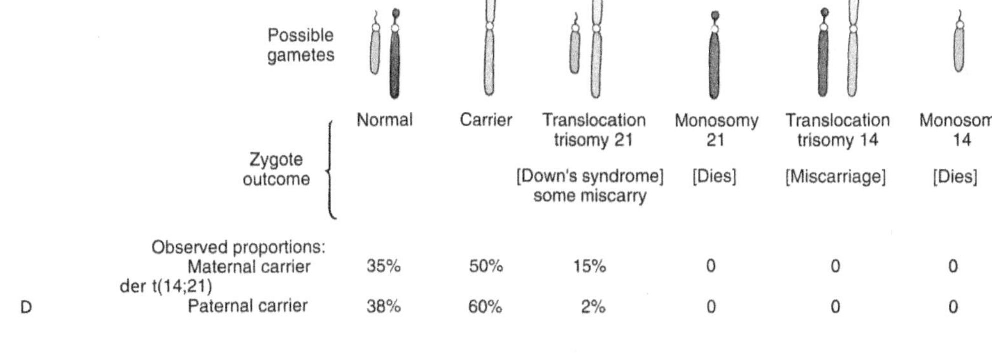

Answer 6: The most important Robertsonian translocations are der(14;21) **(left)** and der(13;14) **(right)** **(A,B)**. A meiosis I configuration formed in a carrier of a der(14;21) is shown in panel **C**, along with the six possible gametic products **(D)**, of which only three are ever observed. Frequency statistics are based on prenatal diagnosis results in carriers.

7 **The answer is D.** The woman is suffering from AIDS, and one class of drugs used to stop the spread of the virus is the dideoxynucleosides (the compound shown in answer D is dideoxyadenosine). The dideoxynucleosides interfere with DNA synthesis after they are activated to the triphosphate level through purine salvage pathway enzymes. Since these compounds lack a 3′-hydroxyl group, once they are incorporated into a growing DNA strand, they cannot form a phosphodiester bond with the next nucleotide, and synthesis stops. Reverse transcriptase, an enzyme carried by HIV but not found in eukaryotic cells, appears to have a higher affinity for these drugs than does normal cellular DNA polymerase, so the agents have a greater ability to preferentially stop virus synthesis and not cellular DNA synthesis, although it does occur to a small extent. Structure A is adenosine, a ribonucleoside which when activated may be used for primer synthesis in DNA replication, but not as part of the DNA structure. Structure B is methotrexate, an agent which inhibits dihydrofolate reductase and blocks the synthesis of thymidine, thereby blocking DNA synthesis. It is used as a treatment for psoriasis and was used, in the past, as a chemotherapeutic agent. Structure C is deoxyadenosine, which is a normal substrate for DNA polymerase after activation. Structure E is 5-fluorouracil (5FU), an inhibitor of thymidylate synthase. 5FU blocks thymidine synthesis and stops overall DNA synthesis. It is used for certain tumors as an anticancer drug, but is not used for HIV infections.

8 **The answer is B: RNA polymerase.** During the life cycle of the HIV, the double-stranded DNA which was produced from the genomic RNA integrates randomly into the host chromosome (see the figure below). Cellular RNA polymerase then transcribes the viral DNA to produce viral RNA, which is used in the translation of viral proteins, and as the genomic material for new virions. RNA polymerase lacks 3′–5′ exonuclease activity, thus the enzyme cannot correct any errors it may make while transcribing the viral DNA. The RNA produced, which carries errors in transcription, is then packaged into a new virus particle, and this mutation may lead to a change that confers a growth advantage to this strain of virus. The lack of proofreading by RNA polymerase is not usually a problem in eukaryotic cells, as many messages are produced from a single gene, and if 1% of those messages produce a mutated protein it will be compensated by the 99% of the messages which produce a normal protein. In the viral case, however, the mRNA turns into the genomic material, which will lead to mutations in all future descendants of that virus. This is why HIV is treated with multiple, different antivirals simultaneously, to destroy any virus which mutates to be resistant to the antiviral agents. DNA polymerase has error-checking

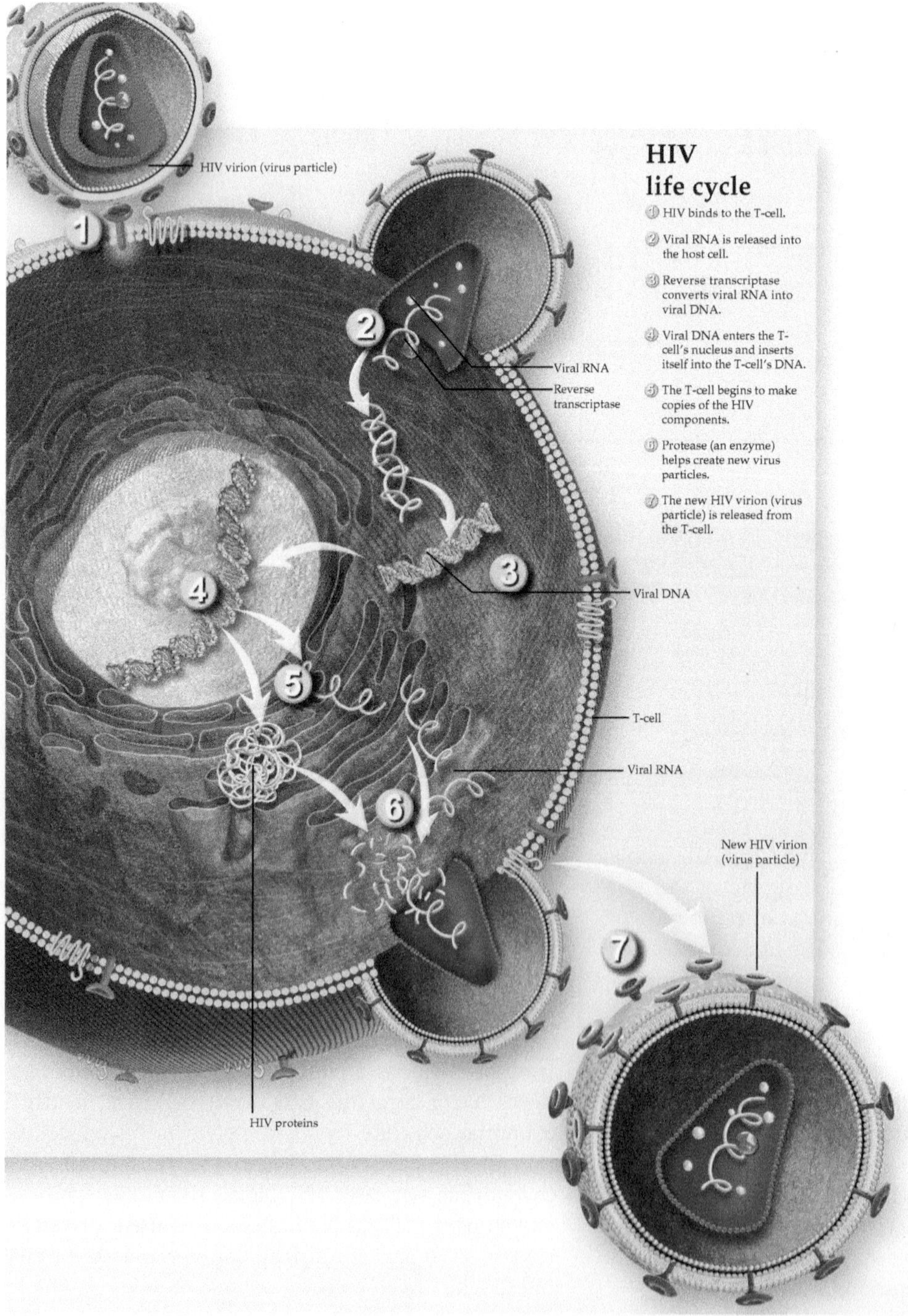

The HIV life cycle.

capabilities, and will not significantly increase the mutation rate of the integrated viral DNA. DNA primase may make errors, but they are corrected when the RNA primer is removed from the DNA. Telomerase only works on the ends of chromosomes, and the viral DNA does not usually integrate at those positions. DNA ligase activity is not required for viral RNA production.

9 **The answer is E: B and C.** The areas labeled B and C are lagging strand synthesis in these two replication forks (see the figure below). This means that the DNA is synthesized in the direction opposite to that of the direction in which the replication fork is moving. Because of this, the DNA must be synthesized in short pieces (as DNA polymerase can only synthesize DNA in the 5′ to 3′ direction, reading the template in the 3′ to 5′ direction) known as Okazaki fragments. These Okazaki fragments need to be sealed together, which occurs with DNA ligase (after the RNA primers have been removed by a DNA polymerase with a 5′–3′ exonuclease activity). The vertical line refers to the origin of replication, and labels A and D are the leading strands of DNA synthesis, which, since synthesis is occurring in the direction that the replication fork is moving, can be synthesized as one continuous piece of DNA.

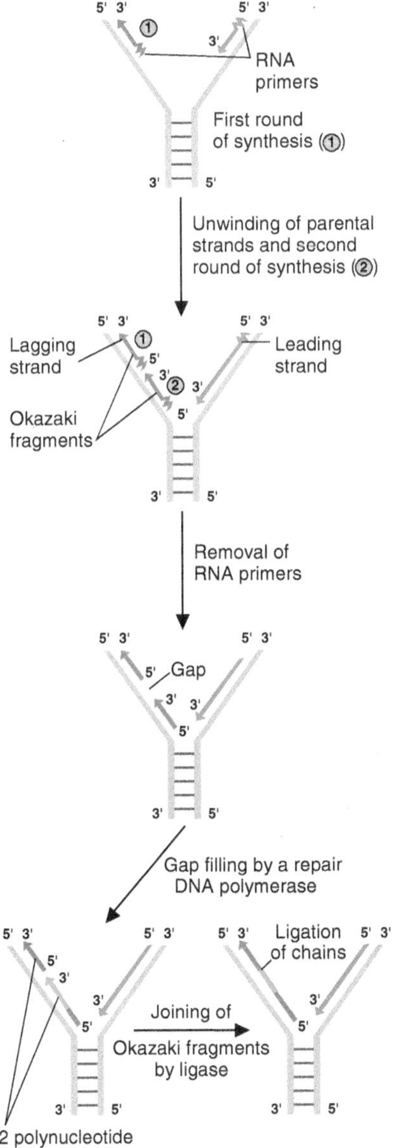

This figure shows one replication fork, moving down the page. As the DNA template must be read in the 3′ to 5′ direction note how the Okazaki fragments are synthesized in pieces, moving opposite to the direction of replication fork movement. It is these Okazaki fragments that must be ligated in later phases of DNA synthesis.

10 **The answer is D: ACGTGGGCAATCGAAT.** The product of DNA replication will be complementary to the template, and antiparallel. Reading from the 5′ end of the template, the product will be 3′-TAAGCTAACGGGTGCA-. When written 5′–3′ (standard notation) one has -ACGTGGGCAATCGAAT-. Recall that uracil (U) is not placed into DNA by DNA polymerase.

11 **The answer is E: A deletion.** The child has Prader-Willi syndrome, which is due to a deletion of a cluster of genes on chromosome 15, on the long arm. When this deletion is inherited from the father, Prader-Willi syndrome is observed. If the same deletion is inherited from the mother, an entirely different syndrome is observed, termed Angelmann syndrome. The diagnosis can be confirmed by FISH analysis using a probe specific for the 15q11–13 region.

12 **The answer is D: DNA helicase.** The child has the symptoms of Bloom syndrome, a disease in which DNA helicase is defective, and DNA replication is compromised. The DNA helicase is necessary to help stabilize the unwinding of the DNA as the replication fork passes through a stretch of DNA. With reduced helicase activity, genomic instability occurs, with increased risk of mutagenic effects and chromosome damage, including chromosome breaks and translocations. These secondary effects lead to the symptoms observed in the patients. The patients also have a higher than normal risk for various malignancies, due to the increased genomic instability. The mutation is in the BLM gene, which is on chromosome 15. This mutation does not alter, in a direct fashion, DNA polymerase or ligase activity nor RNA polymerase activity. Reverse transcriptase is not a normal component of eukaryotic cells (it is introduced to cells when they are infected by a retrovirus).

13 **The answer is C: Transcription-coupled DNA repair.** The child is exhibiting the symptoms of Cockayne syndrome (CS), a defect in transcription-coupled DNA repair. Transcription-coupled DNA repair occurs only on actively transcribed genes; if RNA polymerase is halted

due to damage to DNA on an actively transcribed gene, this repair system fixes the DNA such that transcription can continue. Cells derived from patients with CS have a reduction in RNA synthesis in response to UV irradiation, as transcription-coupled DNA repair is reduced, thereby reducing the rate of RNA produced from genes which did contain thymine dimers. There are at least two forms of CS: CS 1 (or A), the form present at birth, and CS 2 (or B), one that occurs later in life, during early childhood. The two forms are due to mutations in two different genes (ERCC8, on chromosome 5, is responsible for CS-A, and ERCC6, on chromosome 10, is responsible for CS-B). The child's symptoms are not due to defects in base excision repair or in DNA ligase (sealing nicks in DNA). DNA replication is normal in these children, as is the proofreading capability of DNA polymerase.

14 **The answer is B: Topoisomerase.** The quinolone family of antibiotics is targeted toward the bacterial enzyme DNA gyrase, which is the bacterial counterpart of the mammalian topoisomerases. These are the enzymes which break the phosphodiester backbone to allow relief of torsional strain as the DNA helix is unwinding to allow replication to proceed. Through an inhibition of gyrase, DNA replication in the bacteria is inhibited, which leads to bacterial cell death. Since the topoisomerases are not affected by these drugs, there is no effect on eukaryotic DNA synthesis. DNA polymerase α is unique to eukaryotic cells (the bacteria have DNA polymerases I, II, or III). DNA ligase, primase, and DNA helicase are not targets of this class of drugs. The helicase is the enzyme which allows the DNA strands to unwind; however, it needs to work with gyrase (or topoisomerase) such that the tension created by unwinding can be relieved.

15 **The answer is C.** The drug is 3′-deoxyadenosine. This nucleoside will be activated when it enters cells (to the triphosphate level), and will be recognized by RNA polymerase and incorporated into growing RNA chains. Since the compound lacks a 3′-hydroxy group, RNA synthesis is terminated, as the next phosphodiester bond cannot be created. This drug is not recognized by DNA polymerase because it contains a 2′-hydroxy group, and DNA polymerase will only recognize nucleotides which lack 2′-hydroxy groups. This drug does not resemble tRNA, or mRNA, or rRNA, so it will not have a direct effect on protein synthesis. Protein synthesis may be decreased, however, if no mRNA is present to translate. However, the drug does not directly inhibit the mechanisms of translation.

16 **The answer is A: A defect in DNA mismatch repair.** The patient is concerned about HNPCC, hereditary nonpolyposis colon cancer, which is due to mutations in genes which are involved in DNA mismatch repair. This colon tumor does not form large numbers of polyps within the intestine, as does the other form of inherited colon cancer, adenomatous polyposis coli (APC). HNPCC is also a right-sided colon cancer. Defects in base excision repair do not lead to HNPCC. A defect in the Wnt signaling pathway, which controls the action of β-catenin, an important transcription factor, may play a role in APC. Defects in repairing double-strand breaks in DNA are linked to breast cancer. Mutations in telomerase would lead to earlier cell senescence and death due to an inability to maintain the proper length of the chromosomes.

17 **The answer is B: Increase in DNA mutation rates.** p53 is a protein which scans the genome for damage, and when damage is spotted, it induces the synthesis of genes which will stop the cell from continuing through the cell cycle. p53 will also lead to the synthesis of genes involved in repairing the DNA damage. Once the damage has been repaired, the cell will resume its passage through the cell cycle. If the damage cannot be repaired, apoptosis will be initiated in the cell. If p53 is missing, or mutated such that its functions are lost, damaged DNA will be replicated, and at times, the replisome will make errors repairing the damage. This will increase the overall mutation rate of the cell such that eventually mutations will appear in genes which regulate cell proliferation, and a cancer will develop. p53 is not involved in Wnt signaling or activation of MAP kinases. Functional p53 can increase apoptotic events, but the lack of p53 will actually decrease the frequency of apoptosis in cells. This protein is also not involved in transcription-coupled DNA repair.

18 **The answer is E: The need for a primer.** DNA polymerase requires a primer in order to synthesize DNA. The primer is provided by a small piece of RNA, synthesized by DNA primase (an RNA-polymerase). RNA synthesis does not require a primer. Once a small piece of RNA is synthesized, DNA polymerase will begin to add deoxyribonucleotides to the end of the RNA. Later, during DNA replication, another DNA polymerase will come along and remove the RNA, replacing the RNA bases with deoxyribonucleotides. However, as initially synthesized, Okazaki fragments will contain uracil. While the deamination of cytosine can produce uracil, this is much more frequent in the more stable DNA than RNA. Thymine cannot be easily converted to uracil in DNA (it would require a demethylation), and does not contribute to uracil content in Okazaki fragments. Mismatch repair does not operate on DNA:RNA hybrids (which form when the primer is synthesized), and DNA polymerase does not recognize uracil, so it would not make the type of mistake in which uracil were placed into DNA.

19 **The answer is C: Creation of a fusion protein not normally found in cells.** The patient exhibits the Philadelphia chromosome (a translocation between chromosomes 9 and 22), which creates the bcr–abl protein, a fusion protein of two normal cellular proteins. The abl protein is a tyrosine kinase; when the gene is moved from chromosome 9 to 22 and put under the control of the *bcr* gene, it is misexpressed and constitutively active and leads to cellular growth in the blood cells in which the protein is expressed. The patient has chronic myelogenous leukemia (CML). Since this is a dominant activity, there is no loss of a tumor suppressor gene. The translocation does not interfere with DNA repair, so there is no direct increase in mutation rate due to this translocation. There is no loss of tyrosine kinase activity (there is actually a gain of activity), nor is there gain of a ser/thr kinase (as abl is a tyrosine kinase).

20 **The answer is B: Ribonucleoside triphosphates.** DNA synthesis requires the synthesis of primers upon which deoxyribonucleotides will be added. The primers are composed of ribonucleotides (DNA primase is a DNA-dependant RNA polymerase), and the scientist forgot to add NTPs to the reaction mixture (deoxyribonucleotides are not recognized by DNA primase, and cannot be used to synthesize a primer). Reverse transcriptase is not required for DNA synthesis from a DNA template (as in this situation). Sigma factor is a required factor for bacterial RNA synthesis; it is not a required factor for eukaryotic DNA synthesis.

Chapter 4

RNA Synthesis

The questions in this chapter are organized about the process of transcription and diseases and problems associated with transcription. Regulation of gene expression will be covered in more detail in Chapter 6.

QUESTIONS

Select the single best answer.

1 An IV drug user is tested, and found positive, for infection by HIV. If the patient is only placed on one antiviral medication, viral loads will initially be reduced, but will then rapidly increase. The resistance to the drug occurs due to which of the following?

(A) Lack of error checking in DNA polymerase
(B) Lack of error checking in RNA polymerase
(C) Lack of DNA repair enzyme systems in HIV-infected cells
(D) Incorporation of uracil in the RNA genome of HIV
(E) Incorporation of thymine in the RNA genome of HIV

2 A researcher needs to prepare RNA for Northern blot analysis. Initial experiments using total RNA produce no signal when the experiment is completed. A method to increase the sensitivity of the assay would be to do which of the following to the total RNA sample?

(A) Separate by size on agarose gel electrophoresis
(B) Run the RNA through an oligo-dT affinity column
(C) Run the RNA through an oligo-dA affinity column
(D) Separate by size on polyacrylamide gel electrophoresis
(E) Perform a phenol extraction of the total RNA

3 A researcher has obtained an antibody to cytosolic protein X and runs a Western blot using as samples a variety of tissue types. The results of the Western blot are shown below. A potential interpretation of the results is which of the following?

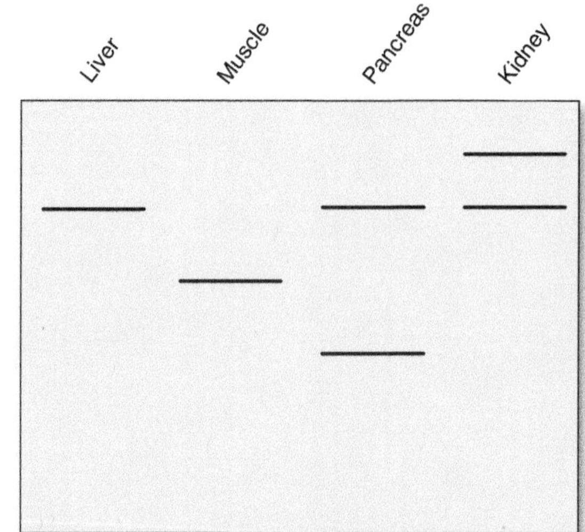

(A) Codon degeneracy within the genetic code
(B) Tissue-specific posttranslational modifications
(C) Tissue-specific alternative splicing of the primary transcript
(D) Polyadenylation is lacking in certain tissues
(E) Differences in location of 5′-cap formation in the tissues

4 An individual having β-thalassemia minor exhibits two bands on a Northern blot using a probe against exon 1 of β-globin. The smaller band is of normal size and "heavier" than the other larger band, which consists of approximately 247 additional nucleotides. One explanation for this finding is which of the following?

(A) The presence of a nonsense mutation in the DNA
(B) A mutation which creates an alternative splice site
(C) A lack of capping of the mRNA
(D) An extended poly-A tail
(E) A loss of AUG codons

5 A careful analysis of cellular components discovers short-lived RNA species in which an adenine nucleotide is found with three phosphodiester bonds (linked to

the 2′, 3′, and 5′ carbons). This transient structure is formed during which of the following processes?
(A) mRNA cap formation
(B) mRNA polyadenylation
(C) Splicing of hnRNA
(D) Transcription of microRNAs
(E) Transcription of rRNA

6 A patient suffering from chills, vomiting, and cramping was rushed to the emergency department. He had eaten wild mushrooms for dinner that he had picked earlier in the day. His symptoms are due to an inhibition of which of the following enzymes?
(A) RNA polymerase I
(B) RNA polymerase II
(C) RNA polymerase III
(D) Telomerase
(E) DNA primase

Questions 7 and 8 refer to the figure of active transcription below.

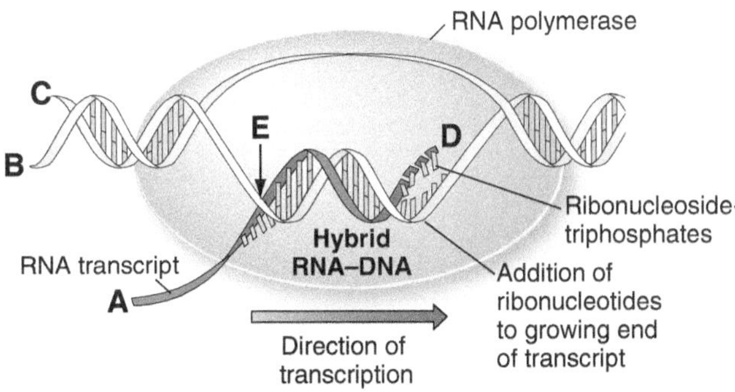

7 The message identical strand is best represented by which letter on the diagram?

8 The 3′ end of the newly synthesized RNA is best represented by which letter on the above diagram?

9 A 22-year-old woman (see the figure below) sees her physician for a variety of complaints over the past year. These include fevers that come and go, fatigue, joint pain and stiffness, a butterfly rash on the face, sores in her mouth, easy bruising, and increased feelings of anxiety and depression. A diagnostic blood test is likely to show autoimmune antibodies directed against which class of molecules?

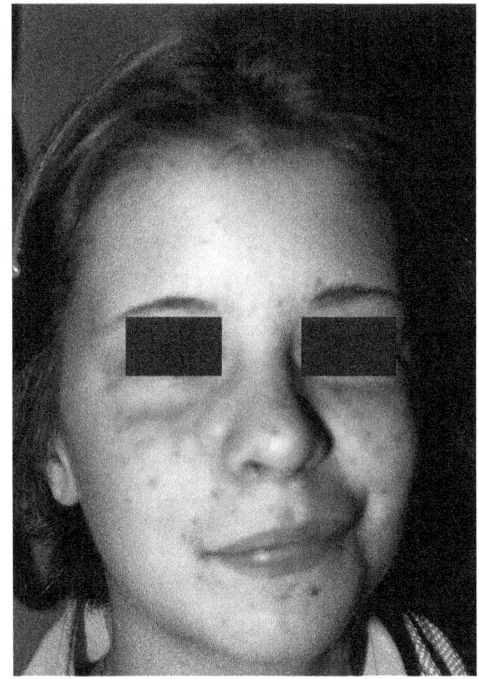

(A) Ribonuclear protein complexes
(B) DNA polymerases
(C) Carbohydrates
(D) tRNA complexes
(E) Peroxisomal proteins

10 When first discovered, introns were not thought to code for a functional product. Recently, however, introns have been found to code for products that can regulate the expression of a large number of genes. This regulation occurs at which stage of gene expression?
(A) Transcription of mRNA
(B) Posttranscriptional processing
(C) Export of mRNA into the cytoplasm
(D) Ribosome biogenesis
(E) Degradation of the mRNA

11 A researcher, while studying a liver cell line, found the following anomalous result. He was studying protein X production within the liver cell. Western blot analysis using a polyclonal antibody showed a normal size, and amount, for protein X. Enzyme assays demonstrated normal levels of activity for protein X. Northern blot analysis, however, yielded two bands of equal intensity: one the expected size and the other 237 nucleotides longer. One possible explanation for this finding is which of the following?

(A) A nonsense mutation in the DNA
(B) A loss of an intron/exon junction
(C) Inefficient transcription initiation
(D) Loss of a transcription termination site
(E) Gain of an alternative splice site

12 A young child of Mediterranean parents was brought to the pediatrician due to lethargy, tiredness, and pallor. Blood analysis revealed a microcytic anemia, although iron levels were normal (see the figure below). What test should be run to determine that the child has a variant of thalassemia?

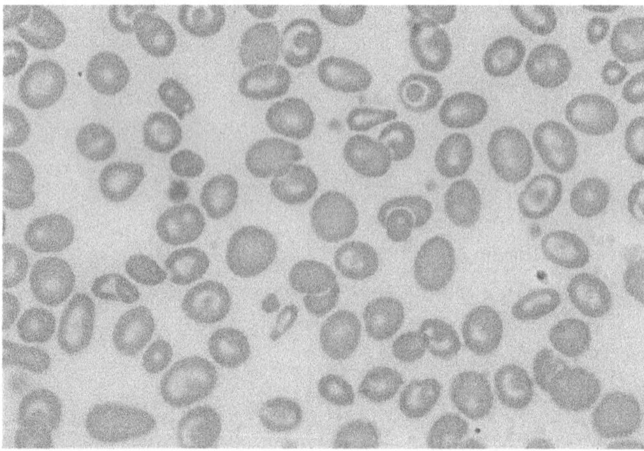

(A) Western blotting of the peptide chains in hemoglobin
(B) PCR of the gene for RNA polymerase
(C) Western blot of snurps in the child
(D) Western blot of TFIID
(E) PCR of the gene for γ-globin in the child

13 An intestinal cell line was being studied for its ability to produce lipid-containing particles. Surprisingly, a mutated variant of this cell line was unable to do so. Western blot analysis yielded a protein with the same size as apolipoprotein B100. A potential mutation in this cell line, which would lead to this result, is which of the following?

(A) Splicing defect
(B) Cap formation altered
(C) RNA editing defect
(D) Inefficient poly-A tail addition
(E) Promoter alteration

14 A patient displays tiredness and lethargy, and blood work demonstrates an anemia. Western blot analysis indicates significantly greater levels of α-globin than β-globin. Molecular analysis indicates a single nucleotide change in an intron of the β-globin gene. How does such a mutation lead to this clinical finding?

(A) A microRNA is produced, which is targeted against the β-globin mRNA, thereby reducing β-globin production
(B) Creation of an alternative splice site, such that β-globin levels are decreased
(C) Creation of a new transcription initiation site, such that the mRNA for β-globin is now out of frame
(D) Creation of a stop codon in the β-globin mRNA
(E) Elimination of the polyadenylation signal, thereby reducing β-globin production

15 Consider two individuals, each with some form of thalassemia. Patient X has a deletion of the α genes on one chromosome but normal expression of all other α and β genes. This person has a mild form of the disease. Patient Y has a normal complement of α genes but has a homozygous mutation in the β genes in which an abnormal splice site is used 80% of the time, producing a transcript with a premature stop codon. Patient Y has a more severe disease than patient X. Why is patient Y's disease more severe than patient X's?

(A) The ratio of α/β in patient X is 1:2, whereas in patient Y it is 1:5
(B) The ratio of α/β in patient X is 1:2, whereas in patient Y it is 5:1
(C) The ratio of α/β in patient X is 2:1, whereas in patient Y it is 1.2:1
(D) The ratio of α/β in patient X is 2:1, whereas in patient Y it is 1:1.2
(E) The ratio of α/β in patient X is 1:2, whereas in patient Y it is 1.2:1

16 Dideoxynucleotides are effective agents against DNA synthesis, but appear to have little, or no, effect on RNA synthesis. This is most likely due to which of the following?

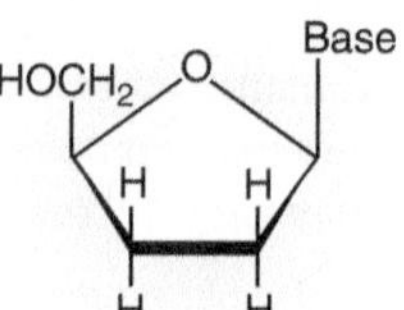

A dideoxynucleoside

(A) Lack of a 3′-OH group
(B) Lack of a 2′-OH group
(C) Presence of a 5′-phosphodiester bond
(D) Presence of an N-glycosidic bond at carbon 1
(E) Factor TFIID does not recognize deoxyribonucleotides

17 TFIIIA is a necessary transcription factor for the synthesis of which class of molecules?

(A) mRNA
(B) rRNA
(C) tRNA
(D) hnRNA
(E) microRNAs

18 A 2-year-old has been diagnosed with a rhabdomyosarcoma and is placed on chemotherapy, including the drug dactinomycin. Dactinomycin exerts its effects by which of the following mechanisms?

(A) Binding of the drug to DNA, thereby blocking RNA synthesis
(B) Binding of the drug to ribosomes, thereby blocking translation
(C) Binding of the drug to transcription factors, thereby blocking RNA synthesis
(D) Binding of the drug to RNA polymerase II, thereby blocking RNA synthesis
(E) Binding of the drug to DNA, thereby blocking DNA synthesis

19 A man with a bacterial infection was prescribed rifampin to resolve the infection. Rifampin does not affect eukaryotic cells due to which of the following?

(A) Differences in ribosome structure between eukaryotes and prokaryotes
(B) Structural differences in RNA polymerase between eukaryotes and prokaryotes
(C) Differences in transcription factors between eukaryotes and prokaryotes
(D) Inability of the drug to bind to DNA containing nucleosomes
(E) Differences in snurp structure between eukaryotes and prokaryotes

20 A cell line was derived, which was temperature sensitive for splicing hnRNA. At the nonpermissive temperature, splicing was unable to occur. A potential activity that is mutated in the splicesome is which of the following?

(A) Ability to carry out RNA synthesis
(B) Ability to carry out DNA synthesis
(C) Loss of 3′–5′ exonuclease activity
(D) Loss of endonuclease activity
(E) Loss of ability for transcription-coupled DNA repair

ANSWERS

1 **The answer is B: Lack of error checking in RNA polymerase.** As part of the life cycle of the virus (see the figure below), the RNA genome of the virus is converted to DNA, which integrates randomly into the host chromosome. Host cell RNA polymerase II then transcribes the viral DNA, producing viral RNA, which is translated to produce viral proteins, and which is also utilized as the genome for new viral particles. RNA polymerase does not contain 3′–5′ exonuclease activity (which DNA polymerase does), so RNA polymerase cannot check its work and cannot fix errors when a mismatch is made. The accumulated effect of these errors increases the mutation rate of the virus much more than organisms containing DNA genomes. Since the enzyme that creates the viral DNA is reverse transcriptase, which also has no error-checking capability, the risk for mutations is greatly enhanced. DNA polymerase does check its work but is not used in the viral life cycle. The DNA repair enzymes are not altered by HIV infection. Uracil is a normal component of the viral RNA genome, whereas thymine is not, but neither of these facts results in an increase in mutation rate.

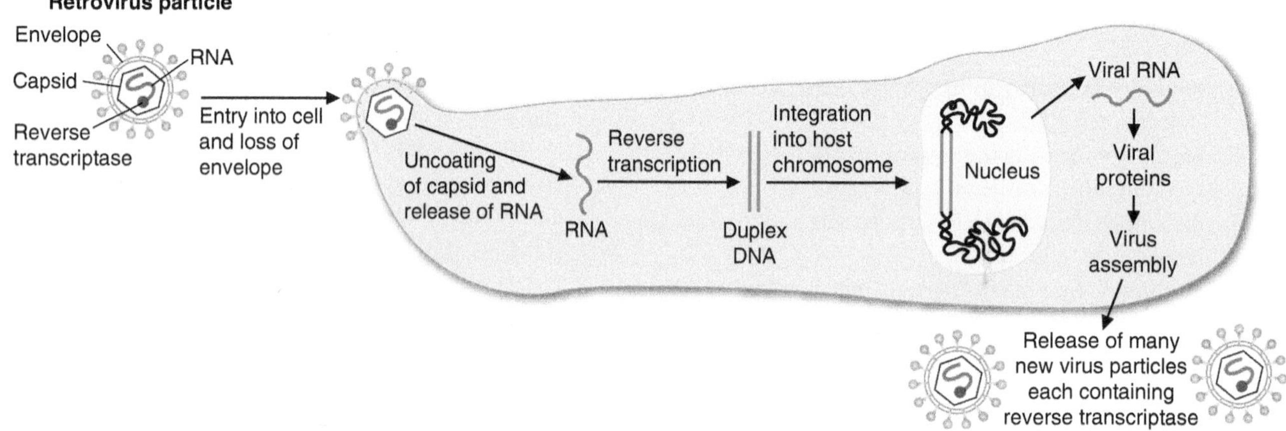

An overview of the retroviral life cycle.

2 **The answer is B: Run the RNA through an oligo-dT affinity column.** Mature mRNA from eukaryotes has a poly-A tail, which is added posttranscriptionally by poly-A polymerase (see the figure below for an overview of eukaryotic mRNA synthesis). The poly-A tail will hybridize to the oligo-dT on a column, thereby allowing the mRNA to bind to the column and other types of RNA to pass through the column. Altering the salt conditions (through a reduction of salt concentration) can then elute the mRNA specifically from the column. Phenol extraction is required for nucleic acid isolation, but it is not specific for mRNA. Electrophoresis, either agarose or polyacrylamide, will separate nucleic acids by size but does not by itself lead to mRNA isolation. An oligo-dA column will not hybridize to the poly-A tail of mRNA.

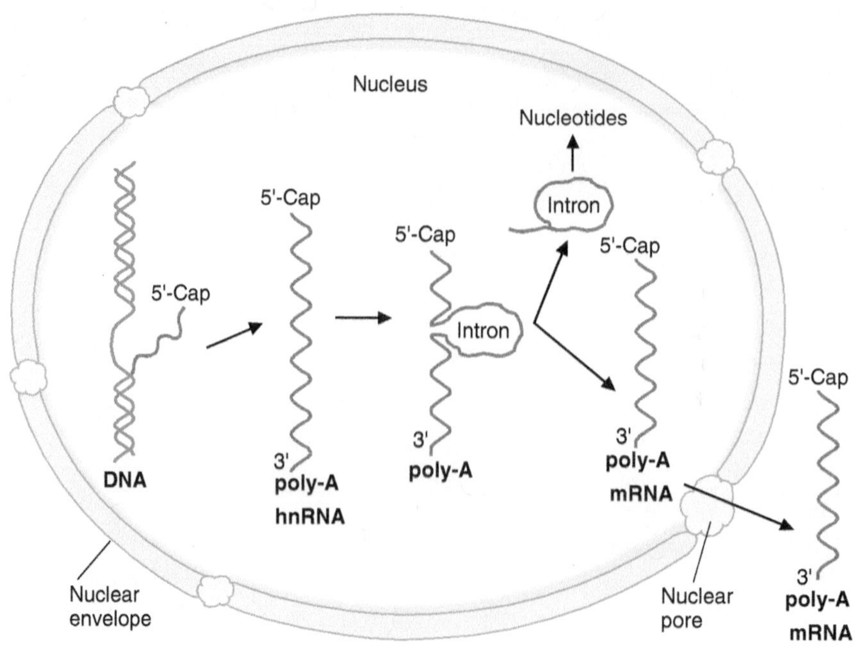

3 **The answer is C: Tissue-specific alternative splicing of the primary transcript.** Tissue-specific alternative splicing of one primary transcript can give rise to a number of distinct mature mRNAs, each of which gives rise to a variant of the parent protein (but all separate proteins in their own right) (see the figure below). Posttranslational modifications are made primarily to membrane bound or targeted proteins, but not cytosolic proteins. Polyadenylation and cap formation do not alter the reading frame of the protein and are required to fully mature the mRNA. Codon degeneracy will allow a number of different codons to specify the same amino acid in the protein's primary sequence; it will not alter the sequence of amino acids in the final protein as will alternative splicing.

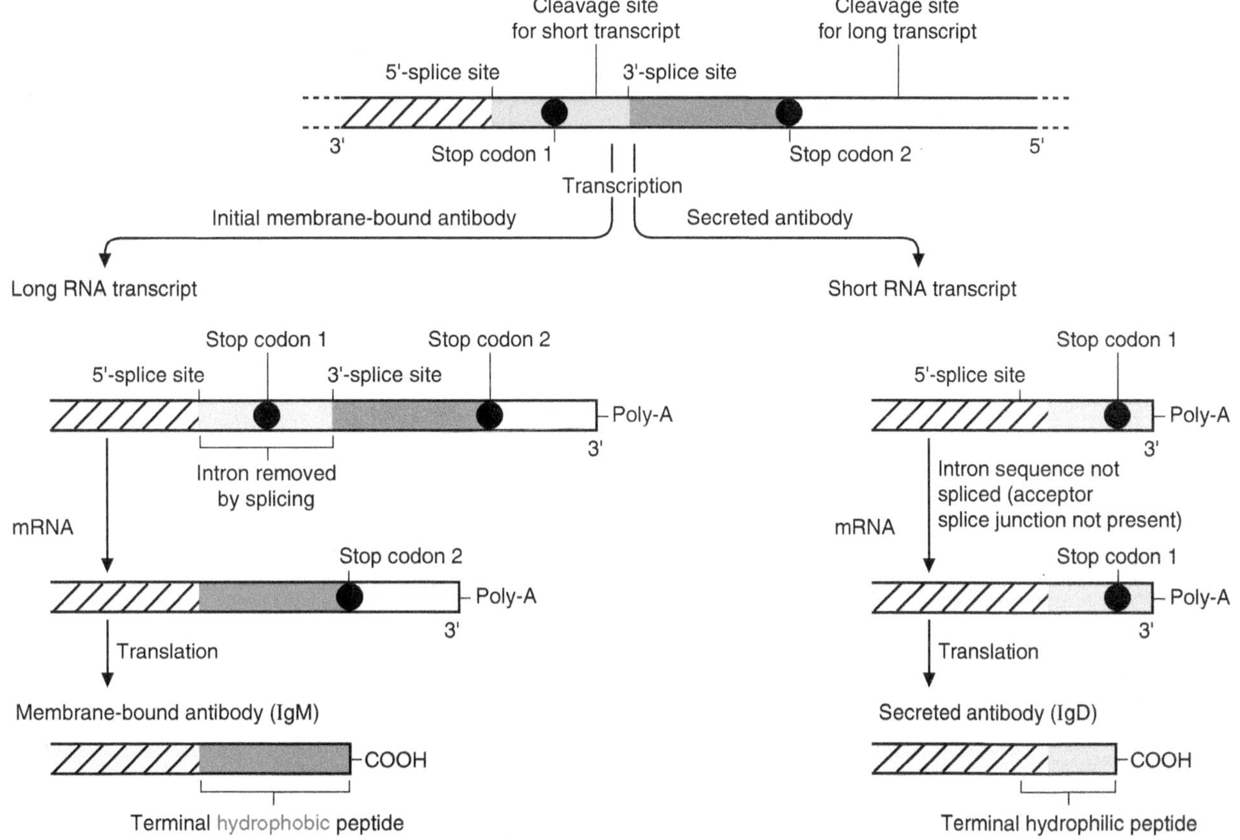

Two different antibodies (IgM and IgD) produced from the same initial RNA transcript as a result of alternative splicing.

4 **The answer is B: A mutation which creates an alternative splice site.** The patient has developed a mutation in an intron which acts, only a small percentage of the time, as a splice donor site instead of the normal site at the intron/exon boundary. Thus, when this site is utilized by the splicesome, a piece of the intron is incorporated into the mRNA product, producing a longer than normal mRNA. This is an infrequent event, however, as judged by the finding that the density of the normal sized mRNA band on the gel is darker than this abnormal band. A nonsense mutation in the DNA will not affect transcription (although it does affect the protein product made from the mRNA). The lack of a cap would result in an unstable mRNA that perhaps would not be translated but would not significantly change the size of the mRNA. Poly-A polymerase adds the poly-A tail and would add the same size tail to both species of mRNA. If the polyadenylation signal were mutated, then the overall mRNA size would be larger, but there would not be two different proteins produced. Since the patient has a β-thalassemia, defective β-globin protein is being produced from the larger mRNA. Loss of methionine codons will affect translation, but not transcription.

5 **The answer is C: Splicing of hnRNA.** As seen on page 34, an adenine nucleotide in the middle of the intron is a required component for splicing to occur, and the sugar residue attached to this adenine is involved in three phosphodiester linkages; the normal 3′ and 5′ and also 2′ to the splice site. The resulting structure resembles a lariat. Such a structure does not form during capping, polyadenylation, or the normal transcription of genes. It is unique to the splicing mechanism.

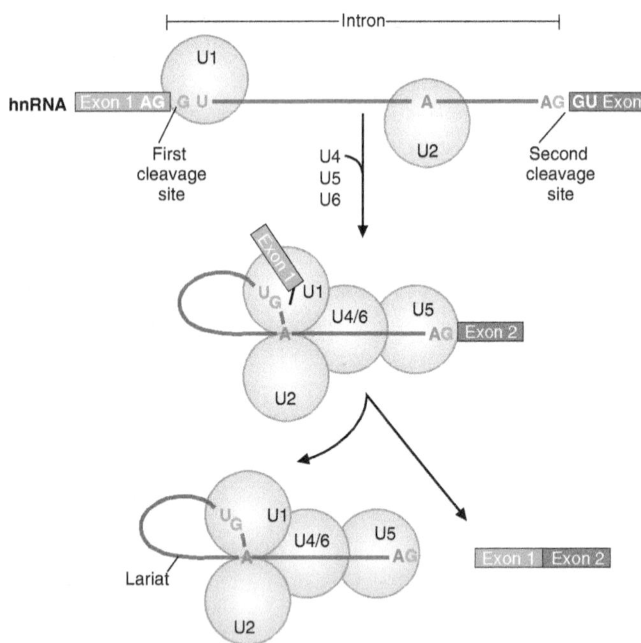

Lariat formation during splicing, showing the required intronic adenine nucleotide with three phosphodiester bonds.

6 **The answer is B: RNA polymerase II.** The patient has ingested α-amanitin, a toxin that, at very low concentrations, inhibits RNA polymerase II and blocks the transcription of single-copy genes. RNA polymerase I and III are more resistant to the effects of amanitin, and this toxin has no effect on telomerase or any type of DNA polymerase. The inability to synthesize new proteins in all cells leads to the symptoms observed. The structure of amanitin is shown below. Amanitin poisoning initially causes gastrointestinal disturbances, then electrolyte imbalance and fever, followed by liver and kidney dysfunction. Death can follow 2 to 3 days after ingestion.

α-Amanitin

7 **The answer is B.** The message-identical strand of DNA is the one that has the same sequence of bases as the mRNA product (with the exception that when there is a U in RNA, there is a T in DNA). Thus, this is the strand that is complementary to the strand that is being used as the template for RNA synthesis (which is designated as C in the figure).

8 **The answer is D.** The newly synthesized RNA strand is made in the 5′–3′ direction, so letter A represents the 5′ end of the newly synthesized RNA and letter D represents the 3′ end. The DNA template is being read in the 3′–5′ direction (letter C would represent the 3′ end of the template strand).

9 **The answer is A: Ribonuclear protein complexes.** The woman has lupus, an autoimmune disorder. One class of antibodies developed is against the snurps, small ribonuclear protein complexes, which are involved in mRNA splicing. Autoantibodies are not developed against DNA polymerase (although antibodies against DNA are often found), carbohydrates, tRNA complexes, or peroxisomal proteins.

10 **The answer is E: Degradation of the mRNA.** Introns have been shown to contain genes for microRNAs, which are processed to small, interfering RNAs, which can regulate gene expression either by binding to and initiating degradation of a particular mRNA or by binding to a particular mRNA and blocking translation of the mRNA. These small RNA molecules do not affect the transcription of the target mRNA, nor posttranscriptional processing (capping and polyadenylation). They also do not affect the export of mRNA into the cytoplasm, nor do they alter ribosome biogenesis. As an example, the miR-17-92 cluster encodes seven microRNAs and resides within an intron of the C13 or F25 gene on chromosome 13. These miRNAs are upregulated in lung cancer, and may contribute to the progression of the disease by downregulating their target genes.

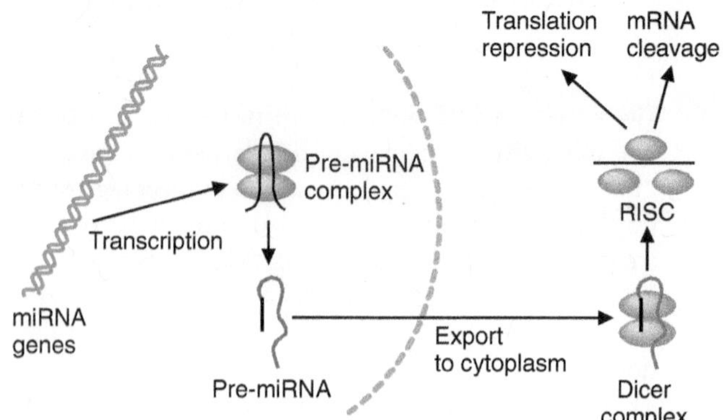

An overview of microRNA transcription, processing, and mode of action. The miRNA genes are transcribed in the nucleus, processed to a pre-miRNA, and exported to the cytoplasm. In the cytoplasm, the pre-miRNA is further processed by an RNase (Dicer), and the resultant double-stranded miRNA forms part of the RISC (RNA-induced silencing complex). A strand selection separation process occurs that allows recognition of the appropriate mRNA to ablate (either by nuclease degradation or inhibition of translation).

11 **The answer is D: Loss of a transcription termination site.** One of the genes that encoded protein X had a mutation at the transcription termination site, which enabled the mRNA to be transcribed into a longer form (237 nucleotides longer). The reading frame of the mRNA was intact, as was the start and stop codons, so the protein produced from this lengthened mRNA was normal. If a nonsense mutation had been created in gene X, a truncated, likely inactive, protein would have been produced. The loss of an intron/exon junction would alter the splicing pattern of the mRNA, and would most likely alter the reading frame of the protein and create a nonfunctional protein. Another possibility is that the loss of an intron/exon junction would produce an elongated protein (due to intronic DNA being transcribed as part of the mRNA), with a concomitant loss of activity. Gaining an alternative splice site would potentially lead to two forms of the final protein being produced, yet only one is seen by Western blot. Inefficient transcription initiation would not produce two distinct mRNAs.

12 **The answer is A: Western blotting of the peptide chains in hemoglobin.** Thalassemias are the result of an imbalance in the synthesis of α- and β-globin genes. If this were to occur, a Western blot analysis of the α and β chains would show a difference in the amount of each in the red blood cells, suggesting either an α- or β-thalassemia (in an α-thalassemia, one would see less α chains or variants of α chains being produced, as compared to just one, normal β chain. The opposite would be true for a β-thalassemia). As many α-thalassemias are caused by gene deletions, FISH might be another way to determine this condition, using a probe specific for the α-globin gene. Most β-thalassemias are not due to gene deletions. PCR for γ-globin (fetal Hb) or RNA polymerase will not address an imbalance in α- and/or β-globin chain synthesis. Similarly, Western blots of snurps or TFIID will not address an imbalance in synthesis (if there was a problem with snurps, all RNA splicing would be affected, not just the α or β-globin gene; similarly, if TFIID were altered, all mRNA synthesis would be altered). Clinical labs will also use hemoglobin electrophoresis to quantitate the levels of globin chains in a patient. The illustration used in the question was obtained from a patient with β-thalassemia.

13 **The answer is C: RNA editing defect.** The intestine contains an RNA editing complex that alters one base in the apo B100 mRNA, which creates a stop codon, such that when the mRNA is translated, protein synthesis stops after 48% of the codons have been translated. This is a unique type of posttranscriptional modification. The initial transcripts for both apo B48 and apo B100 are the same. Mutations that alter splicing, cap formation, or polyadenylation would not produce the full size protein in place of apo B48. Mutations in the promoter would alter initiation of transcription, but not the end product formed. RNA editing in this case is shown in the figure below.

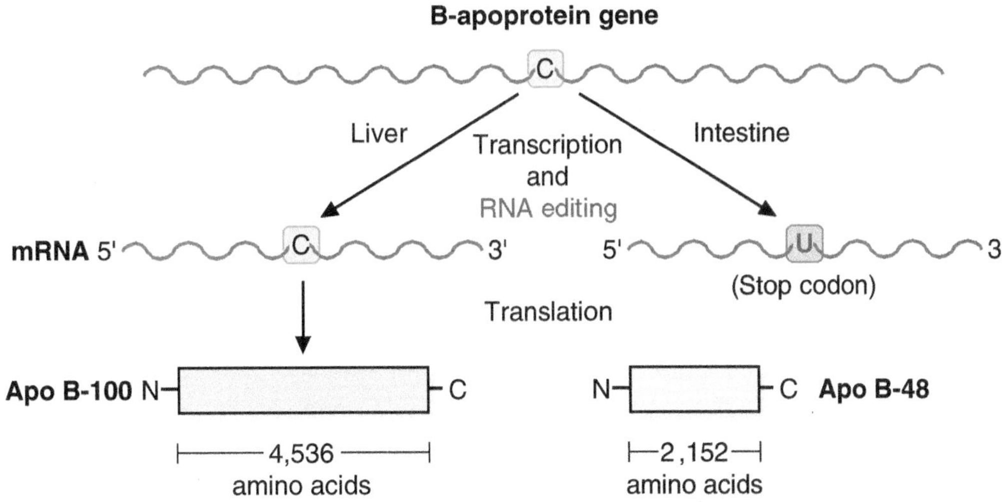

Answer 13: In intestinal cells, RNA editing converts a cytosine (C) to a uracil (U), producing a stop codon. Consequently, the B-apoprotein of intestinal cells (apo B48) contains only 2,152 amino acids. Apo B48 is 48% the size of apo B100, the product synthesized in the liver from the same gene, and which was not edited at the RNA level.

14 **The answer is B: Creation of an alternative splice site, such that β-globin levels are decreased.** If an intronic mutation created an alternative splice site, the spliceosome would utilize this site for splicing a certain percentage of the time, forming an mRNA that would not code for functional β-globin protein. This would lead to a reduction in β-globin synthesis relative to α-globin synthesis, thereby creating a β-thalassemia. If a microRNA were created which targeted the β-globin mRNA, then there would be a drastic reduction in β-globin synthesis as all β-globin mRNA would be targeted for destruction, which is not observed. Since the introns would be normally spliced from the mature mRNA, the creation of a transcription initiation site would have no effect on the mature mRNA. Similarly, the creation of a stop codon in an intron would have no effect on the mature mRNA. The polyadenylation signal is not found in introns, so the mutation could not be at this location within the gene.

15 **The answer is B: The ratio of α/β in patient X is 1:2, whereas in patient Y it is 5:1.** An individual with the genotype of patient X is producing 50% normal α chain (two normal genes, two deleted) and 100% β-globin for a ratio of 1:2 of α to β(each chromosome 11 contains two α-genes, for a total of four α-genes per cell). Such a ratio would lead to little, if any, clinical symptoms. Patient Y is producing 100% α chain and 20% β chain for a 5:1 ratio of α to β. This ratio is big enough to lead to clinical symptoms. Recall, the major biochemical problem in thalassemia is the imbalance in synthesis of α and β chains, leading to nonfunctional α_4 and β_4 tetramers forming from the excess chains produced. The other ratios presented as answers do not represent the mutations present in the patients.

16 **The answer is B: Lack of a 2′-OH group.** RNA polymerase is looking for substrates that contain a 2′-hydroxyl group (recall, DNA polymerase utilized dNTPs, which normally lack a hydroxyl group at the 2′ position). As this substrate lacks a 2′-hydroxyl group, therefore the binding affinity of this drug for RNA polymerase is very low, such that the likelihood that this chain terminator will be incorporated into a growing RNA chain is minimal. DNA polymerase, however, utilizes substrates lacking a 2′-hydroxyl group, and can bind and utilize this substrate.

17 **The answer is C: tRNA.** RNA polymerase III requires transcription factors to bind to promoters, which are labeled as TFIIIx, where x is a variable letter. Polymerase III will synthesize tRNA molecules and 5S rRNA. RNA polymerase II synthesizes mRNA while RNA polymerase I synthesizes primarily rRNA. Accessory factors for the polymerases are labeled TFIIx or TFIx, respectively. MicroRNAs are synthesized by polymerase II. hnRNA is the precursor for mature mRNA, also synthesized by RNA polymerase II.

18 **The answer is A: Binding of the drug to DNA, thereby blocking RNA synthesis.** Dactinomycin binds to DNA and blocks the ability of RNA polymerase to transcribe genes, thereby blocking transcription. The drug does not bind specifically to ribosomes, transcription factors, or RNA polymerase II. It also does not interfere with DNA synthesis.

19 **The answer is B: Structural differences in RNA polymerase between eukaryotes and prokaryotes.** Rifampin binds to prokaryotic RNA polymerase but cannot bind (due to the different structures of the RNA polymerase between prokaryotic and eukaryotic cells) to eukaryotic RNA polymerase. The drug does not bind to ribosomes, DNA, snurps, or transcription factors. Snurps are not present in prokaryotic cells.

20 **The answer is D: Loss of endonuclease activity.** The act of splicing requires the breakage of internal phosphodiester bonds, which is the job of an endonuclease. Splicing does not require new RNA synthesis, DNA synthesis, error-checking (the 3′–5′ exonuclease activity), or DNA repair. The process of splicing is shown again below.

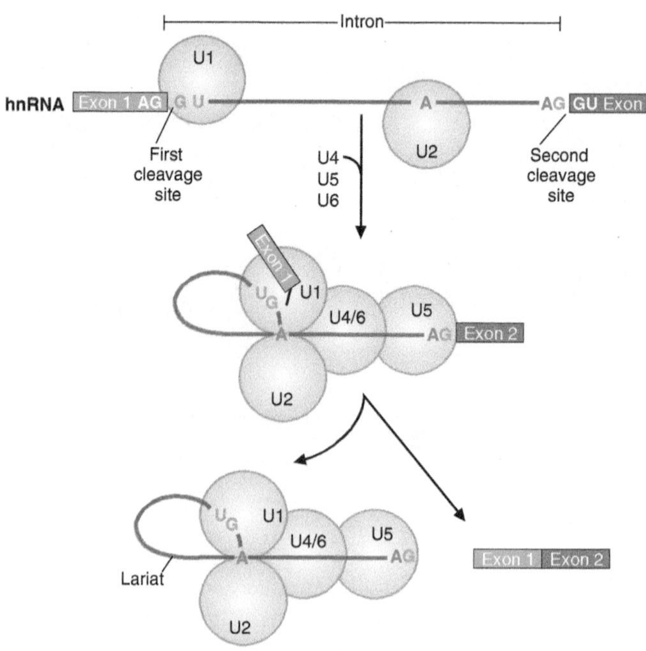

Lariat formation during splicing, showing the required intronic adenine nucleotide with three phosphodiester bonds.

Chapter 5

Protein Synthesis

This chapter covers the basics of protein synthesis (translation), including posttranslational modifications, and how differences between prokaryotic and eukaryotic translation are exploited in the use of antibiotics. A number of questions require reference to the genetic code, which is presented in Table 5-1.

Table 5-1.

First Base		Second Base			Third Base
(5′)	U	C	A	G	(3′)
U	Phe	Ser	Tyr	Cys	U
	Phe	Ser	Tyr	Cys	C
	Leu	Ser	Stop	Stop	A
	Leu	Ser	Stop	Trp	G
C	Leu	Pro	His	Arg	U
	Leu	Pro	His	Arg	C
	Leu	Pro	Gln	Arg	A
	Leu	Pro	Gln	Arg	G
A	Ile	Thr	Asn	Ser	U
	Ile	Thr	Asn	Ser	C
	Ile	Thr	Lys	Arg	A
	Met	Thr	Lys	Arg	G
G	Val	Ala	Asp	Gly	U
	Val	Ala	Asp	Gly	C
	Val	Ala	Glu	Gly	A
	Val	Ala	Glu	Gly	G

QUESTIONS

Select the single best answer.

1 A researcher has discovered a temperature-sensitive cell line that displays an overall reduction in protein synthesis. Analysis of the mRNA produced at the nonpermissive temperature indicated that a key structural feature, normally present on mRNA, was missing. Such a structure is most likely which one of the following?

(A) Intron–exon secondary structure
(B) Pseudouridine
(C) The 5′ cap
(D) Thymine
(E) The poly-A tail

2 Under conditions of active exercise, protein synthesis is reduced in the muscle. Under these conditions, which aspect of translation is inhibited?

(A) Inability to initiate translation
(B) Inability to elongate during translation
(C) Inability to terminate translation
(D) Inability to synthesize mRNA
(E) Inability to produce rRNA

3 A young child exhibits the following symptoms: Coarse facial features, congenital hip dislocation, inguinal hernias, and severe developmental delay. These symptoms are fully evident at the child's age of 1. Cellular analysis demonstrated the presence of inclusion bodies within the cytoplasm of liver cells. The inclusion bodies are the result of which of the following?

(A) Enhanced lysosomal enzyme activity
(B) Reduced lysosomal enzyme activity
(C) Enhanced peroxisomal enzyme activity
(D) Reduced peroxisomal enzyme activity
(E) Enhanced protein secretion

4 A eukaryotic cell line contains an aberrant, temperature-sensitive ribonuclease that specifically cleaves the large rRNA molecule into many pieces, destroying its secondary structure and its ability to bind to ribosomal proteins. This cell line, at the nonpermissive temperature, has greatly reduced the rates of

protein synthesis. This rate-limiting step is which of the following?
(A) Initiation
(B) Termination
(C) Elongation
(D) Peptide bond formation
(E) tRNA activation and charging

5 A cell contains a mutated alanine-tRNA^{ala} synthetase that recognizes glycine instead of alanine as its substrate. The anticodon of the tRNA recognized by this enzyme is IGC. When the cell translates the following portion of an mRNA molecule (presented in frame beginning with the 5′ nucleotide), what will be the amino acid sequence of the protein produced from this stretch of mRNA?
-AUGGCGGACUCGGCUAUG-
(A) M-G-S-D-G-M
(B) M-A-D-S-G-M
(C) M-A-D-S-A-M
(D) M-A-S-D-A-M
(E) M-G-D-S-A-M

Questions 6 and 7 refer to the following case. A 3-year-old boy, whose parents did not immunize him due to fears of postimmunization side effects, exhibited fever, chills, severe sore throat, lethargy, trouble breathing, and a husky voice. Physical exam indicated greatly enlarged lymph nodes, an increased heart rate, and swelling of the palate. A picture of the boy's throat is shown below.

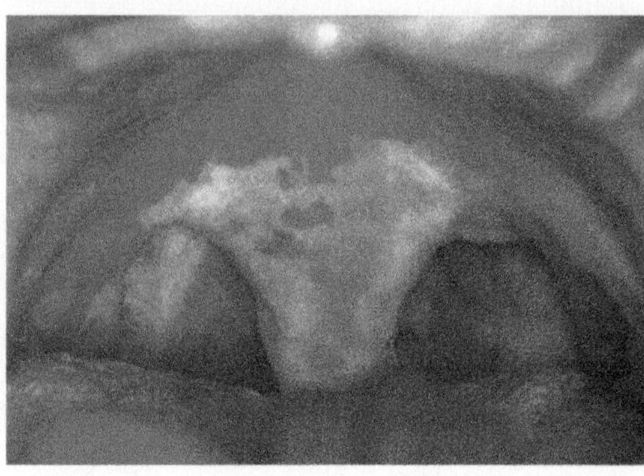

The throat is dull red, and a gray exudate (pseudomembrane) is present on the uvula, pharynx, and tongue.

6 A necessary cofactor for allowing these symptoms to appear in the child is which of the following?
(A) ATP
(B) NAD^+
(C) FAD
(D) Acetyl-CoA
(E) UDP-glucose

7 The molecular mechanism responsible for these physical observations in the boy is which of the following?
(A) Activation of protein kinase A
(B) Activation of an elongation factor for translation
(C) Glycosylation of a G protein
(D) Inhibition of protein kinase A
(E) Inhibition of an elongation factor for translation

8 A 2-year-old girl exhibits a very high fever of sudden onset and complains of a stiff neck. Physical exam reveals a positive Brudzinski and Kernig sign and petechiae on the extremities. The pediatrician, in addition to rushing the child to the hospital, prescribes a drug that blocks prokaryotic peptide bond formation, even though it can have serious side effects. That drug is which of the following?
(A) Rifampin
(B) Rapamycin
(C) Chloramphenicol
(D) Cycloheximide
(E) Puromycin

9 A Russian youngster was prescribed erythromycin for a bacterial infection, but he developed hearing loss due to use of this drug. This occurred due to which of the following?
(A) Inhibition of mitochondrial protein synthesis
(B) Inhibition of mitochondrial RNA synthesis
(C) Inhibition of mitochondrial DNA replication
(D) Weakening and tearing of the eardrum
(E) Increased neuronal signaling in the inner ear

10 While investigating structure–function studies in a membrane transport protein, a researcher discovered a single nucleotide mutation that led to the loss of a key α-helical segment of the protein. The mutation that led to this finding is most likely which of the following?
(A) CUC to CCC
(B) GUU to GCU
(C) UUG to CUG
(D) AUC to GUC
(E) GUG to UUG

11 An adult male is diagnosed with a typical pneumonia. His physician prescribes clarithromycin, which is specific for prokaryotic cells. Which of the following best explains the mechanism of prokaryotic specificity?
(A) The drug binds to the 50S ribosomal subunit of bacteria and inhibits f-met-tRNAi binding
(B) The drug binds to the 30S ribosomal subunit of bacteria and blocks initiation of protein synthesis
(C) The drug binds to the 50S ribosomal subunit of bacteria and blocks translocation
(D) The drug binds to the 30S ribosomal subunit of bacteria and blocks peptide bond formation
(E) The drug binds to both ribosomal subunits and prevents bacterial ribosome assembly

12 A patient underwent a kidney transplant and among the many drugs she received posttransplant was rapamycin. Rapamycin aids in preventing an immune response to the transplant via which of the following mechanisms?

(A) The drug inhibits ribosome subunit assembly
(B) The drug inhibits cap formation
(C) The drug specifically inhibits RNA polymerase III
(D) The drug inhibits initiation of protein synthesis
(E) The drug inhibits antibody-specific transcription factors from binding to DNA

13 You see a very sick patient (vomiting and bloody diarrhea, dehydration, and mental status changes) in the emergency department, who, you are told, was an amateur chef trying out a new creation in which he wanted to experiment with the extracts of castor beans. This person's symptoms are all due to which of the following?

(A) Inhibition of RNA polymerase I
(B) Inhibition of RNA polymerase II
(C) Ribosomal inactivation by covalent modification
(D) Ribosomal disassembly due to covalent modification
(E) Inhibition of amino-acyl tRNA synthetases

14 A 2-year-old boy with an ear infection was given amoxicillin, but it did not clear up the problem. Switching to azithromycin successfully eradicated the infection, and subsequent laboratory work indicated that the offending bacterium was resistant to amoxicillin. Bacterial resistance to antibiotics is often due to which of the following?

(A) Altered ribosome structure
(B) Altered cell wall
(C) Enzymatic destruction of the antibiotic
(D) Inability to transport the drug into the bacteria
(E) A mutation in RNA polymerase

15 A young boy exhibits myopathy, encephalopathy, lactic acidosis, and strokelike episodes. All of his siblings have some aspects of the same symptoms. The boy most likely has which type of mutation?

(A) A defect in mRNA synthesis
(B) A defect in mitochondrial tRNA production
(C) A defect in mitochondrial rRNA production
(D) A defect in cytoplasmic tRNA
(E) A defect in cytoplasmic rRNA

16 Given the serine codons shown below, what is the minimum number of tRNAs which is required to bind to them?

UCU, UCC, UCA, UCG, AGU, AGC

(A) 1
(B) 2
(C) 3
(D) 4
(E) 5

17 A young boy has edema, a protruding abdomen, and very thin arms and legs. The edema has at its origins which of the following?

(A) Lack of muscle protein synthesis
(B) Lack of liver protein synthesis
(C) Lack of intestinal protein synthesis
(D) Excessive water production due to protein hydrolysis
(E) Excessive water production due to triglyceride hydrolysis

18 A patient taking lovastatin and Zetia® for elevated cholesterol was found to produce lower levels of glycosylated proteins. This is most likely due to the unintended consequence of blocking the synthesis of which of the following compounds?

(A) Coenzyme Q
(B) Cholesterol
(C) Dolichol
(D) HMG-CoA
(E) Ketone bodies

19 A patient with type 2 diabetes has been prescribed recombinant insulin to help control his disease. Three months after starting this regime, a blood test is done, which indicates that the patient is still producing endogenous insulin, in addition to the recombinant insulin the patient is taking. The blood test has, at its basis, which of the following?

(A) Posttranslational proteolytic processing
(B) Posttranslational glycosylation
(C) Posttranslational modification of amino acid side chains
(D) Posttranslational acylation
(E) Posttranslational quaternary structure formation

20 A hospital laboratory made an error and mistyped a patient's blood as AB, instead of B. When given type A blood, the patient had an adverse reaction. The major difference between individuals with AB and B type blood is due to which of the following?

(A) The presence of a specific glycosyl transferase
(B) The presence of a specific acyl transferase
(C) The presence of a specific peptidase
(D) The lack of dolichol pyrophosphate
(E) Increased levels of dolichol pyrophosphate

ANSWERS

1 **The answer is C: The 5′ cap.** The 5′ cap of mRNA is recognized by initiation factors (specifically eIF4E) to allow ribosome assembly on the mRNA. The absence of a cap would not allow a translation initiation complex to form (see the figure below for an overview of translation initiation. Factor eIF4e is required for the mRNA binding to the small ribosomal subunit through cap recognition). Introns are not found in mature mRNA (they are removed by splicing in the nucleus); thus, intron–exon secondary structure would not be present. Pseudouridine is found only in tRNA, not in mature mRNA. Thymine, while found in tRNA by posttranscriptional processing, is not found in mRNA (uracil is placed into the mRNA when an adenine is in the template strand), and the poly-A tail, at the 3′ end of the mRNA, adds stability to the mRNA, but it does not play a role in translation initiation.

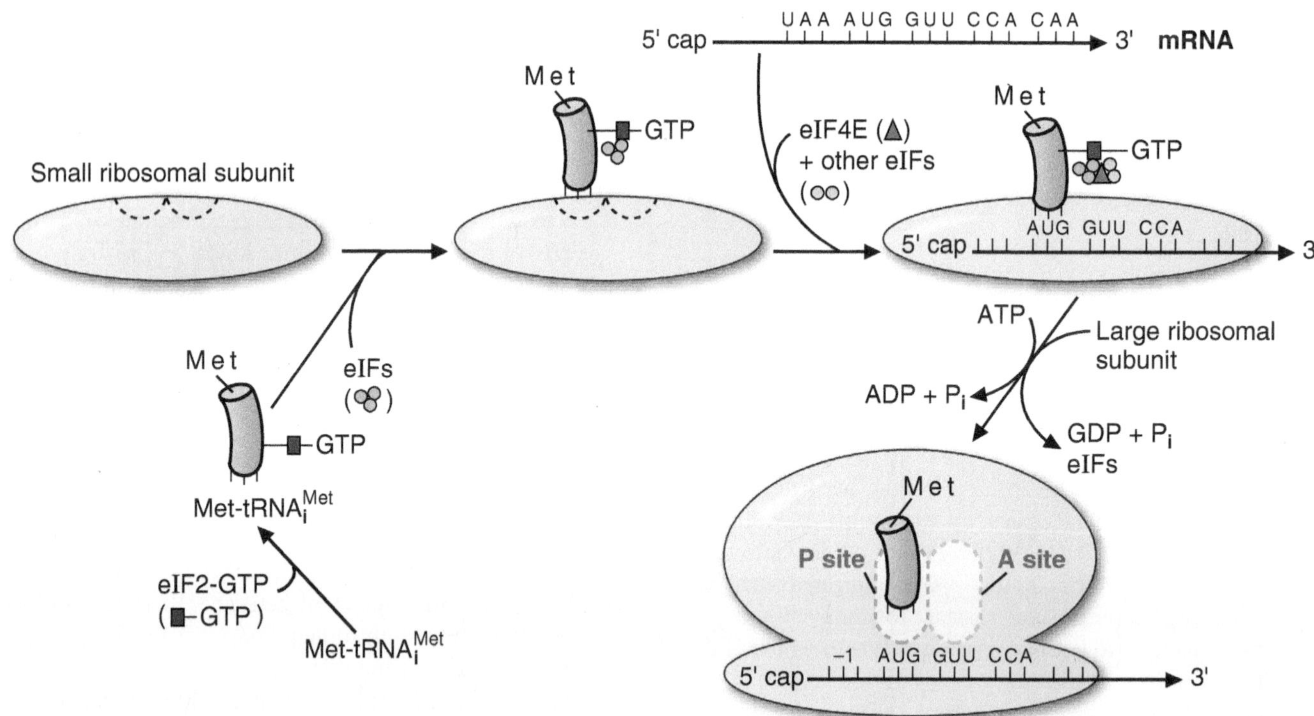

2 **The answer is A: Inability to initiate translation.** As muscle works, and AMP levels rise, the muscle wants to preserve its ATP for muscle contraction, and not to use it for new protein synthesis. The increase in AMP levels leads to the activation of AMP-activated protein kinase, which will phosphorylate and inactivate eIF4E (eukaryotic initiation factor 4E), which is a necessary component in recognizing the 5′ cap structure of the mRNA to allow ribosome assembly on the mRNA (see the figure in the answer to the previous question). The activation of the AMP-activated protein kinase does not alter elongation or the termination of translation. It does not block overall transcription, either of mRNA or rRNA (although it may lead to an inhibition of ribosomal biogenesis as well as the transcription of certain specific genes).

3 **The answer is B: Reduced lysosomal enzyme activity.** The child has I-cell disease (mucolipidosis type II), which is a deficiency in protein sorting, particularly of sending lysosomal enzymes to the lysosome (a lysosomal storage disease). The I of I-cell disease stands for inclusion bodies. If the child develops these clinical and radiologic symptoms later in life, one would consider the diagnosis of Hurler syndrome (mucopolysaccharidosis). Lysosomal enzymes are tagged with mannose-6-phosphate (M6P) during posttranslational modification. Enzymes containing M6P then bind to a M6P receptor, which transports the enzymes to the lysosomes. Lacking such a signal, patients with I-cell disease secrete their lysosomal contents into the plasma and interstitial fluids. This leads to lysosomal dysfunction and cellular and tissue destruction. The enzyme that is defective is shown on page 41. This disease is not peroxisomal, nor does it enhance protein secretion.

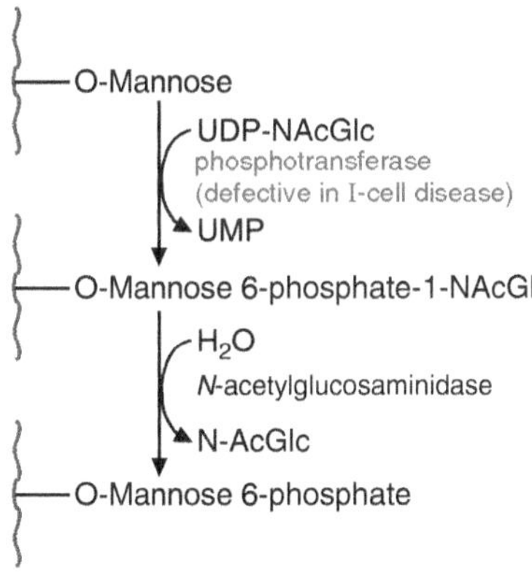

O-Mannose
UDP-NAcGlc
phosphotransferase
(defective in I-cell disease)
UMP
O-Mannose 6-phosphate-1-NAcGlc
H_2O
N-acetylglucosaminidase
N-AcGlc
O-Mannose 6-phosphate

Generation of the mannose-6-phosphate signal on lysosomal proteins within the ER.

4 **The answer is D: Peptide bond formation.** It is the large ribosomal RNA that catalyzes peptide bond formation, using peptides and amino acids in the "A" and "P" sites on the ribosome. Destroying the secondary structure of this rRNA via the aberrant ribonuclease will limit the ability of the ribosome to create peptide bonds. The large, ribosomal RNA molecule is not essential for the initiation, termination, elongation (moving the ribosome along the mRNA after peptide bond formation has occurred), or tRNA activation and charging.

5 **The answer is B: M-A-D-S-G-M.** The variant cell line will mischarge a $tRNA^{ala}$ with glycine, but only the $tRNA^{ala}$ that has, as its anticodon, IGC. IGC will recognize three codons: GCA, GCU, and GCC. Thus, when these codons are present in the mRNA, glycine will replace alanine. Thus, reading the RNA from the 5′ end (as translation reads the mRNA 5′ to 3′) provided in a series of 3, we have AUG (which is methionine), GCG (which is alanine—the anticodon for this codon is CGC; IGC will not recognize the GCG codon), GAC (which is aspartic acid), UCG (which is serine), GCU (which, in this cell line, is glycine and not alanine, since the IGC anticodon will recognize the GCU codon), and AUG (methionine). The answer choices utilize the single-letter codes to represent the amino acids.

6 **The answer is B: NAD^+.** Diphtheria toxin, after entering cells, is cleaved by a protease to form an active enzyme, which, utilizing NAD^+ as a substrate, ADP-ribosylates eEF2, thereby inhibiting protein translation. ATP, FAD, acetyl-CoA, and UDP-glucose are not required for the ADP-ribosylation reaction. The final modified product, an arginine with an ADP-ribose attached, is shown below.

7 **The answer is E: Inhibition of an elongation factor for translation.** The child has diphtheria, which is caused by a bacterium (*Corynebacterium diphtheriae*), which produces a toxin that leads to the inhibition of eEF2 (eukaryotic elongation factor 2), which is required for the movement of tRNA from the "A" site to the "P" site. The toxin catalyzes the ADP-ribosylation (using NAD^+ as a substrate) of eEF2 to bring about this inhibition. If one treats such a child with nicotinamide (the reaction product resulting from the loss of ADP-ribose from NAD^+), one can reverse and block the ADP-ribosylation reaction catalyzed by the toxin. The toxin has no effect on protein kinase A, nor does it glycosylate a G protein. Diphtheria causes sore throat, fever, swollen nodes (bull neck), weakness, hoarseness, painful swallowing, and chills. The hallmark of the disease is a thick, gray membrane covering the pharynx.

8 **The answer is C: Chloramphenicol.** Chloramphenicol blocks peptide bond formation in prokaryotic ribosomes (with no effect on eukaryotic ribosomes). This concept is the basis of certain antibiotic therapy; the differences in ribosome structure between eukaryotic and prokaryotic cells allow selective drug inhibition. The child has meningococcal meningitis, and chloramphenicol, despite its side effects of inhibiting mitochondrial protein synthesis, is a very effective agent for this disorder. Cycloheximide has the same effect as chloramphenicol in eukaryotic cells but has no effect on prokaryotes. Rapamycin leads to the blockage of translation initiation, not peptide bond formation. Puromycin is a chain terminator, stopping protein synthesis but not directly inhibiting peptide bond formation. Rifampin inhibits prokaryotic mRNA synthesis and has no direct effect on translation. Rifampin might be used as prophylaxis for household contacts of meningococcal meningitis but is not as effective a treatment for the actual disease.

9 **The answer is A: Inhibition of mitochondrial protein synthesis.** Ototoxicity (hearing loss) occurs with a subset of antibiotics because, in addition to affecting prokaryotic ribosomes, the drugs also have an effect on mitochondrial ribosomes. Mitochondria contain their own DNA, RNA polymerase, and protein synthesizing apparatus (recall that it is thought that during evolution, bacteria invaded eukaryotic cells

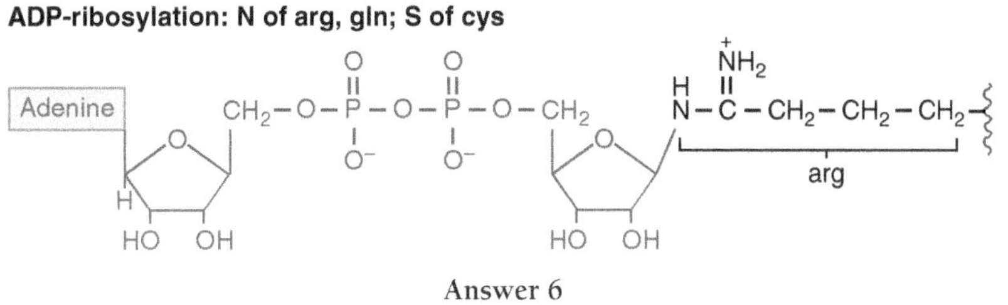

ADP-ribosylation: N of arg, gln; S of cys

Adenine
$CH_2-O-P(=O)(O^-)-O-P(=O)(O^-)-O-CH_2$
HO OH HO OH
$H-N-C(=\overset{+}{N}H_2)-CH_2-CH_2-CH_2-$
arg

Answer 6

and formed a symbiotic relationship, with the bacteria eventually becoming the mitochondria), which is very similar to the prokaryotic apparatus. Thus, certain drugs will affect mitochondrial protein synthesis, and the effects seem to be greatest on those organs that have high energy needs (such as neuronal tissue). Erythromycin does not affect mitochondrial RNA synthesis or DNA replication. It does not affect the ear drum, nor does it increase neuronal signaling in the inner ear.

10 **The answer is A: CUC to CCC.** The most efficient way to destroy an α-helix is to insert a proline into the middle of it, as proline cannot form an α-helix due to the restriction of rotation of certain bond angles. Choice (A) has a leucine going to proline; all of the other substitutions (val to ala, leu to leu, ile to val, and val to leu) would still allow α-helix formation after the substitution took effect as these are conservative substitutions.

11 **The answer is C: The drug binds to the 50S ribosomal subunit of bacteria and blocks translocation.** Clarithromycin (an antibiotic in the macrolide family with erythromycin and azithromycin) is specific for the large ribosomal subunit of prokaryotes (it will not bind to eukaryotic ribosomes). When this drug binds to the large ribosomal subunit, translocation of the ribosome (movement along the mRNA) is blocked, which blocks overall protein synthesis. tRNA binding is not affected by clarithromycin, nor is there a blockage of the formation of an initiation complex. It is the large subunit (50S) that contains the peptidyl transferase activity, which is also not blocked by this agent.

12 **The answer is D: The drug inhibits initiation of protein synthesis.** Rapamycin inhibits the mammalian target of rapamycin (mTOR), which is a protein kinase. One of the many targets of mTOR is eIF4E binding protein (eIF4E is a required initiation factor for protein synthesis). When not phosphorylated, the binding protein binds tightly to eIF4E and prevents it from participating in the formation of the translational initiation complex, thereby blocking protein synthesis. When phosphorylated at multiple locations by mTOR, the binding protein falls off the initiation factor and allows translational initiation complexes to form. In the presence of rapamycin, mTOR has no kinase activity, and the binding protein remains bound to eIF4E, thereby inhibiting protein synthesis. The drug does not affect ribosome assembly. The drug also has no effect on transcription or RNA processing.

13 **The answer is C: Ribosomal inactivation by covalent modification.** Ricin, a toxin found in castor oil beans, specifically cleaves an N-glycosidic bond in the 28S rRNA of the large ribosomal subunit (an adenine base is removed, but the phosphodiester backbone remains intact). The sequence of the rRNA that is altered is required for binding elongation factors during protein synthesis. As ribosomes become inactivated by ricin, protein synthesis in cells stops, leading to cell death. Ricin does not inhibit RNA polymerases or aminoacyl tRNA synthetases. Ricin does not initially affect ribosome assembly. The LD_{50} for ricin is 30 mg/kg body weight.

14 **The answer is C: Enzymatic destruction of the antibiotic.** Bacteria that develop resistance to antibiotics usually do so by containing an enzymatic activity that destroys the structure of the antibiotic so that it cannot effectively inhibit its target within the cell. Amoxicillin works by destroying the bacterial cell wall, by being incorporated into the growing cell wall, which leads to a cessation of cell wall synthesis. It does not alter ribosome structure. Mutations in RNA polymerase will not lead to resistance to drugs. Azithromycin was effective because the bacteria did not produce an enzyme that destroyed the drug.

15 **The answer is B: A defect in mitochondrial tRNA production.** The boy has MELAS (Mitochondrial myopathy, encephalopathy, lactic acidosis, and stroke), a neurodegenerative disorder due to a mutation in mitochondrial tRNA, leading to defective protein synthesis within the mitochondria. The component most often affected is complex 1 of the respiratory chain. The severity of the disease will be dependent on the extent of heteroplasmy (what percentage of the mitochondria codes for the altered tRNA). The more mutant mitochondria present, the more severe the symptoms.

16 **The answer is C: 3.** A tRNA with the anticodon IGA will bind to UCU, UCC, and UCA (with wobbling at the third position of the codon). A tRNA with the anticodon CGA will bind to UCG. And the third tRNA, with

an anticodon of ICU, can base-pair with both AGU and AGC. Recall that I will base-pair with A, C, or U in the wobble position. These codon–anticodon interactions are shown below.

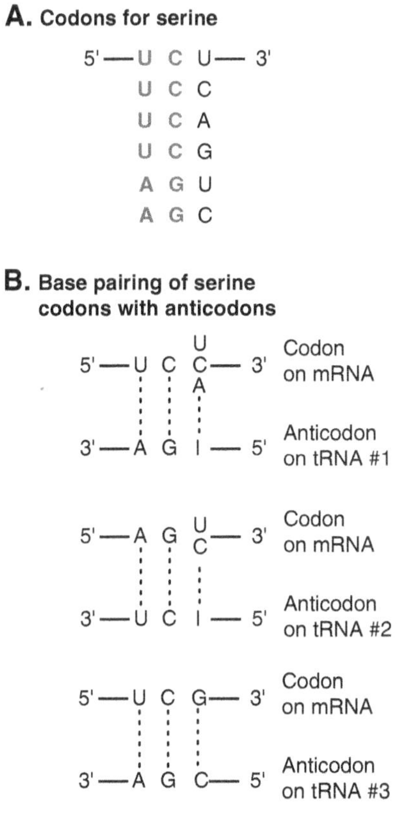

A. Codons for serine

5'—U C U— 3'
U C C
U C A
U C G
A G U
A G C

B. Base pairing of serine codons with anticodons

5'—U C C— 3' (U/A wobble) Codon on mRNA
3'—A G I — 5' Anticodon on tRNA #1

5'—A G C— 3' (U) Codon on mRNA
3'—U C I — 5' Anticodon on tRNA #2

5'—U C G— 3' Codon on mRNA
3'—A G C— 5' Anticodon on tRNA #3

17 **The answer is B: Lack of liver protein synthesis.** The boy is displaying kwashiorkor due to a calorie-deficient diet low in protein. Since the boy is taking in less protein than he needs, he is becoming deficient in the essential amino acids. Thus, to synthesize new proteins, existing proteins need to be degraded such that a pool of essential amino acids is available for the new protein synthesis. This protein degradation occurs in the muscles, leaving the boy with very thin arms and legs. The liver, despite the increased muscle protein turnover, is still deficient in essential amino acids and reduces its level of protein synthesis, including those proteins normally found in the blood, such as serum albumin. The reduced protein content in the blood reduces the osmotic strength of the blood such that when the blood flows through the body, the osmotic strength of the tissues is higher, and fluid leaves the blood and enters the interstitial space around the tissues. This leads to the protruding abdomen seen in these starving individuals. The problem is not related to reduced muscle protein synthesis (which does occur, but does not affect the osmotic strength of the blood), or reduced intestinal protein synthesis, for the same reason as the muscle. Both protein hydrolysis and triglyceride hydrolysis require water; water is not produced when these molecules are broken down.

18 **The answer is C: Dolichol.** The biosynthesis of both coenzyme Q and dolichol is dependent on isoprene units, specifically isopentenylpyrophosphate, which is derived from mevalonic acid in the de novo pathway of cholesterol biosynthesis. Lovastatin inhibits HMG-CoA reductase, which reduces mevalonate production. This can have, then, the unintended consequence of a reduction in dolichol production, thereby leading to underglycosylation of processed proteins. A reduction of coenzyme Q synthesis can lead to muscle weakness (a side effect of the statin class of drugs), but coenzyme Q is not involved in protein glycosylation. Cholesterol, HMG-CoA, and ketone bodies are not required for protein glycosylation as well. The structure of dolichol, in which the isoprene building block is highlighted, is shown below.

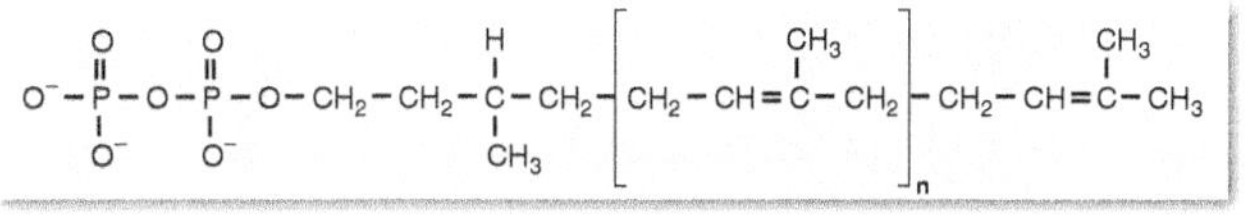

$$O^{-}-\overset{O}{\overset{\|}{P}}(O^{-})-O-\overset{O}{\overset{\|}{P}}(O^{-})-O-CH_2-CH_2-\overset{H}{C}(CH_3)-CH_2-\left[CH_2-CH=\overset{CH_3}{C}-CH_2\right]_n-CH_2-CH=\overset{CH_3}{C}-CH_3$$

19 **The answer is A: Posttranslational proteolytic processing.** As shown on page 44, insulin is synthesized as a preproinsulin. The pre sequence is the signal sequence, which is cleaved when the protein enters the endoplasmic reticulum. Proinsulin contains the C-peptide, which is removed to form mature insulin, and disulfide bonds that hold the A and B chains together. The modification is thus proteolytic processing, and not glycosylation, modification of side chains, acylation, or altered quaternary structure. The test is a C-peptide level. If a person is producing insulin, a C-peptide level can show this. This is also a way to see if a person has type 1 diabetes mellitus (no C-peptide, since they cannot produce endogenous insulin) or type 2 (normal or high C-peptide levels, since this disease is a reduced response to normally produced insulin).

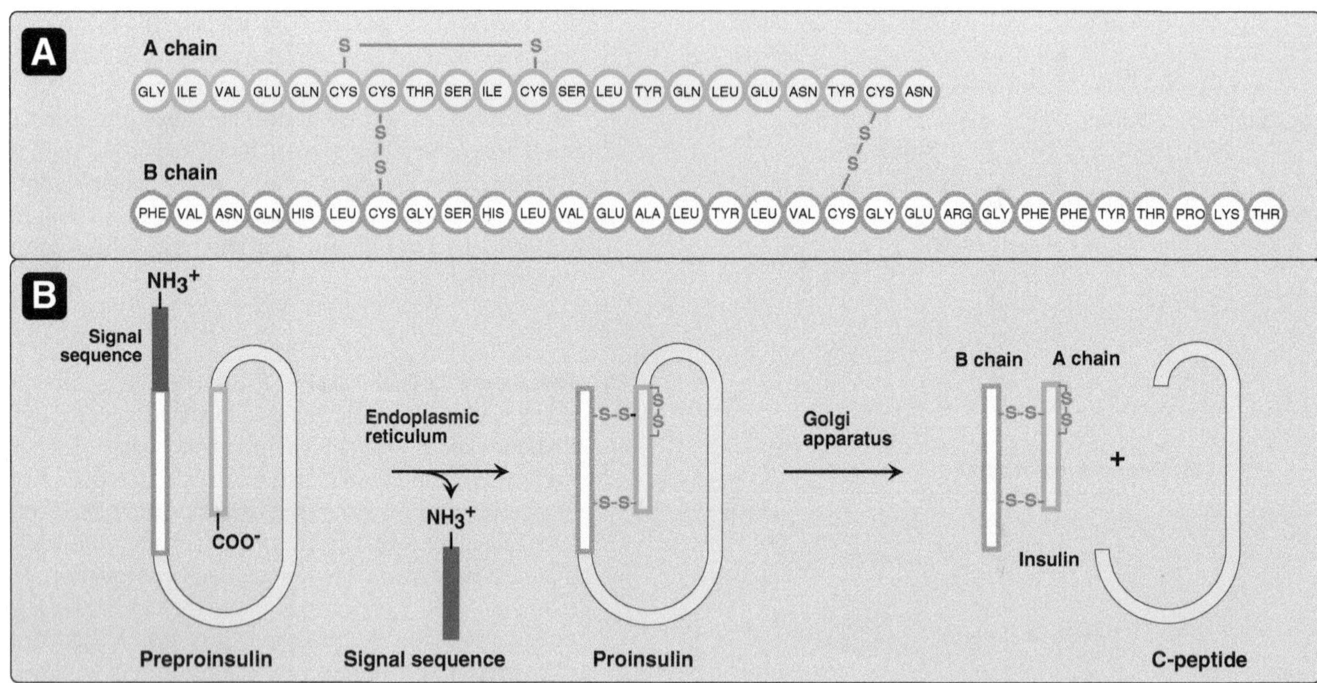

Answer 19: Panel A indicates the amino acid sequence of mature insulin while **panel B** indicates the steps involved in converting preproinsulin to mature insulin.

20 **The answer is A: The presence of a specific glycosyl transferase.** As shown below, type A and B blood differ by the presence of one sugar on glycosylated proteins. Individuals with type A blood add one type of sugar (*N*-acetylgalactosamine), while individuals with type B blood add a different sugar (galactose) due to differences in the specificity of a glycosyl transferase that recognizes the base carbohydrate structure. The differences in blood group antigens are not due to acylation or proteolytic processing on the cell surface. As these carbohydrates are O-linked, dolichol (which is required for N-linked glycosylation) is not required for their synthesis.

Blood type

Type O: Gal, GlcNAc, R, Fuc — H substance

Type A: GalNAc, Gal, GlcNAc, R, Fuc

Type B: Gal, Gal, GlcNAc, R, Fuc

Structures of the blood group antigens.

Chapter 6

Regulation of Gene Expression

In this chapter, the questions will cover various aspects of gene regulation, focusing on the ways in which both prokaryotes and eukaryotes regulate both transcription and translation.

QUESTIONS

Select the single best answer.

1 While studying the lac operon in bacteria, a scientist isolates mutants of *Escherichia coli,* which always express the genes of the lac operon (constitutive synthesis). The scientist creates partial diploids of the regulatory elements of the lac operon in these mutants of *E. coli*. In one partial diploid, expression of the lac operon is still constitutive (synthesis of the genes is observed even in the absence of an inducer). A likely explanation for this result is which of the following?

(A) There is a mutation in cis with the operon
(B) There is a mutation in trans with the operon
(C) Inducer can no longer bind to the repressor
(D) Inducer binds too tightly to the repressor
(E) The transactivation domain of the repressor is mutated

2 An African American patient has displayed vaso-occlusive episodes for most of his life. The incidents are more prevalent under conditions in which blood oxygen levels are low, such as during exercise or taking trips to locations at high altitudes. The patient has been placed on hydroxyurea. The rationale behind this treatment is which of the following?

(A) To prevent vaso-occlusive episodes through hydroxyurea induced protein degradation
(B) To reduce synthesis of a defective protein
(C) To induce synthesis of a functional protein
(D) To enhance oxygen levels in the blood
(E) To activate the enzyme that produces 2,3-bisphosphoglycerate

3 A hematologist is studying an African American family as one of the children was recently diagnosed with sickle cell disease. His sibling shows no symptoms of the disease, although genetic tests showed homozygosity for the HbS gene. An analysis of his red blood cells is likely to show which of the following?

(A) Reduced alpha chain synthesis
(B) Reduced sickle chain synthesis
(C) Increased gamma chain synthesis
(D) Increased zeta chain synthesis
(E) Increased delta chain synthesis

4 A healthy teenage girl has come to her pediatrician for a presports physical. Results of hemoglobin electrophoresis indicated an elevation of fetal hemoglobin. This can come about via which of the following mechanisms?

(A) Overall increased expression of all transcription factors
(B) Overall reduced expression of all transcription factors
(C) Deletions in the locus control region of the β-globin gene cluster
(D) Deletions in the locus control region of the α-globin gene cluster
(E) Inappropriate looping of chromosomal DNA, allowing transcription of previously inaccessible genes to occur

5 In a study with mice exhibiting hypercholesterolemia, cholesterol was affixed to double-stranded RNA, which targeted the dsRNA to enter cells through cholesterol diffusion through the plasma membrane. The dsRNA was targeted to bind to mRNA that encoded the apolipoprotein B gene and resulted in a lowering of circulating cholesterol levels. This result occurs due to which of the following?

(A) Inhibition of apolipoprotein B transcription
(B) Inhibition of apolipoprotein B translation
(C) Inhibition of apolipoprotein B folding
(D) Enhanced degradation of apolipoprotein B
(E) RNA editing of the apolipoprotein B mRNA

6 A woman with a BMI of 16.5 visits her family physician because she always feels tired. The history indicates that the woman is always on a diet, exercises over 3 h/day, and perceives herself as fat. Blood work indicates that her glucose levels are only slightly below normal under fasting conditions. The patient's ability to maintain her blood glucose levels near normal results, in part, from activation of which of the following proteins?

(A) eIF4
(B) eEF2
(C) CREB
(D) Ribosomal subunit S6
(E) Steroid hormone receptor

7 A long-standing patient of yours has developed multiple tumor types during his life (41 years old). You have diagnosed him as having a specific syndrome involving *p53*. The multiple cancers that result from this syndrome are primarily due to which of the following initial direct effects of the inherited mutation?

(A) Impaired gene transcription
(B) Enhanced gene transcription
(C) Impaired protein synthesis
(D) Enhanced protein synthesis
(E) Altered chromosomal structure

8 A patient has been prescribed methotrexate for chemotherapy. After an initial success in reducing tumor growth, the tumor resumes its rapid growth. One potential mechanism for this is which of the following?

(A) Amplification of the dihydrofolate reductase (DHFR) gene
(B) Amplification of the gene for degrading methotrexate
(C) Reduced transcription of the gene allowing methotrexate entry into the cell
(D) Increased transcription of the gene allowing methotrexate efflux from the cell
(E) An inactivating mutation in the gene for DHFR

9 A 16-year-old girl has been losing weight and feeling lethargic over the past 4 months and is taken to the physician by her parents. During the history, the parents expressed concern that their daughter had seemed to eat very little during the day, a claim denied by the patient. Laboratory results indicated an iron deficiency and a microcytic anemia. The cells of the patient have adapted to the iron deficiency in which one of the following ways?

(A) Increased transcription of ferritin mRNA
(B) Reduced transcription of the transferrin receptor mRNA
(C) Increased translation of the ferritin mRNA
(D) Increased translation of the transferrin receptor mRNA
(E) Increased degradation of the transferrin receptor mRNA

10 Theoretically, a disease could result from an increased expression of a particular gene. This can occur in eukaryotes through a single-nucleotide mutation in a promoter-proximal element. This is best explained by which one of the following?

(A) More efficient splice site recognition
(B) Increased opportunity for hydrogen bonding to a transacting factor
(C) Beneficial amino acid replacement derived from the missense mutation
(D) Increased amount of sigma factor binding
(E) Reduced energy need to melt the DNA helix at this position

11 A human genetic condition in which too much of a gene is routinely expressed has been mapped to a locus on a different chromosome from where the gene in question is located. Which one of the following is a potential explanation for the condition?

(A) The activated gene has a TATA box mutation
(B) The locus control region for the gene is deleted
(C) A gene encoding a transcriptional repressor has been mutated
(D) A transcriptional activator sustained a missense mutation, which reduces its affinity for DNA
(E) A variant promoter region is formed owing to a splice site mutation

12 A patient is taking cyclosporin A after receiving a kidney transplant. Cyclosporin A protects against organ rejection by which of the following mechanisms?

(A) Blocking translation of cytokine genes
(B) Activating transcription of cytokine receptors
(C) Stimulating the phosphorylation of transcription factors
(D) Blocking the dephosphorylation of specific transcription factors
(E) Stimulating translation of cytokine genes

13 A patient has asthma, but has become resistant to glucocorticoid inhalation. A potential mechanism for this resistance is which of the following?

(A) Inability of glucocorticoids to enter target cells
(B) Inability to induce histone acetylation
(C) Reduction of levels of transactivating factors in the nucleus
(D) Cytokine induction of protein kinases
(E) Increased dimerization of the glucocorticoid receptor

14 Induction of certain transcription factors leads to a decrease in the expression of certain genes. This occurs through which of the following mechanisms?

(A) Decreasing the rate of RNA polymerase catalyzed phosphodiester bond formation
(B) Inducing the synthesis of a protein that posttranscriptionally edits mRNA such that translation initiation is blocked
(C) By decreasing the rate of RNA polymerase binding to the promoter
(D) Through stimulation of proteins with HAT activity
(E) Increasing enhancer binding to DNA

15 Shown below is a partial map of the promoter region, and promoter-proximal region, for the γ-globin gene. The overlapping binding sites for transcription factors allow for which of the following to occur?

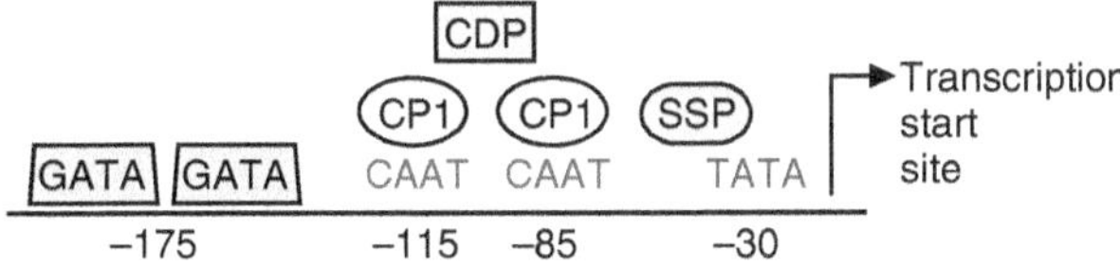

Aspects of the γ-globin gene promoter.

(A) The ability to modulate the binding of positive, or negative, transacting factors to the DNA
(B) The ability to reduce the risk of losing transcriptional control via mutation in this region
(C) Promoting looping of this DNA region
(D) Providing a target for interfering RNAs
(E) Providing ribosome binding sites for translation initiation

16 A hypothetical patient was suffering from excessive free iron in the blood, yet a cellular analysis indicated low intracellular levels of iron, despite high intracellular levels of ferritin, and normal transferrin levels in the blood. The disease was shown to be caused by a single base change in the DNA that led to a dysfunctional protein. The mutation is likely to be in which of the following proteins?
(A) Transferrin
(B) Transferrin receptor
(C) Transcobalamin
(D) Iron response element binding protein
(E) Ceruloplasmin

17 A cell is producing a certain transcription factor that contains a single point mutation, such that N is converted to V. Circular dichroism experiments show that this altered factor has the same secondary structure as the nonmutated factor. Under normal conditions, serum stimulation of quiescent cultures shows strong induction of five genes. When quiescent cells harboring the mutant transcription factor are exposed to serum, the level of expression of those five genes stays at basal levels (there is no increase in mRNA production). This finding is most likely due to which of the following?

(A) Loss of ionic interactions between the transcription factor and DNA
(B) Increase in hydrogen bonding between transcription factor and DNA
(C) Decrease in hydrogen bonding between the transcription factor and DNA
(D) Increase in ionic interactions between the transcription factors and DNA
(E) Inability of the transcription factor to bind to the DNA

The next two questions refer to the following situation. In order to better analyze the promoter region of a particular gene, this cloned region of the gene was placed in front of a reporter gene and the resultant vectors placed in eukaryotic cells to measure the expression of the reporter, using various deleted constructs. The results obtained were as follows:

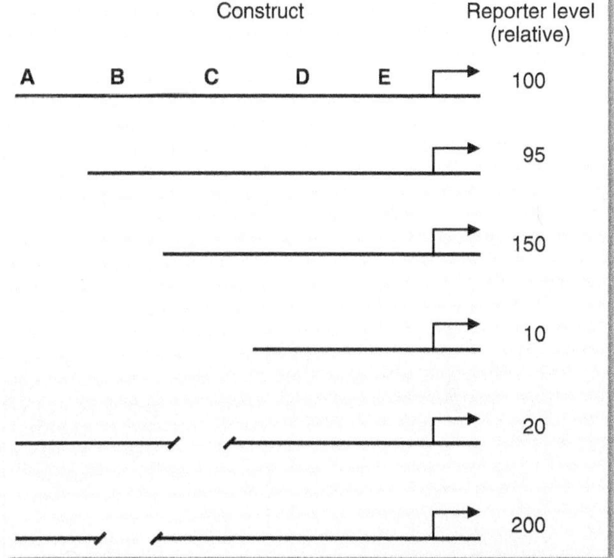

18 Indicate which region (as designated by the letters A, B, C, D, and E) binds an inhibitory transcription factor.

19 Referring to the figure above, which region binds stimulatory transcription factors?

20 A woman developed the following symptoms after taking certain drugs such as barbiturates. The symptoms included severe pain in the abdomen, hallucinations, disorientation, and a reddish tint to the urine. These symptoms appeared due to the induction of genes involved in which of the following pathways?
(A) Cytochrome synthesis
(B) Cytochrome degradation
(C) Ubiquinone biosynthesis
(D) Ubiquinone degradation
(E) Dolichol synthesis

ANSWERS

1 **The answer is A: There is a mutation in cis with the operon.** Constitutive synthesis can occur by either of the two mechanisms. The first is an inability to synthesize lac repressor; the second is to have a mutation in the operator region that renders repressor binding impossible (an o^c mutation; see the figure below). An inability to synthesize lac repressor can be repaired in trans; if the partial diploid contains a functional lac repressor gene, functional protein will be synthesized from the gene, which can bind to the chromosomal operator region, and regulate lac gene expression. If, however, an o^c mutation occurred, the operator region is in cis with the operon and can only regulate regions of DNA that are adjacent to the operator. Thus, if a partial diploid contains a normal operator region on the extrachromosomal region of DNA, that operator region cannot regulate the operon on the chromosomal DNA. Thus, the constitutive mutant that was not rescued in a partial diploid is most likely an o^c mutation. If the inducer could no longer bind to the repressor, then no expression would occur, as the repressor would not leave the operator region. In addition, if this were the case, then adding normal repressor to the cell (via the partial diploid) should allow expression of the operon. Similarly, if inducer bound too tightly to the repressor, the introduction of normal repressor should reverse the effects of the mutated repressor. The lac repressor does not contain a transactivation domain.

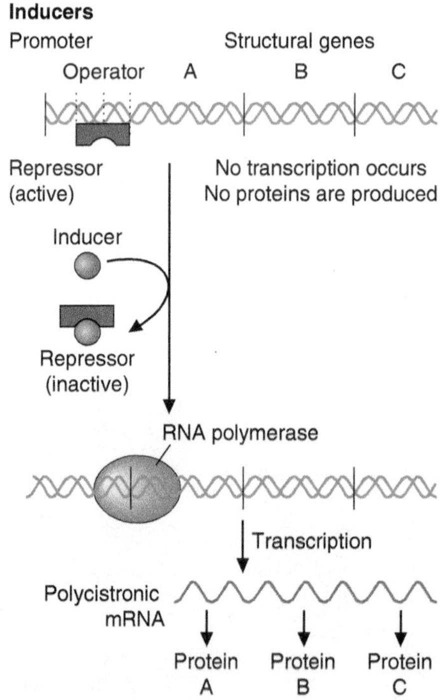

An overview of the regulation of the lac operon (an inducible operon). In the absence of an inducer, the repressor binds to the operator, preventing the binding of DNA polymerase. When the inducer is present, the inducer binds to the repressor, inactivating it. The inactive repressor no longer binds to the operator. Therefore, RNA polymerase can bind to the promoter region. If there is a mutation in the operator region such that the repressor can no longer bind (an o^c mutation), constitutive expression of the operon (expression in the absence of inducer) will result.

2 **The answer is C: To induce synthesis of a functional protein.** The patient has sickle cell anemia, and hydroxyurea treatment is designed to activate transcription of the γ-globin chain, which is normally only expressed during development (fetal hemoglobin). When expressed, the γ-globin gene will form functional hemoglobin tetramers with the α-globin chains, thereby reducing the effects of the mutated β-globin chain. Hydroxyurea does not bind to hemoglobin and denature it; it does not reduce the synthesis of the β-chains, nor does it alter oxygen levels in the blood or 2,3-bisphosphoglycerate levels in the erythrocyte. The γ-chain is normally turned off at birth as part of the hemoglobin-switching pathway (see the figure on page 49). The challenge to scientists at this time is to understand how to reactivate γ-chain synthesis in patients with both sickle cell disease and β-thalassemias.

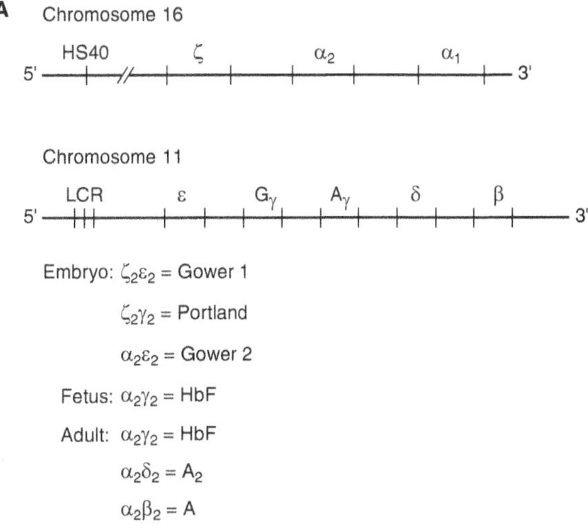

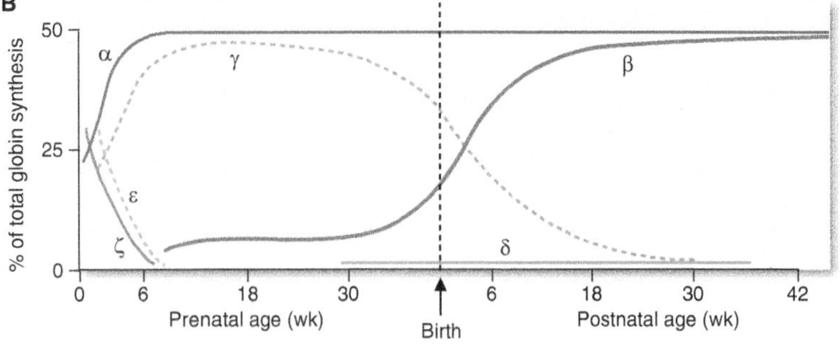

Answer 2: Changes in globin chain expression during development. **Panel A** indicates the chromosomal location of the globin chains while **Panel B** indicates at which stage of development a particular chain is expressed. Note that at birth, γ-chain expression is reduced significantly while β-chain expression begins to increase.

3 **The answer is C: Increased gamma-chain synthesis.** The sibling has, in addition to sickle cell disease, hereditary persistence of fetal hemoglobin (HPFH). Individuals with HPFH express the γ-globin chain throughout their life, and it can be at high levels. Since this child is expressing both the HbS protein and the γ-protein, some normal fetal hemoglobin can be formed in this child, with reduced levels of HbS formed. This reduces the level of sickling and allows oxygen delivery to the tissues. Thus, the HPFH protects against the effects of homozygous HbS expression, and the sibling shows few, if any, symptoms of his HbS mutations. Alterations in the expression of the δ-chain have not been observed. Reduced α-chain synthesis would lead to an anemia, and there is no effective way to reduce the synthesis of HbS chain. Increased ζ-synthesis has also not been observed.

4 **The answer is C: Deletions in the locus control region of the β-globin gene cluster.** The girl is expressing HPFH (hereditary persistence of fetal hemoglobin). This can come about by deletions on the locus control region of the β-globin gene cluster (since fetal hemoglobin is $\alpha_2\gamma_2$, and adult hemoglobin is $\alpha_2\beta_2$, mutations in the locus control region of the α-gene cluster will not affect fetal hemoglobin synthesis). A general loss of transcription factors would not lead to increased transcription of the γ-chains, nor would a general increase in all transcription factor expression in the cell. While inappropriate looping may help to lead to γ-globin gene expression, the looping needs to be modulated by transcription factors for gene expression to occur.

5 **The answer is B: Inhibition of apolipoprotein B translation.** The cholesterol tag on the dsRNA allowed cells to take up the dsRNA, which was processed by intracellular ribonucleases to make a specific silencing RNA for the apolipoprotein B mRNA. Binding of the processed dsRNA to the apoB mRNA will lead to either the destruction of the mRNA or the blockage of translation of the mRNA. In either event, there will be a reduction in apoB translation such that cells can no longer produce apoB100 or apoB48. The dsRNA does not affect the transcription of the apoB gene, nor does it interfere with apoB folding once it becomes transcribed and translated. The dsRNA does not affect the turnover of the apoB protein, nor does it edit the apoB mRNA (other systems in the cell will do that). This situation was first reported in Soutschek J et al. Nature. 2004 Nov 11;432(7014):173–178.

6 **The answer is C: CREB.** CREB (cyclic AMP response element binding protein) is a transcription factor that is activated by protein kinase A and that regulates, in part, the expression of phosphoenolpyruvate carboxykinase

(PEPCK), a necessary protein for gluconeogenesis. Since the patient is anorexic, her blood glucose levels are being maintained primarily by gluconeogenesis, and the enzymes for that pathway need to be upregulated. The release of glucagon and epinephrine, both of which would be elevated in this patient, leads to the activation of protein kinase A and an increase in gene transcription for those genes regulated by CREB. Under these conditions, protein synthesis will be limited, so factors necessary for protein synthesis would not be generally activated (eIF4, eEF2, and ribosomal protein S6). Neither glucagon nor epinephrine works through steroid hormone receptors (they both utilize serpentine receptors on the cell membrane).

7 **The answer is A: Impaired gene transcription.** Individuals with Li–Fraumeni syndrome inherit a mutated copy of *p53*, the product of the *TP53* gene (on chromosome 17). *p53* is a transcription factor whose major job is to monitor the health of DNA; if DNA alterations are found, *p53*, acting as a transcription factor, will initiate new gene transcription to arrest the cell cycle until the DNA damage is repaired and to also induce genes necessary for DNA repair. If the DNA cannot be repaired, *p53* will initiate gene transcription leading to cellular death (apoptosis). In the absence of *p53* activity, damaged DNA will be replicated, which increases the probability of errors, eventually causing a mutation that leads to a cancer. Thus, the initial inactivating event is impaired gene transcription by *p53*, which is the trigger for all other events that follow. Mutations in *p53* do not lead, directly, to enhanced gene transcription (this may occur as a result of secondary mutations, but not directly from the mutations in *p53*) or to alterations in protein synthesis. *p53* mutations also do not alter chromosome structure.

8 **The answer is A: Amplification of the dihydrofolate reductase (DHFR) gene.** Methotrexate resistance most often occurs due to amplification of the gene for DHFR, the target for methotrexate treatment. Through overproduction of DHFR, there is sufficient enzyme available to overcome the effects of the drug given to the patient. Resistance does not come about by altering the rate of entry of the drug into the cell, by inactivating DHFR, or by inducing an enzyme that can degrade methotrexate.

9 **The answer is D: Increased translation of the transferrin receptor mRNA.** Since the patient has an iron deficiency, leading to a microcytic anemia, cells will upregulate their mechanism for acquiring iron, which is through the transferrin receptor. Ferritin is the iron storage protein within cells, and if intracellular iron levels are low, there is no need to upregulate the synthesis of ferritin (its synthesis is actually downregulated under these conditions). The iron travels in the circulation bound to transferrin, so increasing the number of transferrin receptors on the cell surface will enable a more efficient transport of iron and transferrin into the cells. The regulation of transferrin receptor synthesis is at the level of translation, as is the regulation of ferritin synthesis. Thus, cells under these conditions will increase their translation of the transferrin receptor mRNA. This translational regulation is shown below.

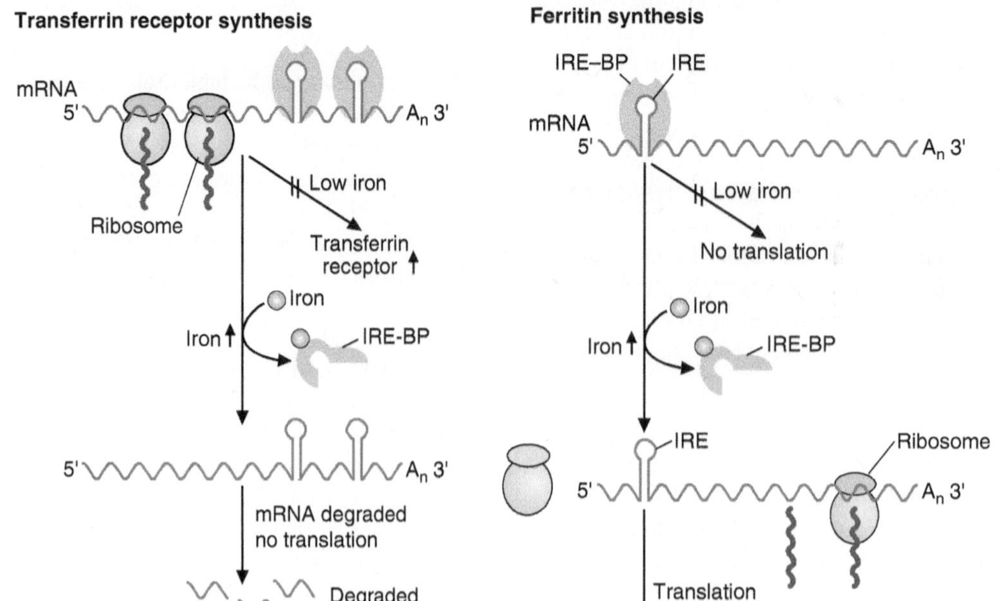

Answer 9: Translational regulation of ferritin and transferrin receptor synthesis via the iron-response element binding protein (IRE-BP). When the IRE-BP binds iron, it will dissociate from the mRNA. When this occurs, the transferrin receptor mRNA is degraded (since there are adequate iron levels within the cell, there is no need to transfer more iron into the cell) and the ferritin mRNA is translated to produce more of this iron-storage molecule.

10 **The answer is B: Increased opportunity for hydrogen bonding to a transacting factor.** A single nucleotide substitution in a promoter-proximal region has the capability of increasing hydrogen bonding to a transacting factor, thereby increasing the interaction between the factor and DNA and enhancing recruitment of RNA polymerase to the promoter. Since the mutation is in the promoter region, it is not involved in splicing (which occurs at exon–intron borders), it does not code for an amino acid (since exons are not in the promoter region), it is not related to sigma (which is prokaryotic specific), and the DNA helix does not have to be significantly melted in this area to allow transcription factor binding.

11 **The answer is C: A gene encoding a transcriptional repressor has been mutated.** For the sake of this answer, let us assume that the overexpressed gene (named *A*) is located on chromosome X and the mutated gene (named *B*) is located on chromosome Y. The gene on chromosome Y is producing a transcriptional repressor that binds to the promoter region of the gene *A* on chromosome X. When the repressor is expressed, gene *A* transcription is reduced. The protein product of gene *B* is acting in trans in regulating gene *A* expression. A mutation that inactivates the protein product of gene *B*, then, would be unable to repress gene *A* transcription, and lead to overexpression of gene *A*. If the promoter for gene *A* had a TATA box mutation, one would expect reduced expression (due to an inability of the basal transcription complex to bind), rather than enhanced expression. Similarly, if the locus control region of the gene is deleted, then reduced expression for gene *A* would be expected, not enhanced expression. If a transcriptional activator (gene *B*) suffered a missense mutation that reduced its affinity for DNA, there would be less transcription of gene *A*, not enhanced expression. And, finally, promoter regions do not undergo splicing.

12 **The answer is D: Blocking the dephosphorylation of specific transcription factors.** Cyclosporin A binds to the protein cyclophilin in immunocompetent lymphocytes, and this protein complex leads to the inactivation of calcineurin. Calcineurin, in response to increases in cytoplasmic calcium, will activate its phosphatase activity and dephosphorylate cytoplasmic nuclear factor of activated T-lymphocytes (NF-AT), a transcription factor. When dephosphorylated NF-AT will translocate to the nucleus, it will interact with nuclear factors and bind to DNA, initiating new gene transcription. When calcineurin is inactivated via cyclosporin–cyclophilin binding, NF-AT cannot translocate to the nucleus, and cytokine synthesis by the cell (second messengers) is compromised. Immunocompetent cells have very low levels of calcineurin, which make them susceptible to cyclosporin treatment. Drug treatment does not directly affect the translation of cytokine genes (it is indirect because the mRNA for these genes is never made), nor does it lead to the activation of transcription of cytokine receptors. Cyclosporin does not lead to the phosphorylation of transcription factors, nor does it stimulate translation of cytokine genes.

13 **The answer is B: Inability to induce histone acetylation.** Glucocorticoids bind to a cytoplasmic receptor and translocate to the nucleus, where they bind to glucocorticoid response elements on the DNA, leading to a complex of proteins at this site. A number of transactivating factors recruited to the DNA contain histone acetyl transferase (HAT) activity, which leads to further unwinding of the DNA from the nucleosome, enabling gene transcription. Patients who become resistant to glucocorticoid treatment show a reduction in histone acetylation in response to the drug for a variety of reasons. The resistance does not appear to be due to inability of the drug to enter target cells. Once inside the cell, the drug will bind to the receptor, and dimerization of the receptor is normal. In some resistant individuals, the dimerized receptor has trouble translocating to the nucleus, which leads to the reduction in HAT activity. In other patients, however, translocation is normal, and the reduction in HAT activity appears to be due to an inability to recruit transactivating factors to the complex, which contain the HAT activity. The levels of transactivating factors are normal, but it has been hypothesized that the receptor is phosphorylated under resistance conditions, leading to an inability to attract the transactivating factors.

14 **The answer is C: By decreasing the rate of RNA polymerase binding to the promoter.** Transcription factors can be either positive or negative acting. In either event, to exert an effect on transcription, the factor must bind to the DNA and then either promote RNA polymerase binding to DNA (in which case, it is a positive-acting factor) or inhibit RNA polymerase binding to DNA (in which case it is a negative-acting factor). Negative acting factors can do so by blocking the binding of positively acting factors to the DNA or by blocking necessary transactivating factors from binding to other factors already bound to the DNA. In either event, the net result is a reduction in the rate at which RNA polymerase binds to the promoter region to initiate transcription. Once initiated, the rate of phosphodiester bond formation is constant. RNA editing is a rare event, and is not used to regulate gene transcription. If HAT activity were stimulated, gene transcription would be increased, as the acetylated histones would have a reduced affinity for DNA, and it would be easier for RNA polymerase to bind to the promoter region. Increasing enhancer binding to DNA would also increase the rate at which RNA polymerase would bind to the promoter, as enhancers increase the association of positive-acting transactivation factors, which would promote RNA polymerase binding to the promoter and transcription.

15 **The answer is A: The ability to modulate the binding of positive, or negative, transacting factors to the DNA.** The recognition of overlapping sequences on DNA by different factors allows either positive-acting or negative-acting effects, depending on which transcription factor is present in higher concentration. The γ-globin gene is turned off after birth, and this has to do, in part, with factors bound to the promoter. When stage selector protein (SSP) is bound, γ-globin synthesis is favored, but when SP1 binds to this area instead, γ-globin synthesis is repressed. A similar story occurs at the CAAT sites; when CP1 is bound, γ-globin synthesis is favored, but when CAAT displacement protein binds, CP1 can no longer bind, and gene transcription is inhibited. Thus, γ-globin expression is regulated by the concentrations of both positive-acting and negative-acting factors available in the cell. The overlapping binding sites were not designed for redundancy in case of mutation, to provide ribosome binding sites (the ribosomes bind to RNA produced from exons, not from the promoter region), or to provide a target for interfering RNAs (the siRNAs are targeted to mRNA). The multiple binding sites, by themselves, do not promote looping of DNA, but once transcription factors have bound to the DNA, looping may occur as the transactivating factors bind to the proteins bound to DNA.

16 **The answer is D: Iron response element binding protein.** As shown in the figure below, the iron-response element binding protein (IRE-BP) binds to loops in RNA (RNA secondary structure), and in the case of ferritin mRNA, the IRE-BP blocks translation when iron levels are low. In the case of the transferrin receptor mRNA, the IRE-BP stabilizes the mRNA when iron levels are low, allowing efficient translation of the mRNA such that transferrin receptors can be synthesized and placed in the membrane. If a patient had a mutated IRE-BP, which could no longer bind to its target sequence in mRNA, then the transferrin receptor mRNA would be unstable and degraded, and cells would not be able to take up iron from the circulation, leading to higher than normal iron levels in the blood yet still would result in cellular depletion of iron. However, the lack of IRE-BP binding would allow ferritin translation and synthesis, leading to high levels of ferritin inside the cell despite the low levels of intracellular iron. Ceruloplasmin is involved in copper transport, not iron. A mutation in transferrin would lead to lower circulating iron levels in the blood as the iron carrier would be mutated. Mutations in the transferrin receptor would not lead to high intracellular levels of ferritin (intracellular iron levels would be low, the IRE-BP would remain bound to the ferritin mRNA, and translation would be blocked). Mutations in transcobalamin would affect vitamin B_{12} transport, not iron.

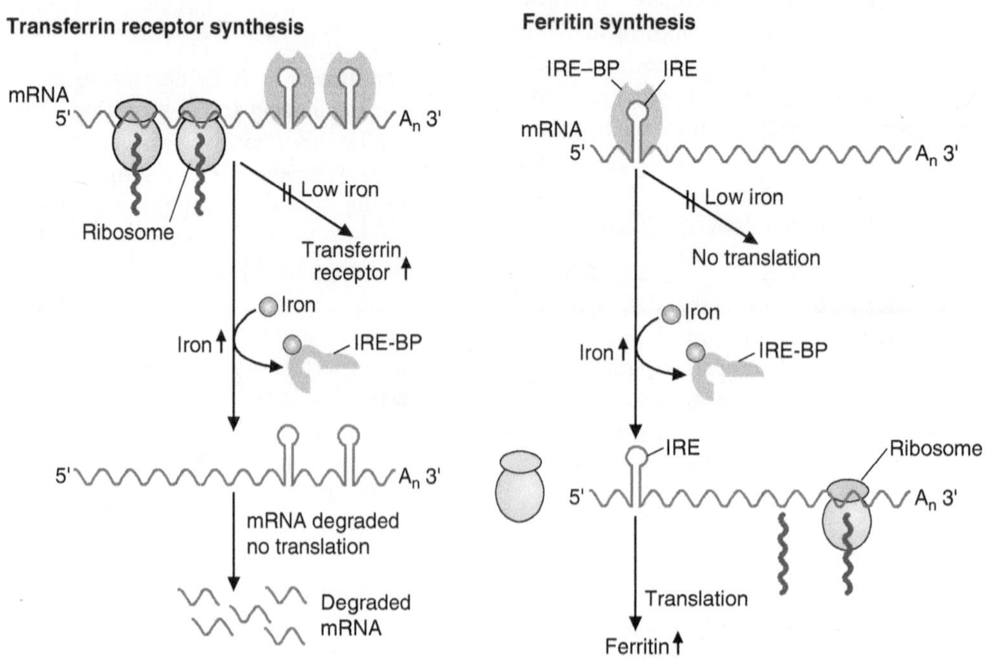

Answer 16: Translational regulation of ferritin and transferrin receptor synthesis via the iron-response element binding protein (IRE-BP). When the IRE-BP binds iron, it will dissociate from the mRNA. When this occurs, the transferrin receptor mRNA is degraded (since there are adequate iron levels within the cell, there is no need to transfer more iron into the cell) and the ferritin mRNA is translated to produce more of this iron-storage molecule.

17 **The answer is C: Decrease in hydrogen bonding between the transcription factor and DNA.** The necessary transcription factor is not binding as well to the DNA, leading to reduced efficiency of transcription. The side chain of aspartic acid can participate in hydrogen bonding with DNA bases, but the side chain of valine (completely carbon–hydrogen bonds) cannot (see the figure below). Transcription factors do not bind to DNA via ionic interactions. An increase in hydrogen bonding between the factor and DNA would lead to enhanced transcription (not reduced transcription). An inability of the transcription factor to bind to DNA would lead to no transcription of the gene; since there is a low level of expression, binding of this factor to the DNA must be occurring, although the affinity for the factor and DNA has been reduced.

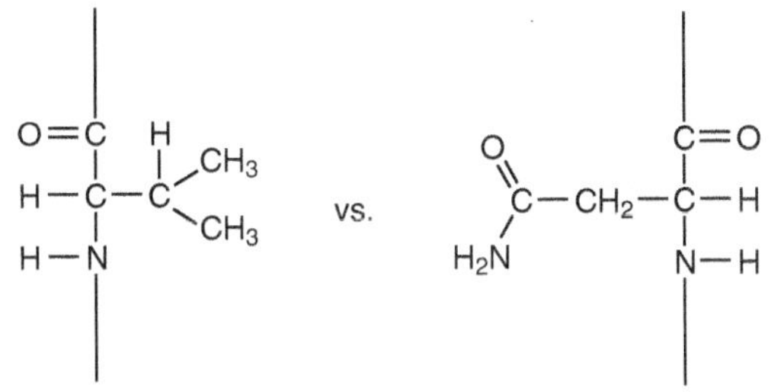

A comparison of valine (V) and asparagine (N) side chains within a protein backbone.

18 **The answer is B.** When region B is deleted from the promoter region, there is an increase in overall expression of the reporter gene (the second and last lines of the figure indicate this). Removal of any other region leads to a decrease in expression, indicating that positive-acting transcription factors bind to those regions of DNA.

19 **The answer is C.** When region C is removed from the DNA, there is a tremendous reduction in the expression of the reporter gene, indicating that this region of the DNA binds important positively-acting transcription factors for the expression of the reporter gene.

20 **The answer is A: Cytochrome synthesis.** The woman has a form of porphyria, an inborn error in the biosynthesis of heme. The buildup of heme intermediates is what generates the symptoms observed. Barbiturates are degraded through the cytochrome P450 series of enzymes, which are induced by the drug. The enzymes require heme, so heme synthesis is also induced, and whenever heme synthesis is induced, the toxic intermediates get accumulated. The end product of heme degradation is bilirubin, and if excessive bilirubin accumulates, jaundice is the result. Both dolichol and ubiquinone synthesis are from isoprenoids, and not related to the heme pathway.

Chapter 7

Molecular Medicine and Techniques

The future of diagnostic medicine is in molecular medicine and the analysis of DNA and RNA for mutations and susceptibility genes. This chapter will test your knowledge of the application of these techniques.

QUESTIONS

Select the single best answer.

1 A patient displays increasing muscle weakness and delayed muscle relaxation. He shows a slack jaw and drooping eyelids. The physician has noted a loss of muscle mass in the calves over the years. A molecular analysis by Southern blot using a probe against the suspected disease gene shows the following. The molecular reason for the difference between the normal and disease gene is which of the following?

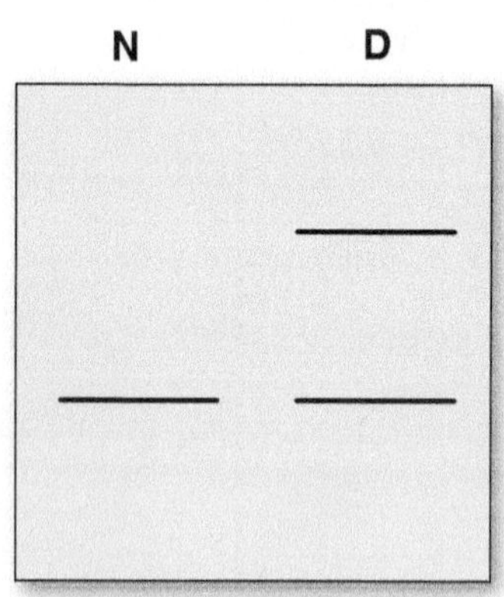

(A) Gene duplication
(B) Gene deletion
(C) Triplet repeat expansion
(D) Increased SNPs in the disease state
(E) Differences in restriction fragment length polymorphisms (RFLPs)

Questions 2 and 3 are based on the following diagram. Shown below is a vector plus insert, with restriction endonuclease sites also shown. The insert was obtained from a gene, and exon 1 of the gene is indicated by the black box.

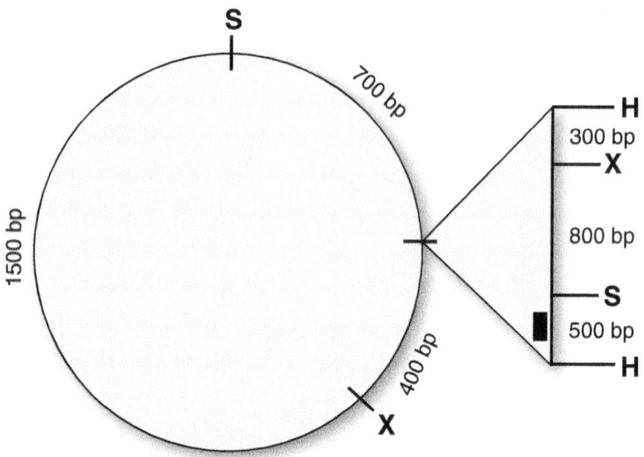

2 If this vector plus insert were to be cleaved to completion with enzymes S and X simultaneously, what size bands would be observed?
(A) 1,600 bp, 2,600 bp
(B) 400 bp, 1,500 bp, 2,300 bp
(C) 400 bp, 1,000 bp, 1,300 bp, 1,500 bp
(D) 800 bp, 1,500 bp, 1,900 bp
(E) 800 bp, 900 bp, 1,000 bp, 1,500 bp

3 Which labeled DNA fragment would work best for a Northern blot analysis?
(A) The 300 bp HX restriction fragment
(B) The 1,100 bp HS restriction fragment
(C) The 500 bp HS restriction fragment
(D) The 1,800 bp SS restriction fragment
(E) The 800 bp XS restriction fragment

4 You are studying a family that exhibits a rare autosomal recessive disease. The disease is caused by a point mutation which abolishes an EcoR1 restriction site in the genome. To genotype the family, one can amplify a 1.8 kb region of this area of the genome using polymerase chain reaction (PCR), restrict the PCR products with EcoR1, and then separate the restricted DNA on an agarose gel. The results of such an experiment are shown below, using DNA obtained from each of the five family members. Which family members have the disease?

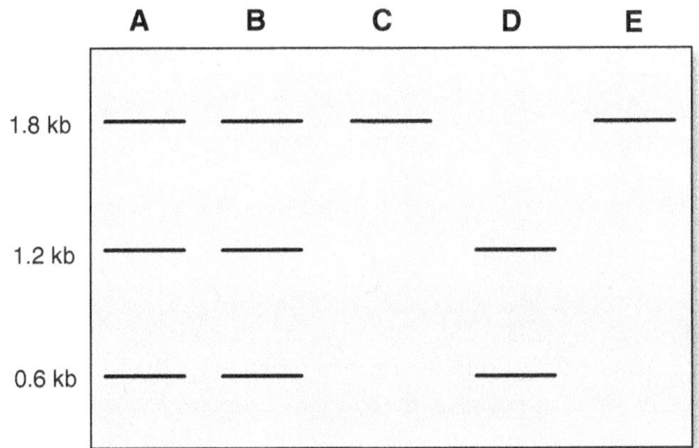

(A) A and B
(B) C and E
(C) D
(D) A, B, and D
(E) C, D, and E

5 A difficult step in the engineering of recombinant insulin was which of the following?
(A) Expressing the entire insulin cDNA in bacteria
(B) Expressing the entire insulin gene in bacteria
(C) Finding bacteria to properly cleave the insulin preproprotein
(D) Allowing the A and B chains to come together appropriately
(E) Finding the appropriate eukaryotic cell in which to express the gene

6 A 6-month-old has had recurrent bouts of pneumonia, and a chest X-ray shows a greatly reduced thymus. Gene therapy would successfully treat this disorder if the gene is placed in which cell type or organ?
(A) Muscle
(B) Liver
(C) Lung
(D) Bone marrow
(E) Kidney

7 A patient has been diagnosed with a particular form of cancer. Appropriate treatment of this cancer, however, requires knowledge of which molecular markers are being expressed by the tumor as compared to normal cells of the same tissue. This is most easily accomplished by which of the following techniques?
(A) Southern blot
(B) Southwestern blot
(C) MicroRNA analysis
(D) Microarray analysis
(E) ELISAs

8 A patient was given an initial ELISA screening test for HIV, which was positive. A second, more specific test was then undertaken, which consisted of a Western blot. The samples that were run through the polyacrylamide gel for this test consisted of which of the following?
(A) Patient sera
(B) Patient plasma
(C) HIV RNA
(D) HIV proteins
(E) Extracts of patient white blood cells

9 A patient has been diagnosed with abetalipoproteinemia. Such a disorder can be determined by which of the following techniques using samples obtained from the blood?
(A) Western blot
(B) Northern blot
(C) Southern blot
(D) PCR analysis
(E) Microarray

10 The DNA sequence represented by the gel shown below, which was generated using the Sanger dideoxy sequencing technique, is which of the following?

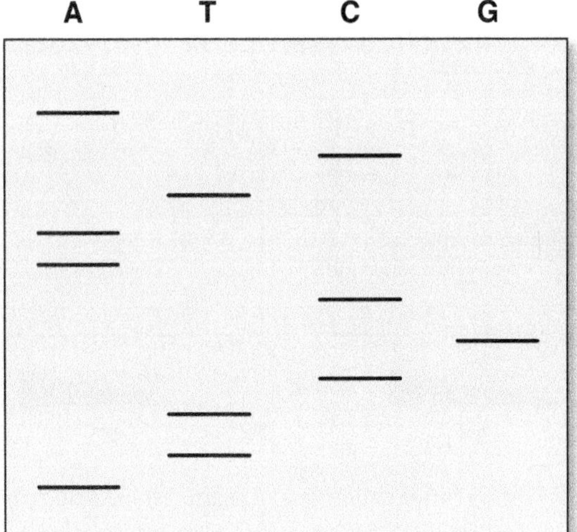

(A) ACTAACGCTTA
(B) ATTCGCAATCA
(C) ATCTATCGATC
(D) GCCCTTTAAAA
(E) AAAATTTCCCG

11 A patient has seen her physician for a variety of complaints over the past several years. These include fevers which come and go, fatigue, joint pain and stiffness, a rash on the face (see the figure below), sores in her mouth, easy bruising, and increased feelings of anxiety and depression. A molecular technique to provide a confirmation of the suspected diagnosis is which of the following?

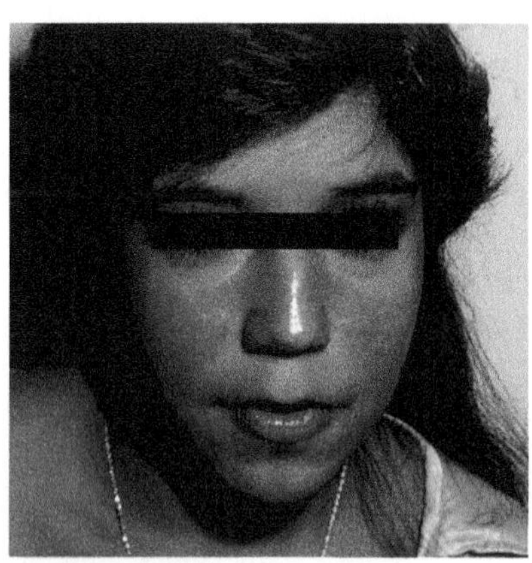

(A) Western blot
(B) Southern blot
(C) Northern blot
(D) DNA sequencing
(E) RFLP analysis

12 Two-dimensional PAGE gels were run on cells from normal tissue, and also on the same tissue which has been affected by a certain disease. Which of the following best describes spot A in the disease state, as compared to spot B in the normal state?

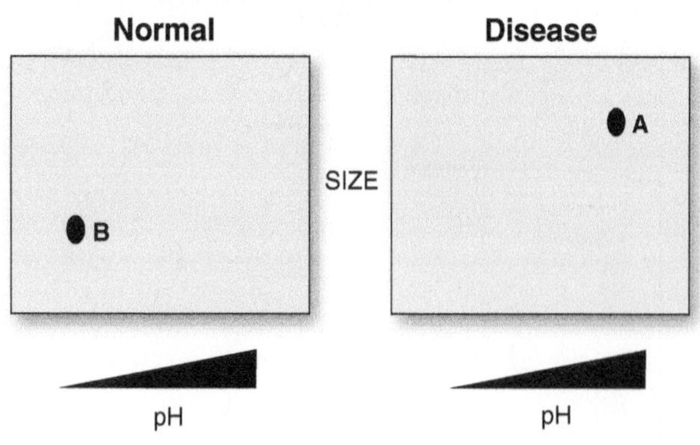

(A) Lower molecular weight, same isoelectric points
(B) Higher molecular weight, more acidic protein
(C) Higher molecular weight, more basic protein
(D) Same molecular weight, more basic protein
(E) Lower molecular weight, more acidic protein

13 The region of DNA shown below is to be amplified by PCR. The appropriate pair of primers to use is which of the following?

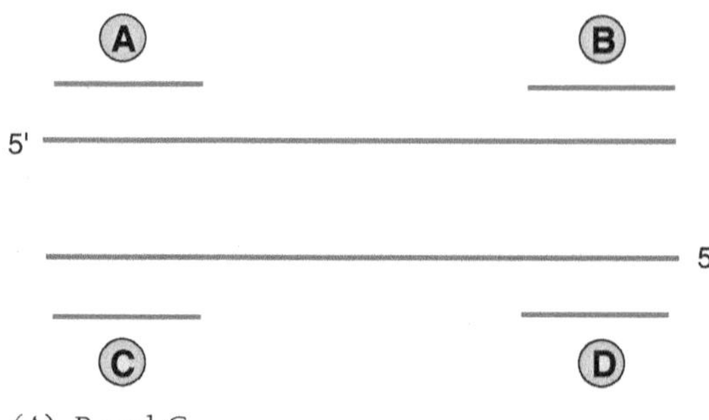

(A) B and C
(B) A and D
(C) A and C
(D) B and D
(E) C and D

14 Having cloned the cDNA for mouse gene X, one wants to use this cDNA as a probe to screen a human cDNA library and isolate the human homolog of this gene. Hybridization conditions should be which of the following for the initial screening of the library?

(A) High temperature, low salt
(B) Low temperature, low salt
(C) High temperature, high salt
(D) Low temperature, high salt
(E) Low temperature, no salt

15 A researcher has isolated the cDNA for gene Y. He performs the following Northern blot experiment using samples prepared from different tissues. A potential explanation for this finding is which of the following?

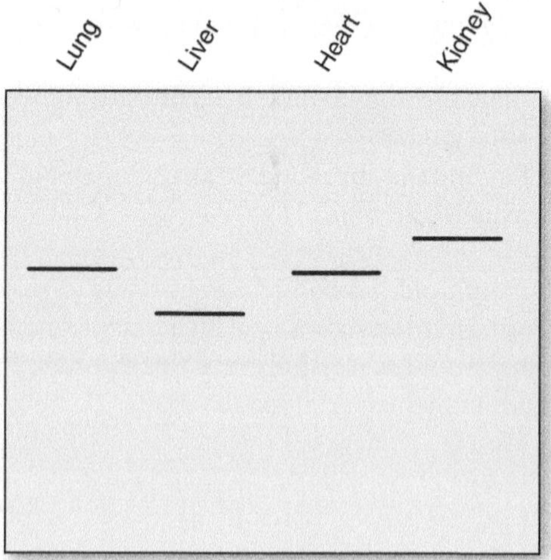

(A) Alternative splicing
(B) mRNA instability
(C) RNA editing
(D) Different AUG start codons in different tissues
(E) Differential polyadenylation

16 Two babies were born at the same time in the hospital, but their nametags may have been mixed up.

DNA fingerprinting was done to determine the parentage of the children, using Southern blots of restricted DNA and a specific probe. The basis for seeing differences between individuals using this technique is which of the following?

(A) Chromosomal deletions
(B) RFLPs
(C) Chromosomal translocations
(D) Triplet repeat expansions
(E) DNA methylation

17 A microarray experiment looking at genes expressed by a cell line both before and after differentiation of the line indicated 15 potential genes which were upregulated. A simple technique to enable the scientist to determine the temporal order of induced gene expression is which of the following?

(A) Southern blot
(B) Northern blot
(C) Western blot
(D) RFLP analysis
(E) Microarray analysis

18 A genomic clone has been isolated and is going to be used for chromosome walking to obtain more clones of the gene. The regions of the clone to be used as probes in chromosome walking are which of the following?

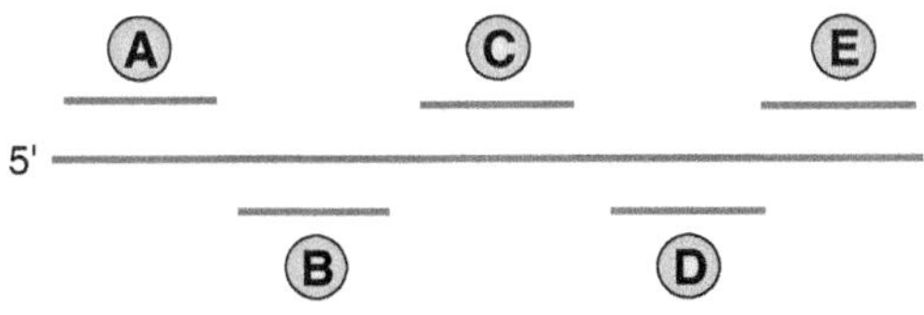

(A) B and C
(B) A and D
(C) A and E
(D) D and E
(E) B and D

19 One studies a disease caused by a single point mutation in which a restriction enzyme site is gained by the mutation. To determine if someone is a carrier of the disease, PCR primers were generated which allowed a 1.8 kb fragment to be amplified across both X restriction sites in the normal gene. After treatment of the amplified DNA by enzyme X, a carrier of the disease would be expected to exhibit which size fragments, as determined by ethidium bromide staining of an agarose gel?

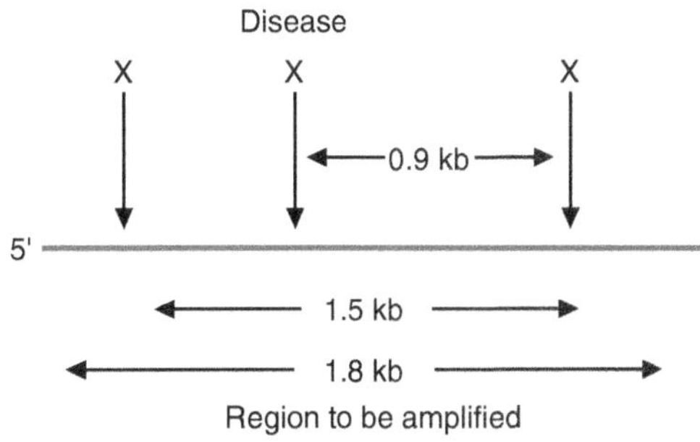

(A) 1.5 kb only
(B) 0.6 and 0.9 kb
(C) 0.6 and 1.5 kb
(D) 0.6, 0.9, and 1.5 kb
(E) 0.9 and 1.5 kb

20 Consider the following map of a genomic region of DNA, showing restriction endonuclease sites for enzymes X and Y. You have a probe to this region (as indicated on the figure). A certain disease maps to this region of DNA, and creates a new restriction site, Z, which is cut with restriction enzyme Z. As a diagnostic tool, a carrier would exhibit which bands when DNA that has been completely restricted with enzyme X is run through a gel and a Southern blot is performed utilizing the indicated probe?

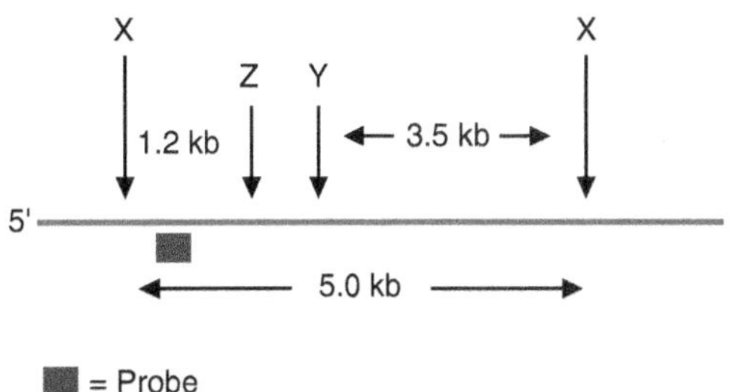

(A) 5.0 kb
(B) 1.0 and 5.0 kb
(C) 1.5 and 5.0 kb
(D) 1.5 and 3.5 kb
(E) 0.5 and 1.0 kb

ANSWERS

1 **The answer is C: Triplet repeat expansion.** The patient has the symptoms of myotonic dystrophy, an autosomal dominant disorder brought about by a triplet repeat expansion in the myotonic dystrophy gene. The presence of this expansion increases the size of DNA observed in Southern blots, and since it is autosomal dominant, only one of the two chromosomes has to contain this expansion for the patient to have the disease. Myotonic dystrophy is due to a CTG triplet repeat expansion in the 3′ untranslated region of the DM1 gene. The DM1 gene codes for a serine/threonine kinase and is located on chromosome 19, band q13. Myotonic dystrophy is not caused by a gene duplication, gene deletion (as would by muscular dystrophy), a change in SNP patterns, or differences in restriction length polymorphisms (although one may be created by the triplet repeat expansion).

2 **The answer is E: 800 bp, 900 bp, 1,000 bp, 1,500 bp.** Starting with the S site at the "top" of the figure, the next restriction cut would be at the X site in the insert, generating a DNA fragment of 1,000 bp (700 + 300). The next site is the S site in the insert, which is 800 bp long. Moving along the DNA the next cut site is the X site in the vector, 900 bp from the previous S site. This leaves, then, a 1,500 bp piece of the vector. The total size of the vector plus insert is 4,200 bp, and the pieces generated, 800 bp, 900 bp, 1,000 bp, and 1,500 bp, add up to the total, 4,200 bp.

3 **The answer is C: The 500 bp HS restriction fragment.** Since the probe is going to be used in a Northern blot, the DNA for the probe must be obtained from an exon, as mRNA will only contain sequences which are complementary to exonic DNA. The exonic DNA is represented by the black box in the figure, which is within the 500 bp SH restriction fragment of the insert. The other parts of the insert represent introns and would not hybridize to mRNA in a Northern blot.

4 **The answer is B: C and E.** Since the disease is autosomal recessive, both chromosomes must carry a mutated gene for the person to have the disease, so only one band should be seen on the gel. Since the mutation which leads to the disease destroys a restriction endonuclease site, the disease-carrying allele will have a larger size on the gel than the normal allele, which will be cleaved by the restriction enzyme. Thus, for individual A, for example, the 1.8 kb band corresponds to the mutant allele, while the 1.2 kb and 0.6 kb bands correspond to the normal allele, which contains the restriction site that enables the DNA to be cut into two pieces. Individual A is a carrier of the disease, as is individual B. Individual D has two normal copies of the gene and is not a carrier of the disease.

5 **The answer is D: Allowing the A and B chains to come together appropriately.** Expression of cDNA in bacteria does not allow for posttranslational events to occur (bacteria do not carry out such events). Thus, the cleavage of insulin (removal of the C-peptide) to form mature insulin would not occur in bacteria. Thus, in making recombinant insulin, the A and B chains are produced separately in bacteria, purified, and then mixed together under appropriate conditions to allow the disulfide bonds to form between the chains to form mature insulin. One cannot express the entire insulin gene in bacteria, as bacteria do not splice mRNA. It has been less expensive to synthesize insulin in bacteria than to try and find a eukaryotic cell line which would process insulin appropriately, and at high levels.

6 **The answer is D: Bone marrow.** The child has adenosine deaminase (ADA) deficiency, or SCID (severe combined immunodeficiency disease). The circulating blood cells pick up deoxyadenosine, which is toxic in the absence of adenosine deaminase, a necessary enzyme for the metabolism of deoxyadenosine. By incorporating functional ADA in bone marrow cells, the stem cells for the production of the circulating blood cells now express ADA, and the mature cells produced from the stem cells will now express ADA, and be resistant to the toxic effects of deoxyadenosine. Placing the gene in other tissues will not address the problem of the death of blood cells.

7 **The answer is D: Microarray analysis.** Microarray experiments allow for rapid screening of many genes in one experiment. The technique is based on hybridizing cDNA samples from cells to an array of known DNA sequences, which correspond to a battery of genes (about 1,000 can fit on one DNA chip; this is further explained in the figure on page 59). Thus, in a single experiment, one can determine the expression levels of 1,000 genes in both the disease and normal state. Southern blots cannot do this, as one would have to probe the blot with 1,000 different probes to try to obtain similar results. Southwestern blot, in which protein binding to DNA is measured, is not relevant to this situation. MicroRNAs regulate gene transcription, but will not tell you about the expression of the bulk of genes in the cell (and microarray genes can also be analyzed in a microarray experiment). ELISAs examine one protein through

antibody binding and cannot give rapid data on over 1,000 different gene products.

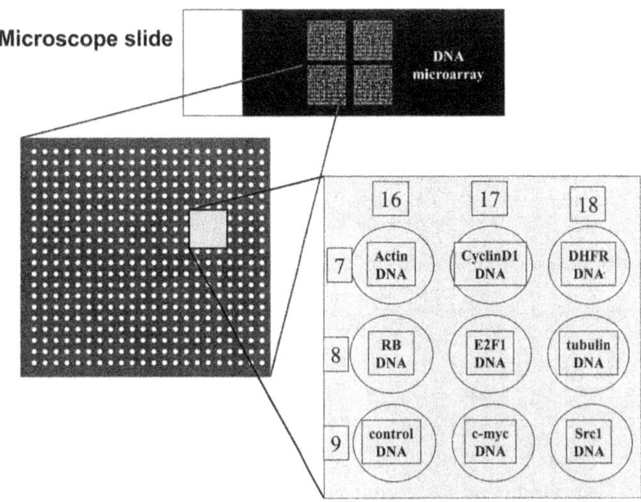

A typical microarray experiment. Note how DNA sequences corresponding to known genes (actin, cyclin D1, etc.) are spotted in an array on a microscope slide. Labeled cDNA from cell samples will be hybridized to the DNA on the slide, and the results analyzed by computer to determine the level of gene expression at each spot of DNA.

8 **The answer is D: HIV proteins.** The HIV tests are looking for the presence of antibodies in the patient's sera against HIV proteins. So, in the confirming Western blot, HIV proteins are separated by size on a polyacrylamide gel, the proteins transferred to filter paper, and the filter paper treated with the sera sample. If the sera contain antibodies to HIV proteins, they will bind to the proteins on the filter paper, and the presence of antibodies on the filter paper is then detected using second antibodies. None of the other answers are appropriate for this type of test.

9 **The answer is A: Western blot.** Abetalipoproteinemia results from the absence of apolipoprotein B in chylomicrons and very low density lipoprotein (VLDL), caused by a mutation in MTTP, the microsomal triglyceride transfer protein. If one isolates plasma (removing the cells), and performs a Western blot for the presence of apolipoprotein B, one would see greatly reduced levels as compared to normal individuals. As apoB is made either in the intestine (apoB48) or the liver (apoB100), apoB mRNA would not be present in blood cells, so a Northern blot would not be informative. Southern blot of DNA would only work if there was a specific probe for MTTP which would distinguish a disease gene from a normal gene. Microarray, which measures mRNA levels, would not show any difference between normal and disease states, as the apoB protein is still made in the liver and intestine; however, it cannot be incorporated into chylomicrons or VLDL due to the lack of functional MTTP activity. PCR analysis suffers from the same problem as Southern blotting.

10 **The answer is B: ATTCGCAATCA.** In the Sanger technique, the sequence is read from the bottom of the gel to the top of the gel (5′ to 3′), going from one size of DNA to the next largest size. This is due to the way in which the fragments are generated, as indicated in the figure below.

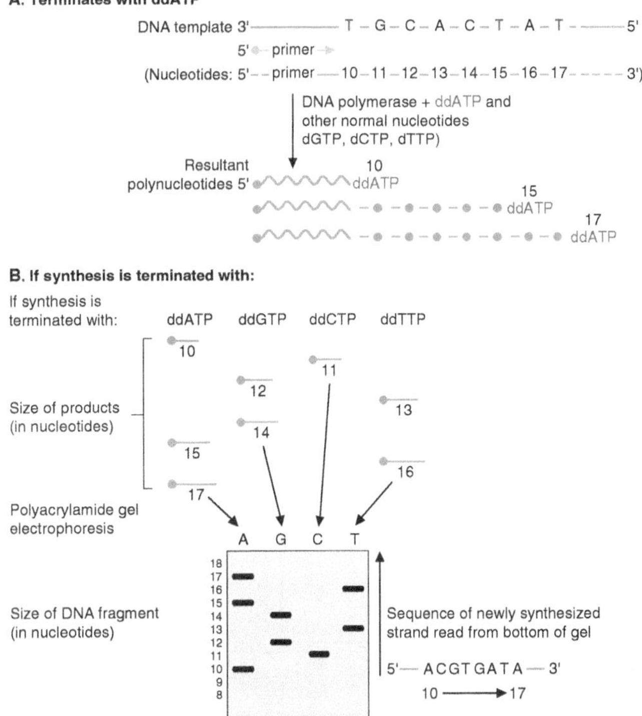

11 **The answer is A: Western blot.** The patient has lupus, which is an autoimmune disorder. To test for the presence of antibodies in the patient's sera, one can use a Western blot, and run typical antigens (such as spliceosome proteins) on the gel, and then determine if the patient's sera contain antibodies against the proteins. ELISAs will also work for this assay. All of the other techniques mentioned require examining nucleic acids, which would not help in determining if autoimmune antibodies were being generated in the patient.

12 **The answer is C: Higher molecular weight, more basic protein.** In two-dimensional electrophoresis, proteins are separated first by charge (they are run through a pH gradient, and when they reach their isoelectric point, they stop migrating), and then by size. As indicated in the figure to the question, larger sizes migrate more slowly and would be closer to the "top" of the figure. Thus, spot A is of a larger molecular weight than spot B, as spot B migrates farther in the sizing portion of the two-dimensional electrophoresis. The horizontal positions are related to the isoelectric points of the proteins, and spot A reaches its isoelectric point at a higher pH than does spot B. This means that protein B is more acidic than protein A. Overall, then, the protein expressed by spot A is larger and more basic than the protein represented by spot B.

13 **The answer is A: B and C.** For a PCR experiment, one requires primers that will allow DNA synthesis to occur across the region of DNA to be amplified. Since DNA polymerase always synthesizes DNA in the 5′ to 3′ direction, the 3′ ends of the primers must face each other and bracket the region of DNA to be amplified. Primers A and D will only allow DNA synthesis away in the opposite direction from the region of interest, due to their orientation on the DNA template strand. The principal behind PCR reactions is shown in the figure below.

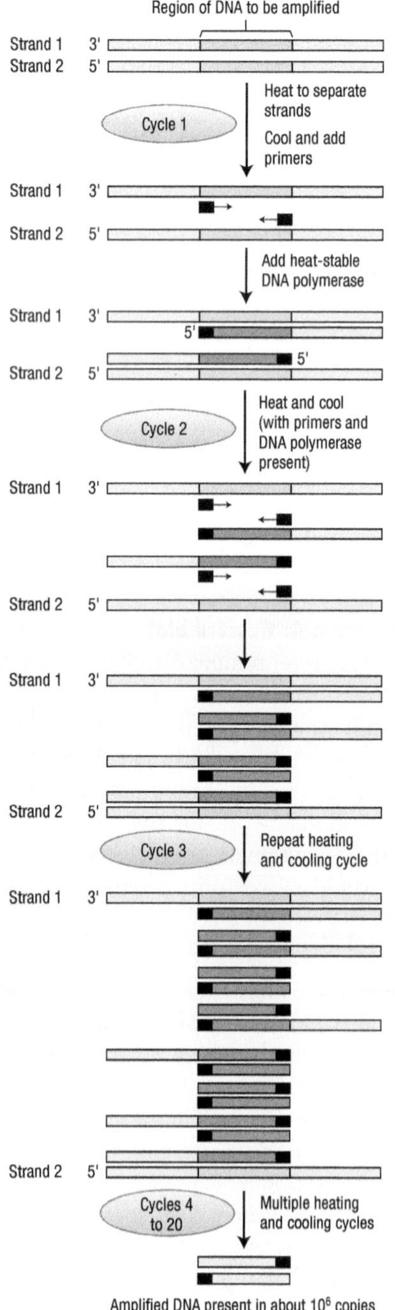

14 **The answer is D: Low temperature, high salt.** Since the probe is from mouse DNA, and the sample is human DNA, low stringency conditions need to be used to allow slight mismatches in hybridization to be tolerated. Thus, low temperature reduces thermal motion, and allows for mismatches, and high salt will reduce the potential disruptive ionic interactions that might result from mismatches and alterations in backbone structure. The combination of low temperature and high salt will provide the highest probability of hybridization between mouse and human DNA.

15 **The answer is A: Alternative splicing.** Since a Northern blot is being run, RNA from the various tissues is run through the gel to be separated based on size. Seeing different sizes of hybridizing bands, depending on the tissue of origin, with the same probe, and from the same animal, indicates that alternative splicing of the mRNA has occurred between the tissues. mRNA instability would lead to reduced levels of signal and not differences in sizes. RNA editing would not alter the overall size of the mRNA; it would just alter the sequence of the mRNA. Start codons are within the mRNA; utilizing different start codons would not alter the size of the mRNA. Differential polyadenylation is only correct if it is a part of differential splicing, which is the best answer.

16 **The answer is B: RFLPs.** RFLPs can be detected with a straightforward Southern blot. Chromosomal translocations are too rare in the population to be used for general DNA fingerprinting. DNA methylation patterns are epigenetic and can be variable amongst individuals, so they are not sufficiently reliable to be used for DNA fingerprinting. Deletions and triplet repeat expansions are too rare and variable in the population to be used as a general screen for DNA identification purposes.

17 **The answer is B: Northern blot.** Once individual genes have been identified as being either upregulated or downregulated after differentiation, the DNA corresponding to the gene can be used as a probe in Northern blots using mRNA obtained at various times after differentiation is induced. In this manner, the time course of increase, or decrease, in mRNA expression can be determined. None of the other techniques will allow this information to be easily obtained. Western blots require antibodies to the proteins produced from the genes identified, which most likely are not available. A microarray analysis is too complex to easily determine the temporal order of gene expression. RFLP analysis does not address the question of temporal gene expression.

18 **The answer is C: A and E.** Chromosome walking involves taking the "ends" of a probe (the DNA at the 5′ and 3′ ends of a probe) and using those as new probes in another library screen. The clones identified in this second screening of the library will hybridize to the "end" of the already identified clone, and should extend the DNA both in the 5′ and 3′ directions from that already represented by the first clone, as indicated in the figure below.

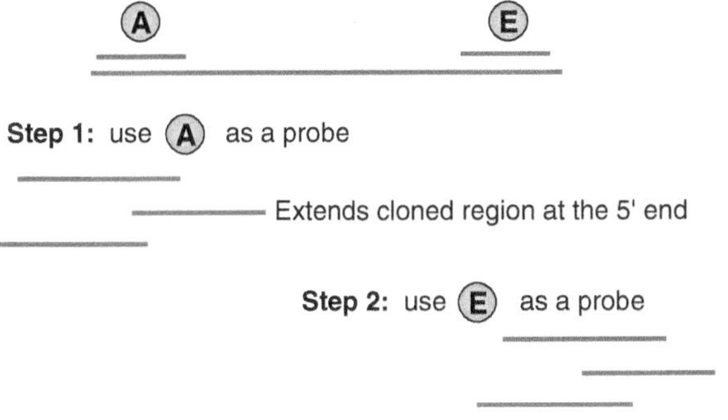

19 **The answer is D: 0.6, 0.9, and 1.5 kb.** A carrier would have one normal gene, and one disease gene, which contains the new restriction enzyme site. After amplifying this area of DNA by PCR, and then cutting with the appropriate restriction enzyme, this individual would show a 1.5 kb band from the normal gene, and both 0.6 and 0.9 kb bands from the disease gene.

20 **The answer is A: 5.0 kb.** This would be a noninformative result. Enzyme X would not cut at site Z, so there would be no difference between the normal and disease gene when the DNA is cut with enzyme X, so both genes would give rise to a 5 kb piece of DNA. In order to distinguish between the normal and the disease gene, one needs to cut with two enzymes, X and Z; using the probe indicated in a Southern blot, the disease gene would then show a piece of DNA that is 1.2 kb in size, while the normal gene would show a piece of DNA that is 5.0 kb in size.

Chapter 8

Energy Metabolism Overview

The use of energy is a key for biochemical pathways to proceed. This chapter covers the basic tenets of biochemical energy utilization, storage, and production, as well as the body's energy needs.

QUESTIONS

Select the single best answer.

Questions 1 to 4 concern the following case. You see in your office a thin, anxious woman who is concerned about her weight. She is worried that she may have a parasite causing her to lose weight. She stands 5′5″ tall (1.67 m) and weighs 101 lb (45.85 kg).

1 An estimate of her body mass index (BMI) is which of the following?
(A) 14
(B) 16
(C) 18
(D) 20
(E) 22

2 The same patient then describes to you a typical day of eating, which consists of 250 g of carbohydrates, 10 g of fat, and 100 g of protein. She denies any ethanol intake. She also exercises about 2 h/day. Her daily caloric intake is about which of the following?
(A) 1,250
(B) 1,500
(C) 1,750
(D) 2,000
(E) 2,250

3 For the same patient, her daily caloric needs can be estimated to be which of the following?
(A) 1,250
(B) 1,500
(C) 1,750
(D) 2,000
(E) 2,250

4 Given this same patient's eating habits and lifestyle, which of the following best describes her metabolic state?
(A) She is gaining weight
(B) She is in caloric balance
(C) She is in the healthy range of BMI but is losing weight
(D) She is in an unhealthy range of BMI and is losing weight
(E) She has a tapeworm and needs lab testing

5 Given the following reaction:
$A + B \leftrightarrows C + D \ \Delta G^{o\prime} = +15.5$ kcal/mol
And [A] = 5 mM, [B] = 4 mM, [C] = 0.5 mM, and [D] = 2.5 mM under cellular conditions, what is the overall Gibbs free energy change for the reaction at 25°C ($R = 1.98 \times 10^{-3}$ kcal/mol/°K) (in kcal/mol)?
(A) +13.86
(B) −13.86
(C) +15.50
(D) −15.50
(E) +17.13

6 Consider the following reaction sequence:
$A \leftrightarrows B \ \Delta G^{o\prime} = +0.50$ kcal/mol
$B \leftrightarrows C \ \Delta G^{o\prime} = -15.50$ kcal/mol
$C \leftrightarrows D \ \Delta G^{o\prime} = -12.15$ kcal/mol
$D \leftrightarrows E \ \Delta G^{o\prime} = +21.15$ kcal/mol
Under standard conditions, which intermediate would accumulate?
(A) A
(B) B
(C) C
(D) D
(E) E

Questions 7 and 8 refer to an unusual bacterium that has been shown to have a five-component electron transfer chain. Table 8-1 shows the $E^{o\prime}$ values for these five components.

Table 8-1.

$A + 2e^- + 2H^+ \rightarrow AH_2$	+0.55V
$B + 2e^- + 2H^+ \rightarrow BH_2$	+0.12V
$C + 2e^- + 2H^+ \rightarrow CH_2$	+0.03V
$D + 2e^- + 2H^+ \rightarrow DH_2$	−0.22V
$E + 2e^- + 2H^+ \rightarrow EH_2$	−0.47V

7 The order of electron flow in this bacterium is which of the following?
(A) A transfers to B, which transfers to C, which transfers to D, which transfers to E
(B) E transfers to D, which transfers to C, which transfers to B, which transfers to A
(C) C transfers to D, which transfers to E, which transfers to B, which transfers to A
(D) A transfers to E, which transfers to B, which transfers to D, which transfers to C
(E) E transfers to C, which transfers to A, which transfers to D, which transfers to B

8 For the bacterial strain referenced in the previous question, the amount of energy available from transporting a pair of electrons across this chain is which of the following? ($R = 1.98 \times 10^{-3}$ kcal/mol/K and $F = 23$ kcal/mol-V)
(A) 2.3 kcal/mol
(B) 23 kcal/mol
(C) 47 kcal/mol
(D) 70 kcal/mol
(E) 100 kcal/mol

9 A sedentary male medical student is 5′9″ tall and weighs 175 lb. Which of the following diets will allow maintenance of the current weight and also falls within current nutritional guidelines?
(A) About 100 g fat, 50 g of ethanol, 100 g of protein, and 300 g of carbohydrate
(B) About 80 g fat, 125 g of protein, and 310 g of carbohydrate
(C) About 125 g fat, 85 g protein, and 350 g of carbohydrate
(D) About 80 g fat, 60 g ethanol, 100 g protein, and 310 g carbohydrate
(E) About 50 g fat, 25 g protein, and 225 g carbohydrate

10 Which one of the following diets provides for the largest number of calories?
(A) 100 g protein, 100 g fat, 100 g carbohydrate, 25 g ethanol
(B) 50 g protein, 100 g fat, 150 g carbohydrate, 25 g ethanol
(C) 75 g protein, 125 g fat, 50 g carbohydrate, no ethanol
(D) 150 g protein, 75 g fat, 125 g carbohydrate, 20 g ethanol
(E) 150 g protein, 50 g fat, 125 g carbohydrate, no ethanol

11 Ivan Applebod is an overweight accountant, with a height of 5′9″ (1.77 m) and a weight of 245 lb (111.4 kg). As a sedentary individual, his daily caloric need approximates which of the following?
(A) 2,500 cal
(B) 3,000 cal
(C) 3,500 cal
(D) 4,000 cal
(E) 4,500 cal

12 Which of the following diet plans will allow Mr Applebod to lose approximately 5 lb/month assuming he does not increase his activity?
(A) 2,000 cal/day
(B) 2,450 cal/day
(C) 2,900 cal/day
(D) 3,350 cal/day
(E) 3,800 cal/day

Questions 13 and 14 refer to the following figure indicating an energy curve for an enzyme-catalyzed reaction:

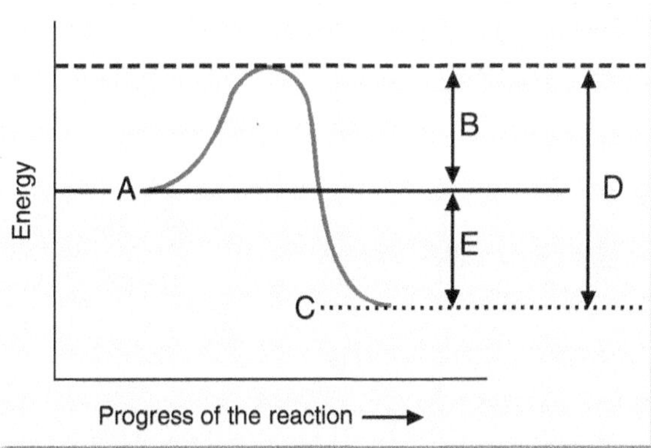

13 Which letter represents the Gibbs free energy of activation?

14 Which letter best represents the difference in energy between the substrates and products?

15 Consider the reaction shown below. If [A] = 5.00 mM, [B] = 2.50 mM, and [C] = 1.25 mM, what would the concentration of D have to be to allow this to be a favorable reaction under these conditions?
$A + B \leftrightarrows C + D \quad \Delta G^{o\prime} = +8.65$ kcal/mol
(A) <0.125 μM
(B) <0.43 μM
(C) <4.3 nM
(D) <43 nM
(E) <5.0 μM

Questions 16 and 17 refer to the following case. A 15-year-old girl has gone to the nutritionist as she is concerned about losing weight. She is 5′7″ tall and weighs 128 lb, down from 135 lb 3 weeks ago. She explains that she had made the cross-country team at her high school, and over the past 3 weeks her running has increased from about 1.5 miles/day to 10 miles/day.

16 Assuming that the patient's weight loss over the past 3 weeks was equally distributed over that time period, how many calories per day was she deficient in her diet?
(A) 800
(B) 1,000
(C) 1,200
(D) 1,400
(E) 1,600

17 After learning that her diet was deficient in calories, the runner decided to make up the deficit by eating equal amounts (in term of calories) of carbohdyrates and proteins, but no fat or alcohol. How many grams of carbs and proteins would she have to add to her diet in order to stop losing weight?
(A) 100 g of each
(B) 150 g of each
(C) 200 g of each
(D) 100 g of carbohydrates, 200 g of protein
(E) 100 g of protein, 200 g of carbohydrate

18 Calculation of the basal metabolic rate (BMR) for morbidly obese individuals using standard methodology is often incorrect due to which of the following?
(A) Underestimation of calories consumed
(B) Overestimation of calories consumed
(C) Preponderance of metabolically active adipocytes
(D) Preponderance of inert adipocytes
(E) Reduced metabolic need of the muscles

19 The BMI is most likely to yield incorrect data for which of the following?
(A) An anorexic 25-year-old woman
(B) An obese 50-year-old man
(C) A normal appearing 30-year-old man
(D) A 30-year-old female bodybuilder
(E) A slightly overweight 42-year-old biochemistry professor

20 Assume that beer contains 5% wt./vol. ethanol. How many calories derived from alcohol would 500 mL (about 17 ounces) of beer contain? Choose the closest answer to your calculated value.
(A) 100
(B) 140
(C) 180
(D) 220
(E) 260

ANSWERS

1 **The answer is B: 16.** The BMI is calculated as the weight of the person (in kg) divided by the height squared (in meters). Thus, for this patient, the BMI is equal to 45.85 divided by $(1.67)^2$, which is 16.44. The BMI stands for body mass index, and can be used to estimate body fat content. A value of <18.5 is considered underweight, values between 18.5 and 24.9 are considered in the normal range, values of 25 through 29.9 are considered overweight, and values of 30 or greater are considered obese. Values of 40 or more are considered morbidly obese, whereas values between 35 and 40 are considered clinically obese. The formulas in order to perform these calculations are summarized in a figure above. The second figure allows one to utilize a graph to calculate the BMI.

Calculation of body mass index (BMI)

Formula:

$$\text{BMI} = \frac{\text{Weight (kg)}}{\text{Height (m)}^2}$$

Conversion:

Kilograms = pounds ÷ 2.2

Meters = inches ÷ 39.4

Example:

A woman who is 5′4″ tall and weighs 134 lb has a BMI of 23.5.

Weight: 134 lb ÷ 2.2 = 61 kg

Height: 64 in. ÷ 39.4 = 1.6 m; $(1.6)^2 = 2.6$

$$\text{BMI} = \frac{61\text{ kg}}{2.6\text{ m}} = 23.5$$

How to calculate the BMI.

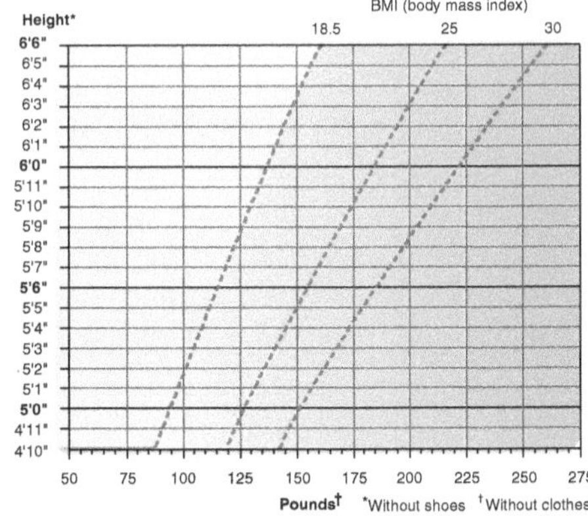

A nomogram used to calculate BMI, knowing the height in inches, and the weight in pounds.

2 **The answer is B: 1,500.** Carbohydrates contain 4 cal/g, protein also contains 4 cal/g, and fat contains 9 cal/g (because it is more reduced than either protein or carbohydrates). Given the patient's diet, she is consuming (250 × 4) + (10 × 9) + (100 × 4), or 1,490 cal/day.

3 **The answer is C: 1,750.** The BMR can be estimated by multiplying the weight (in kg) times 24 cal/kg, which is assuming an energy use of 1 cal/h/kg. Multiplying 45.85 times 24 yields 1,100 cal/day. Her metabolic need can be estimated by multiplying her BMR times an acitivty factor (how active the individual is). For someone who exercises 2 h/day (moderately active) the activity factor is 1.6, so her daily caloric needs are 1,100 × 1.6, or 1,760 cal/day. More accurate representations of the BMR can be obtained from using the formulas in Table 8-2, although for the purposes of this textbook the approximation of 24 cal/kg/day will be utilized for both males and females of all ages.

Table 8-2. Equation for predicting BMR from body weight (W) in kg

Males		Females	
Age Range (years)	**BMR kcal/day**	**Age Range (years)**	**BMR kcal/day**
0–3	60.9W – 54	0–3	61.0W – 51
3–10	22.7W + 495	3–10	22.5W + 499
10–18	17.5W + 651	10–18	12.2W + 746
18–30	15.3W + 679	18–30	14.7W + 496
30–60	11.6W + 879	30–60	8.7W + 829
>60	13.5W + 487	>60	10.5W + 596

Source: Energy and protein requirements: Report of a Joint FAO/WHO/UNU Expert Consultation. Technical report series no. 724. Geneva World Health Organization. 1987:71. See also Schofield et al. Hum Nutr Clin Nutr. 1985;39 (suppl).

4 **The answer is D: She is in an unhealthy range of BMI and is losing weight.** The BMI of 16.4 places the individual in an underweight situation, and she is currently consuming fewer calories (1,490) per day than she requires (1,760), which will lead to weight loss, and further exacerbate her underweight condition. You have a diagnosis, there is no reason to pursue further testing. She can be counseled on how to gain weight.

5 **The answer is A: +13.86.** Recall, $\Delta G = \Delta G^{o\prime} + RT\ln([C][D]/[A][B])$, so for this reaction, $\Delta G = 15.5 + (1.98 \times 10^{-3})(298)\ \ln (1.25/20)$. Thus, $\Delta G = 15.5 + (0.59)\ \ln (0.0625)$. $\Delta G = 15.5 - 1.64 = 13.86$ kcal/mol. As ΔG is a positive number, under these conditions, the reaction is still an unfavorable reaction.

6 **The answer is D: D.** The conversion of A to B is slightly unfavorable, but as soon as B is produced it will be converted to C due to the highly favorable B to C conversion (a high negative ΔG). The conversion of C to D is also highly favorable, which will lead to accumulation of D. The conversion of D to E, however, is highly unfavorable (high positive ΔG), such that D will accumulate under standard conditions.

7 **The answer is B: E transfers to D, which transfers to C, which transfers to B, which transfers to A.** The order of electron flow goes from the lowest standard redox potential (E/EH_2, with a value of −0.47 V) to the highest redox potential (A/AH_2, with a value of +0.55 V). Redox pairs with low redox potentials are good reducing agents (they like to give up their electrons), whereas redox pairs with high redox potentials are good oxidizing agents (they love to accept electrons). Thus, the order of electron transfer would be E to D to C to B and then to A as the terminal electron acceptor.

8 **The answer is C: 47 kcal/mol.** In order to answer this question, one needs to use the Nernst equation, which equates overall changes in redox potential to Gibbs free energy. The Nernst equation is $\Delta G^{o\prime} = -nF\Delta E^{o\prime}$, where n is the number of electrons transferred, F is Faraday's constant, and $\Delta E^{o\prime}$ is the change in redox potential. In this case, $\Delta E^{o\prime}$ is equal to 1.02 V (the difference between −0.47 and +0.55), and $n = 2$ for a pair of electrons traveling through the chain. The equation thus becomes

$$\Delta G^{o\prime} = -(2)(23)(1.02) = -47\ \text{kcal/mol}$$

9 **The answer is B: About 80 g fat, 125 g of protein, and 310 g of carbohydrate.** In order to answer this question, one first needs to calculate the basic daily energy needs of the student. At 175 lb (79.55 kg) one can estimate his BMR as 1,910 cal/day (79.55 kg multiplied by 24 cal/day/kg). Being sedentary, the activity factor is 1.3, for a total daily caloric need of 2,480 cal/day. Current nutritional guidelines indicate that no more than 30% of one's daily calories should be fat, so the maximum caloric intake for fat should be 750 cal, which is about 80 g of fat (fat contains 9 cal/g). These data alone eliminate answers A and C. Answer E has insufficient total calories (450 from fat, 100 from protein, and 900 from carbohydrates, for a total of 1,450) for the needs of the student, and can also be eliminated. Answer D contains too much ethanol (420 cal out of a total of 2,780) and too many calories. Thus, answer B is correct, in which the 80 g of fat provide 720 cal, the 125 g of protein provides 500 cal, and the 310 g of carbohydrates provides 1,240 cal, for a total of 2,460 cal/day.

10 **The answer is D: 150 g protein, 75 g fat, 125 g carbohydrate, 20 g ethanol.** To answer this question, one needs to recall that fat contains 9 cal/g, ethanol 7 cal/g, and protein and carbohydrates 4 cal/g each. Using these numbers, diet A contains 1,875 cal, diet B contains 1,875 cal, diet C contains 1,625 cal, diet D contains 1,915 cal, and diet E contains 1,550 cal.

11 **The answer is C: 3,500 cal.** Mr Applebod's BMR can be approximated as 24 × 111.4, or 2,673 cal/day. Since he is sedentary, his activity factor is 1.3, and has a daily caloric need of 3,475 cal/day.

12 **The answer is C: 2,900 cal/day.** To lose one pound of weight, a reduction in intake of approximately 3,500 cal is required; thus, a loss of 5 lb will require a reduction of 17,500 cal over the next 30 days (one month). Dividing 17,500 by 30 yields 583 cal/day. Since his normal intake (to maintain weight) is 3,475 cal/day, 3,475 − 583 yields 2,892 cal/day.

13 **The answer is B.** The energy required to increase the energy state of the starting material (indicated by A in the diagram) is the Gibbs free energy of Activation. The change in energy states of reactants and products is indicated by E, while D shows the maximal energy change from the energy of activation to the energy level of the products.

14 **The answer is E.** The energy required to increase the energy state of the starting material (indicated by A in the diagram) is the Gibbs free energy of activation. The change in energy states of reactants and products is indicated by E, while D shows the maximal energy change from the energy of activation to the energy level of the products.

15 **The answer is C: <4.3 nM.** Recall, $\Delta G = \Delta G^{o\prime} + RT\ln([C][D]/[A][B])$. In order for the reaction to be favorable,

ΔG must be negative. If one solves for the concentration of D required for $\Delta G = 0$, then any concentration lower than the one calculated will be sufficient to allow for a negative ΔG. Thus, when ΔG is set to zero, $\Delta G^{o\prime} = -RT \ln ([C][D]/[A][B])$. Therefore, $8.65 = -(1.98 \times 10^{-3})(298) \ln ([1.25D]/[12.5])$. This reduces to $-14.66 = \ln (D/10)$, or $(10)(e^{-14.66}) = [D]$ in mM. $[D] = 4.3 \times 10^{-6}$ mM, or 4.3 nM.

16 **The answer is C: 1,200.** Each pound of weight is equivalent to about 3,500 cal. The runner had lost 7 lb, for a total deficit of 24,500 cal. As she lost that weight over 21 days, her daily deficit, if evenly distributed over the course of the three weeks, was 1,167 cal/day.

17 **The answer is B: 150 g of each.** Both proteins and carbohydrates contain 4 cal/g, so to make up approximately 1,200 cal/day the total intake of proteins and carbohydrates would have to be 300 g/day. Since the runner wants to split the calories equally between protein and Carbohydrates, 150 g of each is a better answer than splitting the 300 g into 100 g of one nutrient, and 200 g of another nutrient.

18 **The answer is D: Preponderance of inert adipocytes.** All estimates of the BMR utilize the weight of the individual, however, adipose tissue is primarily metabolically inactive, and if an individual has a lot of adipose tissue, the contribution of the adipose tissue to the overall BMR will lead to an overestimate of the energy needs of the individual. It is not related to the amount of calories consumed, nor does it relate to use of the muscles, since the BMR is estimated for energy use during rest.

19 **The answer is D: A 30-year-old female bodybuilder.** The BMI is an estimate of the "fitness" of an individual, and is calculated by taking the weight, in kilograms, and dividing by the square of the height, in meters. Values between 18.5 and 24.9 are considered the normal range, while values above 24.9 fall into the preobese and obese categories. Body builders, whether male or female, have an increased muscle mass for their height, which adds weight. Thus, body builders will have an inflated BMI which is not indicative of their fat content (it reflects their muscle mass instead). The other individuals listed will mostly fit the criteria for a valid BMI determination.

20 **The answer is C: 180.** With alcohol at 5% wt./vol., 500 mL of beer would contain 25 g of alcohol (5 g/100 mL). Alcohol contains 7 cal/g, so $7 \times 25 = 175$ cal. Beer also contains some carbohydrates, so its total caloric content would be even higher than the 175 due to the ethanol alone. In contrast, 12 ounces of a cola product typically contains 150 cal (none from ethanol).

Chapter 9

Hormones and Signaling Mechanisms

This chapter covers the basics of signal transduction, including second messengers, insulin, glucagon, phosphatidylinositol, and steroid hormone signaling. Because there is another chapter on cancer, signal transduction pathways specifically relating to cancer are discussed in that chapter. This chapter covers the more general aspects of signal transduction.

QUESTIONS

Select the single best answer.

1 A middle-aged female has developed darkened, smooth, velvety skin patches on the neck and in her axillary folds (see the figure below). The molecular basis for this disease can be which of the following?

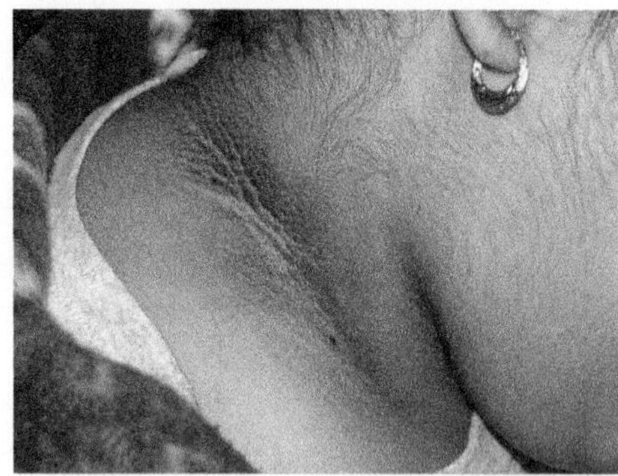

Note the darkened skin along the neck.

(A) Dysfunctional glucagon receptors
(B) Dysfunctional EGF receptors
(C) Persistently stimulated insulin receptors
(D) Persistently inhibited insulin receptors
(E) Dysfunctional thyroid hormone receptor

2 A 4-year-old boy went to the shore with his family and ate clams for dinner, but shortly thereafter developed severe watery diarrhea, vomiting, and leg cramps. The molecular basis of his disorder is which of the following?
(A) Inhibition of protein synthesis
(B) Inhibition of a stimulatory G protein
(C) Activation of a stimulatory G protein
(D) Inhibition of an inhibitory G protein
(E) Activation of an inhibitory G protein

3 A 40-year-old man, with a BMI of 37, has a fasting blood glucose level of 165 mg/dL, a value that has been steadily increasing over the past 5 years. His HbA1c level is 8.9. Analysis of his blood, using Western blot technology, demonstrates the presence of antibodies against the insulin receptor. One consequence of these antibodies is which of the following?
(A) Downregulation of the insulin receptors
(B) Upregulation of the insulin receptors
(C) Enhanced release of pancreatic glucagon
(D) Enhanced glucose uptake into muscle cells
(E) Activation of adenylate cyclase

4 Considering the patient in the previous question, which of the following medical disorders would you expect this patient to also have?
(A) Low blood pressure
(B) Polycystic ovary syndrome (PCOS)
(C) Fatty liver-nonalcoholic hepatitis (NASH—nonalcoholic steatohepatitis)
(D) Hypouricemia
(E) High HDL cholesterol

5 Considering the patient in question 3, which of the following body types would you expect this patient to have?
(A) Body builder
(B) Central obesity
(C) Obesity mostly centered in the hips and breasts
(D) Tall and slender
(E) Ideal body weight

6 A patient with a good appetite has been losing weight and has developed lesions and blisters on his feet and legs. Lab analysis demonstrates hyperglycemia under both fed and fasting conditions. A possible explanation for these symptoms is which of the following?

(A) A glucagon-secreting tumor of the pancreas
(B) An insulin-secreting tumor of the pancreas
(C) Loss of glucose-6-phosphatase activity
(D) Defective glucagon receptors
(E) Destruction of the α cells of the pancreas

7 A cell line has been generated in which a protein important in signal transduction was mutated such that its SH2 domain was no longer functional. After adding insulin to this cell line, protein kinase B could no longer be activated. The protein which was mutated is which of the following?

(A) Ras
(B) Raf
(C) GAP
(D) PI-3′-kinase
(E) GRB2

8 A researcher was studying a tumor in mice that was induced by transfection of a vector, which led to overproduction of c-ras within the tumor. The researcher wanted to now add a second expression vector that would counteract the effects of the overexpressed c-ras. Which one of the following genes should be investigated?

(A) GAP
(B) SOS
(C) Raf
(D) Fos
(E) PKA

9 A 2-year-old boy had frequent infections and a number of pneumonia episodes. Blood work showed greatly reduced levels of both T and B lymphocytes. X-rays showed normal thymus development. The primary mutation in this patient is likely to be which of the following?

(A) Mutated JAK proteins
(B) Mutated STAT proteins
(C) Defective cytokine receptor component
(D) Mutated SMAD proteins
(E) Mutated ubiquitin ligase

10 A world-class sprinter, while in the starting blocks waiting for the race to start, stimulates which of the following muscle proteins in response to hormone release?

(A) A tyrosine kinase
(B) A Gαs protein
(C) A Gαi protein
(D) A Gq protein
(E) cAMP phosphodiesterase

11 A researcher was investigating the mechanism of action of steroid hormone receptors. He created a chimeric receptor that contained the estrogen ligand-binding domain, and also the testosterone DNA-binding domain. The transactivation domain was also from the testosterone receptor. When this chimeric receptor was expressed in eukaryotic cells lacking estrogen receptors, which of the following would you expect to occur when estrogen is added to the cells?

(A) Increase in tyrosine kinase activity
(B) Activation of PKA
(C) Induction of estrogen-specific genes
(D) Induction of testosterone-specific genes
(E) Inhibition of estrogen-specific genes

12 A 17-year-old girl was seen by her family physician due to a lack of menses. On physical exam the girl appeared to be well-developed, but with a striking lack of pubic hair. Blood work indicated very high levels of testosterone, with elevated estradiol levels as well. A karyotype of the patient is shown below. The underlying biochemical defect in this patient is which of the following?

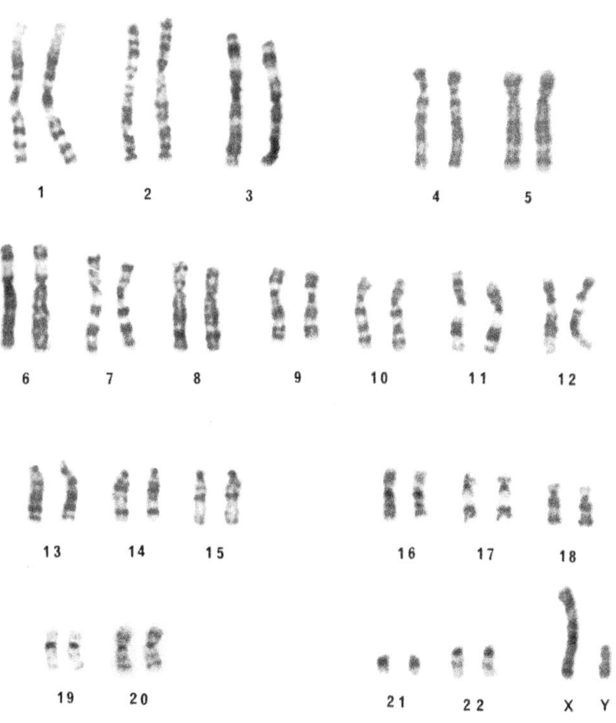

The karyotype from the patient.

(A) Inability to synthesize estrogen
(B) Lack of estrogen receptor
(C) Lack of cortisol receptor
(D) Lack of androgen receptor
(E) Inability to synthesize aldosterone

13 A variant cell line was discovered that would not respond to any form of TGF-β, yet both type I and type II receptors were present and functional on the cell surface, as determined by in vitro experiments. A potential mutation in which one of the following proteins can lead to this phenotype?

(A) SMAD2
(B) SMAD3
(C) SMAD4
(D) JAK1
(E) TYK1

14 A 62-year-old man visits his physician for feeling fatigued. It is noticed that the spleen is enlarged and slightly tender when palpated. He has abdominal pain and echymoses on his skin. His blood pressure is high. Blood work indicates an abnormally high red blood cell, white blood cell, and platelet counts. A bone marrow sample from the patient is shown below. The suggested treatment is phlebotomy to reduce the thickness of the blood. This disorder can result from which of the following?

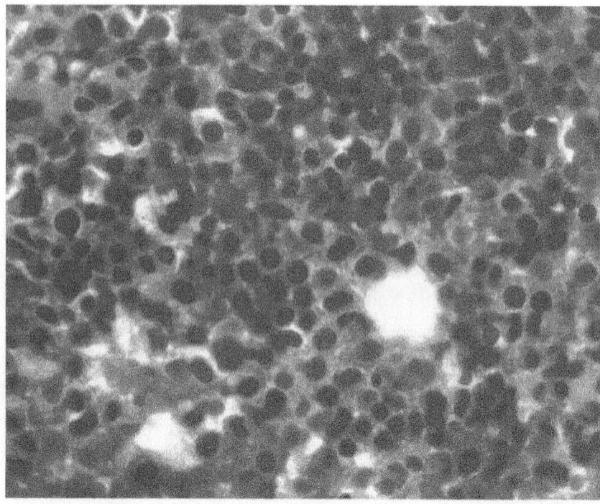

(A) A loss of function of JAK2
(B) A gain of function of JAK2
(C) A loss of function of SMAD4
(D) A gain of function of SMAD4
(E) Constitutive Her2 activity

15 A 3-month-old child of normal parents presents with shortened arms and legs, a large head with a prominent forehead, a curved lower spine, and bowed lower legs. The child is in the fifth percentile for height. The child's condition is most likely the result of which of the following?

(A) Constitutive activation of the EGF pathway in bone
(B) Inactivation of the TGF-β pathway in bone
(C) Constitutive activation of the FGF pathway in bone
(D) Inactivation of the FGF pathway in bone
(E) Constitutive activation of the JAK/STAT pathway in bone

16 A 52-year-old man suddenly collapses and is rushed to the hospital, where it is found that his blood troponin-C levels are elevated. An angiogram indicates an 87% blockage of three major arteries to the heart. If these arteries were examined at a molecular level, excessive smooth muscle cell proliferation would be noticed. This proliferation has occurred over the past 25 years due to the secretion and action of which of the following factors?

(A) VLDL
(B) HDL
(C) FGF
(D) PDGF
(E) EGF

17 A mouse fibroblast cell line is treated with an siRNA targeted toward MEK. When such cells are treated with a growth factor which works through a tyrosine kinase receptor, which one of the following effects would occur?

(A) Activation of ERK
(B) Activation of myc
(C) Activation of phospholipase (PLC-γ)
(D) Activation of fos
(E) Activation of STAT

18 Treatment of fibroblasts with TGF-β and TGF-α will allow such cells to grow in soft agar, a property of transformed cells. This occurs due to which of the following?

(A) Activation of cell growth
(B) Activation of oxidative phosphorylation
(C) Activation of collagen synthesis
(D) Inhibition of ras expression
(E) Inhibition of LETS synthesis

19 An example of an autocrine stimulatory pathway is which of the following?

(A) Blood vessel growth within a tumor
(B) Glucagon release from the pancreas
(C) Insulin stimulation of glucose transport into adipocytes
(D) Injured smooth muscle cells producing PDGF
(E) Platelets secreting PDGF at internal blood vessel injuries

20 A signaling protein is activated by phosphorylation. The site of phosphorylation within the protein falls within the sequence–S–A–T–; either the serine or threonine residue can be phosphorylated. Phosphorylation of either residue results in an active protein. In certain tumors, however, an activating mutation is found in this region that renders the protein active in the absence of any phosphorylation event. Which one of the following amino acid mutations is most likely an activating mutation?

(A) A to E
(B) S to A
(C) T to A
(D) A to T
(E) S to Y

ANSWERS

1 **The answer is D: Persistently inhibited insulin receptors.** The patient has acanthosis nigricans, which results from insulin resistance. One way in which insulin resistance can be obtained is through a persistent inhibition of insulin receptor activity. Alterations in the glucagon, EGF, or thyroid hormone receptors will not lead to insulin resistance.

2 **The answer is C: Activation of a stimulatory G protein.** The boy has contracted cholera. The bacterium which causes cholera (*Vibrio cholerae*) produces a toxin that ADP-ribosylates a stimulatory G protein, leading to permanent activation of the G protein (via inhibition of the intrinsic GTPase activity). This leads to constant cAMP production, which in turn leads to the secretion of sodium and water into the lumen of the intestine, producing watery diarrhea. If not treated, dehydration rapidly results, and death can occur. The figure below outlines the action of cholera toxin in intestinal epithelial cells.

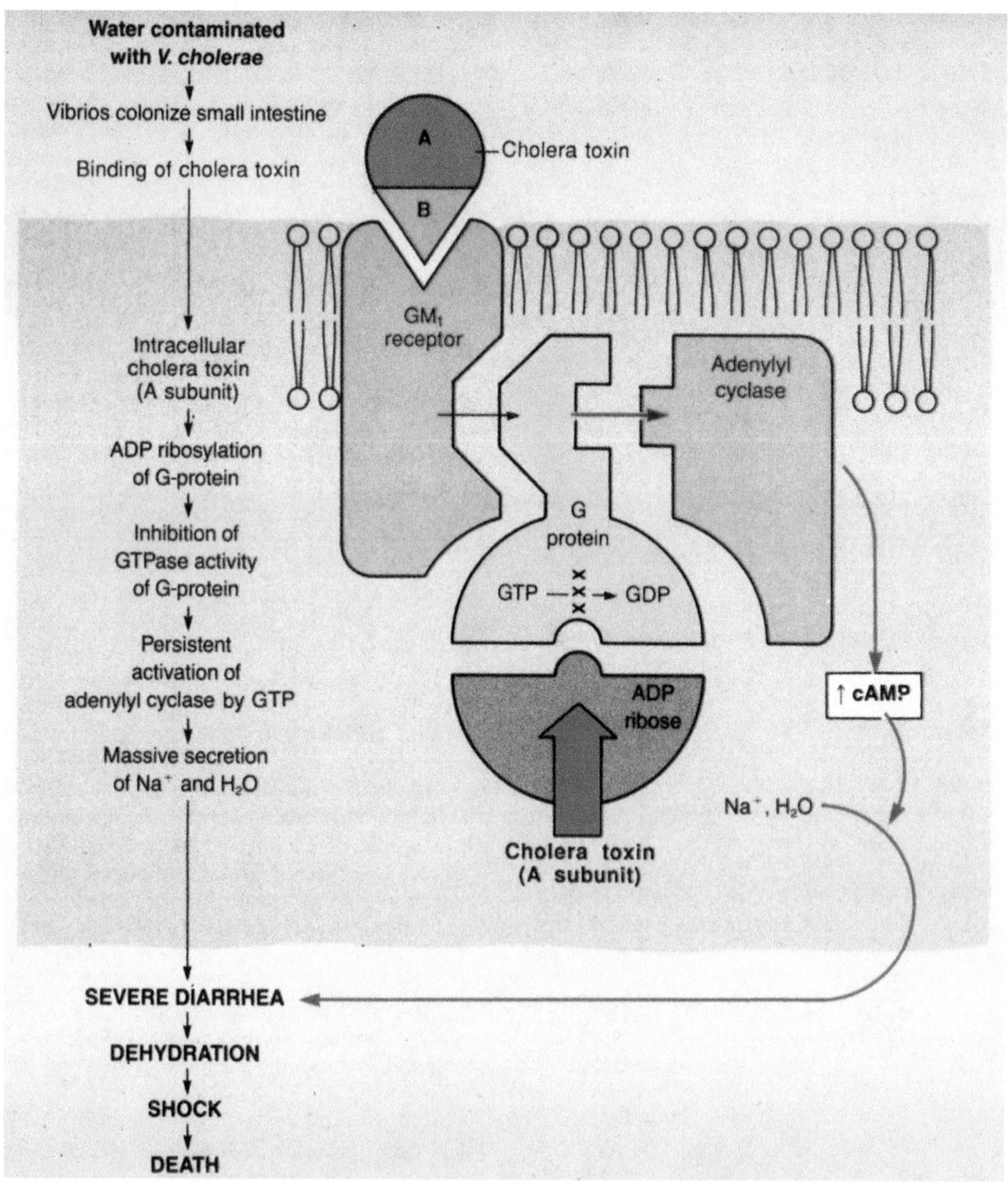

The bacteria containing the cholera toxin are ingested and travel through the digestive system, and within the intestine their toxin exerts its effects, which leads to severe water and electrolyte loss. Dehydration and hypovolemic shock can result.

3 **The answer is A: Downregulation of the insulin receptors.** The patient is exhibiting insulin resistance (persistently elevated blood glucose levels), most likely due to antibody binding to the receptor, leading to downregulation of the receptor. Cells are thus kept in a persistently low insulin receptor state, blunting their ability to be stimulated by insulin. The lack of insulin signaling leads to elevated blood glucose levels. These alterations are not due to changes in glucagon secretion or activation of adenylate cyclase. Since muscle cells have downregulated insulin receptors, the muscle cells are not stimulated to remove glucose from the circulation. The antibodies also do not allow for upregulation of insulin receptors.

4 **The answer is C: Fatty liver-nonalcoholic hepatitis (NASH—nonalcoholic steatohepatitis).** The full insulin resistance syndrome consists of diabetes mellitus 2, central obesity, hypertension, low HDL, high triglycerides, high PAI-1 (plasminogen activator inhibitor-1, a marker of inflammation), high uric acid, and NASH. All of these lead to total body atherosclerosis. PCOS is part of this constellation of symptoms, but occurs only in women. These insulin-resistant patients most likely also have sleep apnea, but this is probably from the obesity and not from the insulin resistance. The causes of NASH (fatty liver, leading to cirrhosis) are multifactorial, but insulin resistance is one factor that can lead to the development of NASH.

5 **The answer is B: Central obesity.** The patient has insulin resistance syndrome, which is a polygenetic disorder usually brought on by gaining weight. Classically, insulin resistance syndrome has a central obesity pattern. The patient's BMI is 37 (clinically obese), so he would not be tall and slender and is not in the ideal body weight range. A body builder could have a BMI of 37 but this would be due to muscle mass and not due to adipose tissue, so he would most likely not be insulin resistant.

6 **The answer is A: A glucagon-secreting tumor of the pancreas.** The patient has a glucagonoma in which the pancreas is constantly secreting glucagon, leading to constant gluconeogenesis and fatty acid oxidation, despite the presence of adequate glucose levels in the blood. This leads to weight loss and hyperglycemia, as the liver is pumping out glucose despite normal blood glucose levels. An insulin-secreting tumor would lead to hypoglycemia (stimulation of glucose uptake from the blood even when blood glucose levels are low). As glucagon is released from the α-cells of the pancreas, loss of α-cells would not allow for glucagon secretion, and these symptoms would not appear. A lack of liver glucagon receptors would not allow hyperglycemia to occur (hypoglycemia would be observed instead), as would a lack of glucose-6-phosphatase. The lesions on the feet and legs are due to nonenzymatic glycosylation of nerves and small blood vessels in the periphery, leading to reduced circulation and feeling in the extremities.

7 **The answer is D: PI-3′-kinase.** Protein kinase B is recruited to the membrane, along with the phosphoinositide-dependant kinase, through binding to PIP_3 in the membrane. The PIP_3 is generated from PIP_2 through the actions of PI-3′-kinase. If PI-3′-kinase had lost its SH2 domains, this protein would no longer be able to bind to phosphorylated IRS-1, and in turn be activated by the insulin receptor tyrosine kinase activity. Proteins containing SH2 domains are capable of binding to other proteins which contain phosphotyrosine residues. In the absence of PI-3′-kinase activity, protein kinase B could not be activated (see the figure below), as both PKB and PDK1 (phosphoinositide-dependant kinase 1) require phosphatidylinositol trisphosphate in the membrane as a docking station, through the proteins pleckstrin homology domain. None of the other choices listed (ras, raf, GAP, GRB2) require PI-3′-kinase activity in order to be activated.

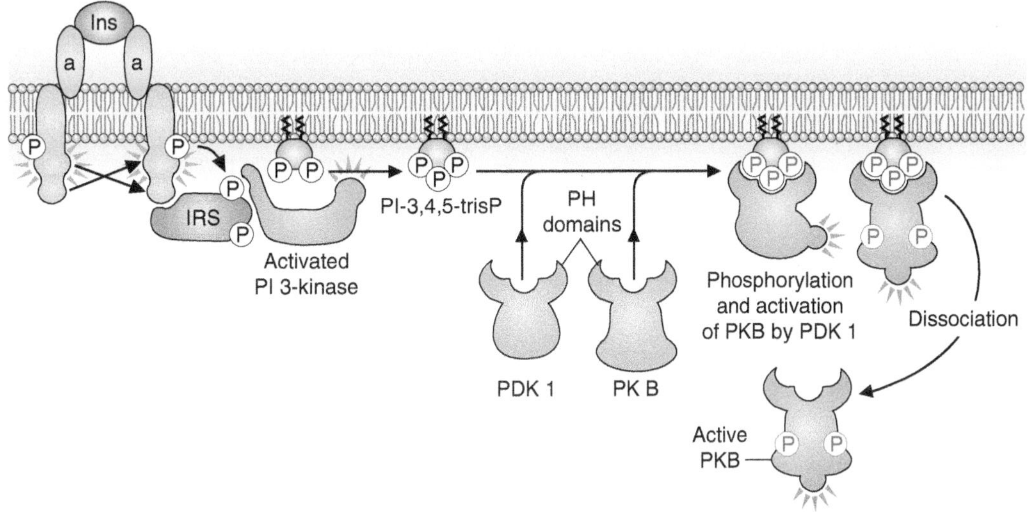

Answer 7

8 **The answer is A: GAP.** Overexpression of ras leads to transformation because there is insufficient GAP (GTPase-activating protein) to inactivate the ras in the cell. This can be overcome by adding GAP to the cells, such that the ras to GAP ratio is closer to one. GAP can thus inhibit ras activity and block transformation. This will not work with oncogenic ras, as oncogenic ras has obtained a mutation which has inactivated its built-in GTPase activity. Thus, GAP cannot activate oncogenic ras and cannot block ras function. SOS is a guanine nucleotide exchange protein that leads to ras activation; it cannot turn off activated ras. Raf, fos, and PKA do not play a role in regulating ras activity. A summary of these activities is shown in the figure above.

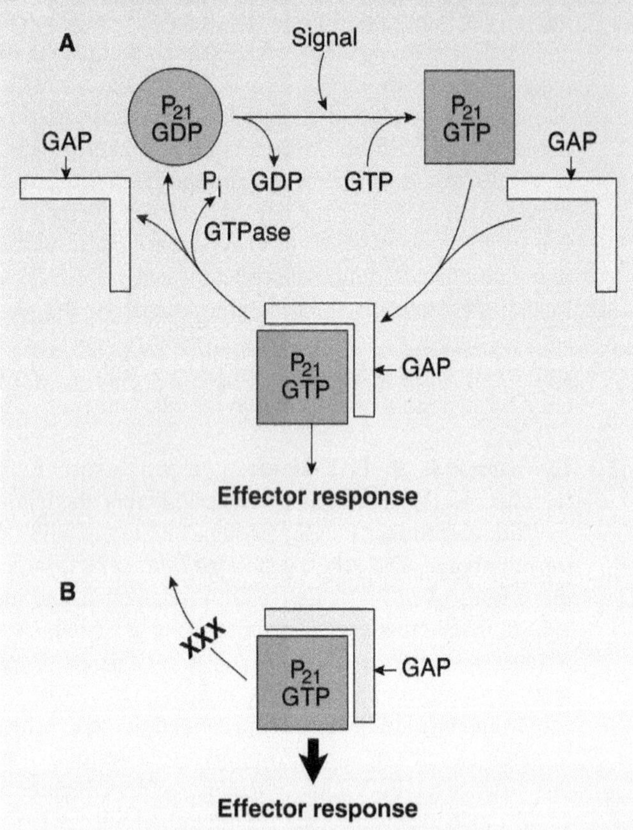

Panel A indicates the regulation of the normal ras protein (p21). **Panel B** indicates the lack of regulation of the oncogenic form of the ras protein, whose GTPase activity has been ablated, such that GAP binding to p21 cannot reduce the activity level of the mutated ras protein.

9 **The answer is C: Defective cytokine receptor component.** Many cytokine receptors contain multiple subunits, and some subunits are shared by multiple receptors. The boy has X-linked severe combined immunodeficiency syndrome (SCID), which is a defect in a cytokine receptor component, the γ-chain, common to a large number of cytokine receptors. Lack of this component renders most cytokine receptors inoperable, leading to lack of response to cytokines and inability to mount defenses against an immune attack. The defect is not in the TGF-β/SMAD pathway, nor in the JAK/STAT family of proteins. It is also not related to a ubiquitin ligase, which targets proteins for proteolysis by the proteasome.

10 **The answer is B: A Gαs protein.** The sprinter has released epinephrine in anticipation of the race. Epinephrine binds to a heptahelical receptor, which is linked to a stimulatory G protein. Upon epinephrine binding the G protein is activated, and the Gαs subunit binds GTP and travels to, and activates, adenylate cyclase, which raises intracellular cAMP levels. Epinephrine binding to such muscle receptors does not result in an increase of tyrosine kinase, inhibitory G protein, phospholipid-specific G protein (G_q), and cAMP phosphodiesterase activities. A summary of different types of heterotrimeric G protein subunits is given in Table 9-1.

Table 9-1. Subunits of heterotrimeric G proteins

Gα subunit	Action	Some Physiologic Uses
α_s; Gα(s)[a]	Stimulates adenyl cyclase	Glucagon and epinephrine to regulate metabolic enzymes, regulatory polypeptide hormones to control steroid hormone and thyroid hormone synthesis, and some neurotransmitters (e.g., dopamine) to control ion channels
$\alpha_{i/o}$; Gα(i/o) (signal also flows through βγ subunits)	Inhibits adenylyl cyclase	Epinephrine, many neurotransmitters including acetylcholine, dopamine, and serotonin
α_t;G_α(t)	Stimulates cGMP phosphodiesterase	Has a role in the transducin pathway, which mediates detection of light in the eye
$\alpha_{q/11}$; Gα (q/11)	Activates phospholipase C_β	Epinephrine, acetylcholine, histamine, thyroid-stimulating hormone (TSH), interleukin 8, somatostatin, angiotensin
$\alpha_{12/13}$; Gα (12/13)	Alters cytoskeletal elements	Thromboxane A2, lysophosphatidic acid

[a]There is a growing tendency to designate the heterotrimeric G protein subunits without using subscripts so that they are actually visible to the naked eye.

11 **The answer is D: Induction of testosterone-specific genes.** The chimeric receptor was created such that when estrogen bound to the receptor, the receptor would then bind to testosterone response elements in promoters in the genome (the DNA-binding domain was specific for the testosterone receptor). The steroid hormone receptors do not have tyrosine kinase activity, nor do they activate PKA. Since the cells being used for this experiment lack the estrogen receptor, there would not be any effect of adding estrogen on estrogen-specific gene expression. The chimeric receptor is shown in the figure below.

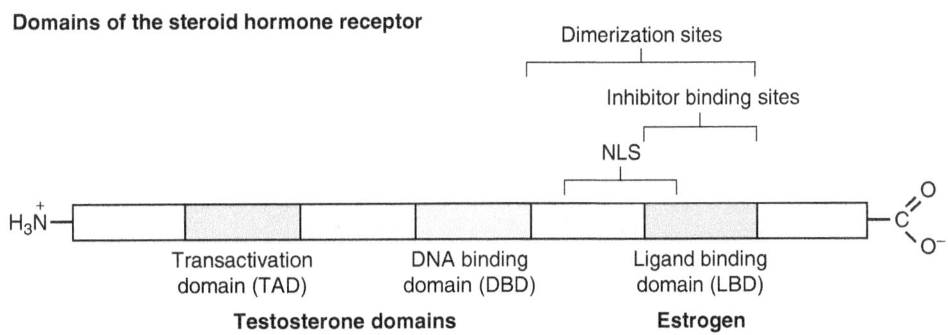

12 **The answer is D: Lack of androgen receptor.** The patient is exhibiting complete androgen insensitivity syndrome (CAIS), an inability to respond to androgens due to a lack of the androgen receptor. Thus, while genotypically a male, and producing normal levels of male hormones, the body cannot respond to the hormones, and female sexual characteristics develop. Androgen synthesis remains normal, however, which leads to high circulating testosterone levels in the patient.

13 **The answer is C: SMAD4.** The TGF-β receptors work together to initiate phosphorylation of SMAD transcription factors. Once phosphorylated, the specific SMAD factor dimerizes with a common SMAD, SMAD4, for transport to the nucleus and binding to the appropriate response elements in DNA. A lack of SMAD4 would account for the total lack of response to TGF-β, as all signaling through TGF-β requires this component. JAK and TYK work with cytokine receptors, not with TGF-β receptors, and SMAD1 and -2 are specific receptor SMADS; loss of either of them would diminish certain types of responses to TGF-β, but not all responses to TGF-β. The pathway of TGF-β signaling is shown below.

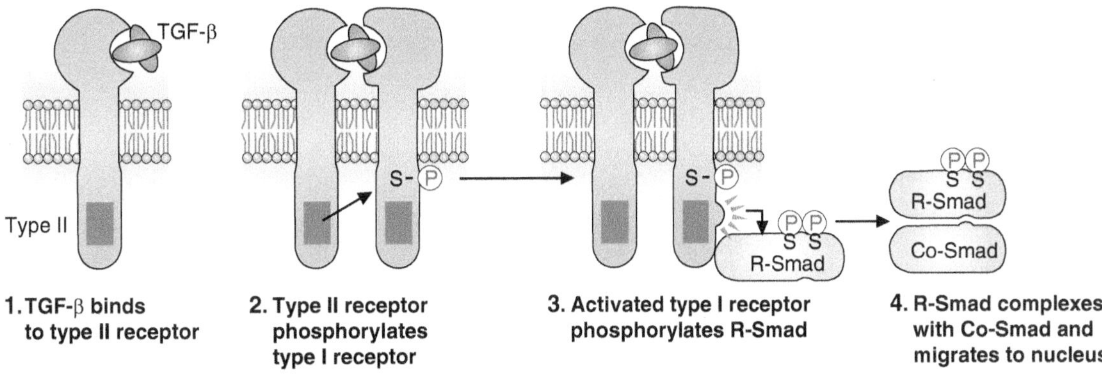

14 **The answer is B: A gain of function of JAK2.** The patient has polycythemia vera, a myeloproliferative disorder, which has recently been shown to result from constitutive JAK2 activity. Under normal conditions, JAK2 is only activated when an appropriate cytokine binds to its receptor. Once activated, JAK2 phosphorylates STAT proteins, which translocate to the nucleus and initiate gene transcription, leading to a proliferative response. In this disorder, JAK2 is always active, and the cells proliferate even in the absence of a signal. SMAD proteins transmit signals from TGF-β signaling and are not involved in this disorder. Her2 is the EGF receptor, which also does not play a role in this disorder. (For more about this case see Kralovics R et al. N Engl J Med 352:1779–2005). JAK–STAT signaling is outlined in the figure below.

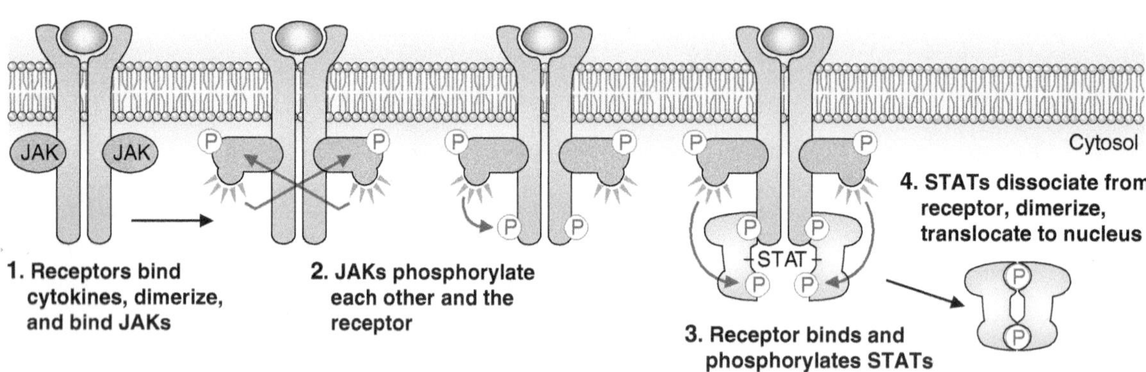

15 **The answer is C: Constitutive activation of the FGF pathway in bone.** The patient has achondroplasia, the most common form of short limb dwarfism in humans. This disorder is due to constitutive activation of FGFR3 (a receptor for FGF), which particularly plays havoc with the cartilaginous growth plate in limbs. Full details of how constitutive activation of this pathway leads to all of the phenotypic effects of this form of dwarfism are not yet fully appreciated. This disorder is not related to alterations in the EGF, TGF-β, or JAK/STAT pathways; it is unique to constitutive activation of the FGF pathway via FGF receptor 3. (For more on this case see Horton, WA, Hall, JG and Hecht, JT, Lancet 2007;370:162)

16 **The answer is D: PDGF.** During the development of an atherosclerotic plaque, PDGF is released by platelets at the site of injury, which aids in the stimulation of smooth muscle cell proliferation as the damage is being repaired. PDGF is also synthesized by smooth muscle cells, in an autocrine fashion, to further stimulate their own proliferation. FGF and EGF do not appear to play a role in the development of such plaques. HDL is a cholesterol carrier that removes cholesterol from tissues, and VLDL is the lipid carrier released by the liver for delivery of triglyceride to the tissues. (See Raines EW. Cytokine Growth Factor Rev 2004;15:237.)

17 **The answer is C: Activation of phospholipase (PLC-γ).** The silencing RNA will ablate MEK expression in this cell line. Effects which are upstream to MEK activation will still occur; effects downstream of MEK activation will be blocked. MEK activates ERK, which leads to alterations in gene transcription, such as myc and fos. Tyrosine kinase receptors do not activate STAT proteins (that occurs with cytokine receptors). PLC-γ activation occurs upon receptor tyrosine kinase activation, and binding of the phospholipase to the receptor via its SH2 domains. Activation of PLC-γ does not require MEK activation. The ras–raf pathway leading to the activation of myc and fos is shown below.

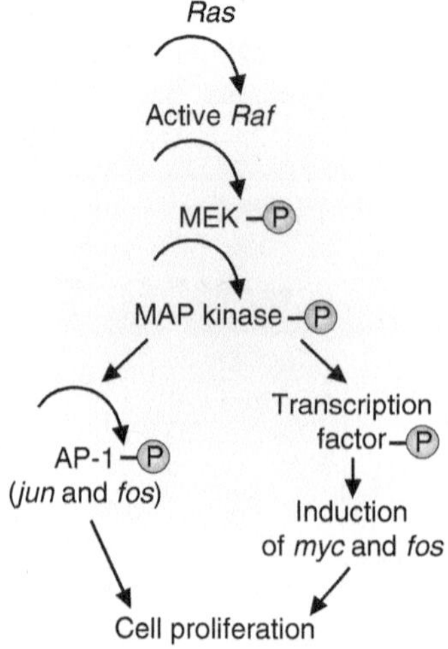

18 **The answer is C: Activation of collagen synthesis.** The combination of TGF-α and TGF-β leads to collagen production in fibroblasts. The collagen is secreted into

the soft agar and provides an adherence point for the fibroblasts, which allows them to proliferate. The cells will not grow if this adherence point is not present. The effects of TGF-α and TGF-β do include activation of cell growth, but this can only occur in soft agar if collagen has been synthesized and secreted. The factors do not block ras expression or inhibit LETS (fibronectin) synthesis. Oxidative phosphorylation is also not directly affected by these growth factors.

19 **The answer is D: Injured smooth muscle cells producing PDGF.** Autocrine stimulation is defined as one cell both secreting and responding to a growth factor. During the development of an atherosclerotic plaque, the smooth muscle cells both secrete and respond to PDGF. When tumors secrete FGF, they stimulate endothelial cell proliferation, which aids in angiogenesis (the tumor cells are not responding to the FGF—the endothelial cells are). Glucagon release from the pancreas is an endocrine process (the target for glucagon are cells far from the pancreas), as is insulin stimulation of glucose transport in muscle. Platelets secreting PDGF is not autocrine, as the platelets do not respond to PDGF. The difference between endocrine, paracrine, and autocrine stimulations is shown in the figure above.

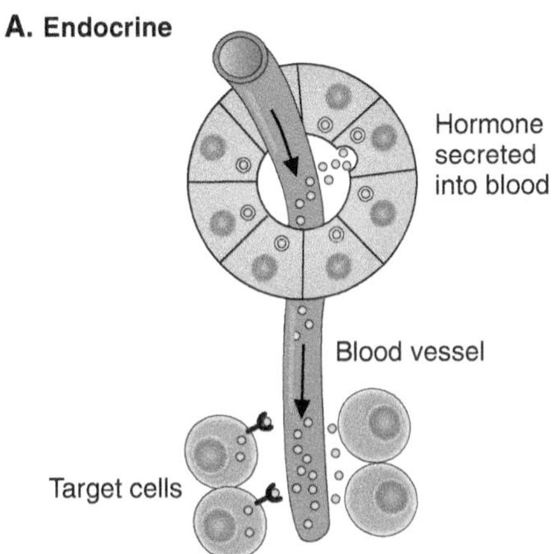

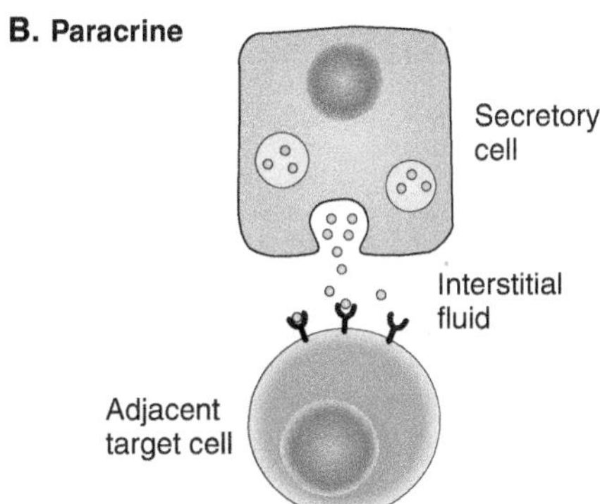

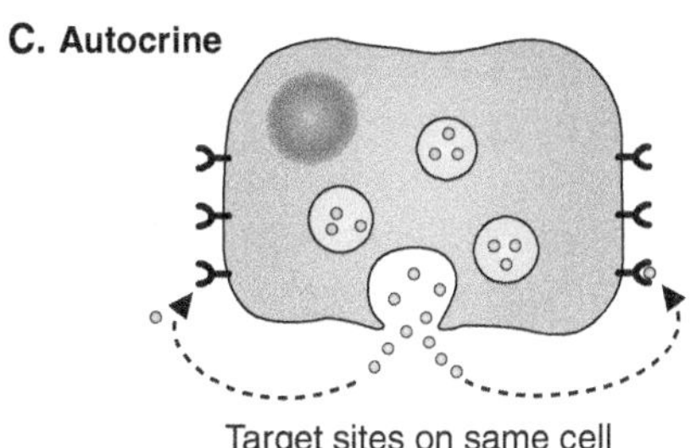

Y Receptor ∘ Hormone or other signal messenger

20 **The answer is A: A to E.** The conversion of an alanine residue to a glutamate residue results in the insertion of a negative charge into this region of the protein (the same overall effect that phosphorylation has). The introduction of the negative charge would lead to similar conformational changes that occur when a phosphate is introduced in this part of the protein. Thus, the glutamate side chain will mimic the effects of phosphorylation. Converting a serine to an alanine does not insert a negative charge into this area of the protein (the side chain of alanine is a methyl group); thus, the required conformation changes cannot occur. The same rationale applies for conversion of a threonine to an alanine; the alanine side chain cannot be modified to contain negative charges. Conversion of the alanine to a threonine introduces a hydroxyl group to the region, but the hydroxyl group has a high pK_a and will not deprotonate at physiological pH. This is similar to the serine to tyrosine conversion; tyrosine also has a hydroxyl group, but the pK_a is too high to lead to significant deprotonation and introduction of a negative charge into this area.

Chapter 10

Glycolysis and Gluconeogenesis

This chapter quizzes the student on the metabolic aspects of glycolysis and the synthesis of glucose, gluconeogenesis. Various aspects of diseases related to carbohydrate metabolism are also reviewed in this chapter.

QUESTIONS

Select the single best answer.

1 Anaerobiosis leads to lactate formation in muscle due to which one of the following?
(A) Inhibiting hexokinase by glucose-6-phosphate
(B) Providing 2,3-bisphosphoglycerate for the phosphoglyceromutase reaction
(C) Inhibiting pyruvate kinase by pyruvate
(D) Providing substrate for glyceraldehyde-3-phosphate dehydrogenase
(E) Inhibiting phosphofructokinase-1 by AMP

2 In muscle, under anaerobic conditions, the net synthesis of ATP starting from one mole of glucose derived from muscle glycogen is which one of the following?
(A) 1 mole of ATP
(B) 2 moles of ATP
(C) 3 moles of ATP
(D) 4 moles of ATP
(E) 5 moles of ATP

3 A 2-week-old newborn was brought to the pediatrician due to frequent vomiting, lethargy, and diarrhea. Family history revealed that the child never seemed to eat well, and had only been breast-fed. Physical examination revealed an enlarged liver and jaundice. The pediatrician was suspicious of an inborn error of metabolism and referred the child to an ophthalmologist for a slitlamp exam, the result of which is shown below. An enzyme that may be defective in this child is which one of the following?

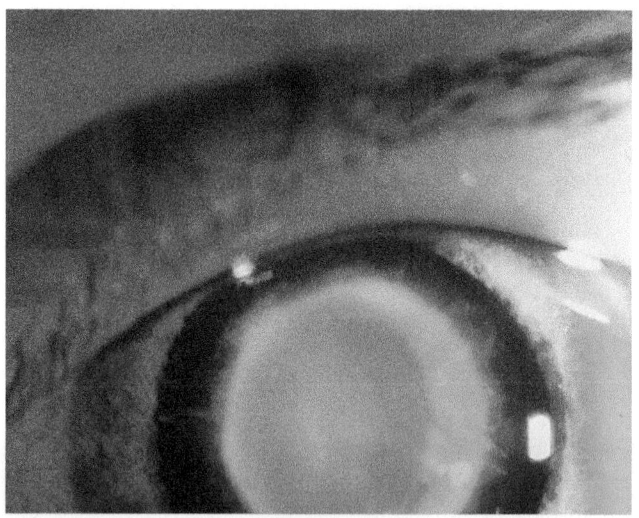

(A) Fructose-1,6-bisphosphatase
(B) Galactose-1-phosphate uridylyltransferase
(C) Galactokinase
(D) Glycogen synthase
(E) Fructokinase

4 A 7-year-old girl, who lives on a farm, started to have shaking and sweating episodes. Upon physical examination, she was found to be hypoglycemic under fasting conditions (fasting blood glucose was 50 mg/dL) and positive for ketones in her blood and urine. Her growth curve is normal. Further analyses showed no other metabolic abnormalities. Probing further into her history, in the absence of her parents, revealed that one of her chores was to collect eggs from the chicken coop every morning, and she had gotten into the habit of eating one or two raw eggs every morning. This had been going on for the past 6 weeks or so. A reasonable explanation for her laboratory results is which one of the following?

(A) Reduced levels of electron acceptors in her system, leading to reduced glucose production
(B) Reduced effectiveness of carboxylation reactions, leading to reduced glucose production
(C) Reduced effectiveness of acyl activation, leading to reduced glucose production
(D) Reduced effectiveness of protein hydroxylation, leading to reduced enzymatic activity and reduced glucose production
(E) Reduced levels of electron donors in her system, leading to reduced glucose production

5 Mr Smith recently had a bout of five days of severe nausea, vomiting, low-grade fever, and diarrhea. This condition had afflicted a number of people in Mr Smith's office. After recovering from this disorder, Mr Smith found that he could no longer drink milk before going to bed as he became flatulent, his stomach hurt, and he would develop diarrhea. If he did not drink milk, these conditions did not occur. He had never experienced these problems before the affliction. A possible explanation for Mr Smith's problem is which one of the following?
(A) Mechanical disruption of the intestinal epithelial cells, leading to reduced transcription of the galactokinase gene
(B) Mechanical disruption of the intestinal epithelial cells, leading to reduced transcription of the fructokinase gene
(C) Mechanical disruption of the intestinal epithelial cells, leading to loss of lactose transport into the cells
(D) Mechanical disruption of the intestinal epithelial cells, leading to loss of the glucoamylase complex from their surface
(E) Mechanical disruption of the intestinal epithelial cells, leading to loss of lactase from their surface

6 Paramedics bring a patient to the emergency department because he was found unconscious in an alley by passers by. The man was unshaven and dishevelled, and appeared to be about 40 years old. Blood alcohol levels were found to be 0.25% and blood glucose levels 32 mg/dL. IV glucose was initiated, and this enabled the man to regain consciousness, although he was still inebriated. While conscious, a history revealed that the man was a chronic alcoholic, and as far as he could remember, he had been only drinking for the past 2 weeks, with nothing to eat. Analysis of liver enzyme levels in his blood revealed normal readings. Assuming that his liver is still functioning normally, why is this patient hypoglycemic?
(A) Liver glycogen stores were depleted by the high $NAD^+/NADH$ ratio
(B) Liver glycogen stores were depleted by the high $NADH/NAD^+$ ratio
(C) The high $NAD^+/NADH$ ratio impaired gluconeogenesis
(D) The high $NADH/NAD^+$ ratio impaired gluconeogenesis
(E) The high $NAD^+/NADH$ ratio impaired glycolysis

7 A 3-month-old girl is brought to the pediatrician due to fussiness and lethargy. According to the parents, the baby was just fine until the mother needed to return to work, and the baby was being switched from breast milk to baby foods, formula, and fruit juices. At that time, the child cried while feeding, sometimes vomited, and had been lethargic. The baby's appetite seemed to have worsened. The parents thought that if only formula was used, the baby was better, but they really could not remember. Which possible enzyme defect might lead to this case presentation?
(A) Galactokinase
(B) Fructokinase
(C) Aldolase
(D) Hexokinase
(E) Glucokinase

8 A thin, anxious woman, who is 5′ 6″ tall, weighs 92 lb. Blood work indicates a glucose level of 70 mg/dL under fasting conditions. Her liver is using which of the following as precursors for glucose production under these conditions?
(A) Glycerol, lactate, and leucine
(B) Fatty acids, alanine, and glutamine
(C) Glycerol, lactate, and glutamine
(D) Glycerol, fatty acids, and glutamine
(E) Lactate, heme, and lysine

9 A 50-year-old man has been trying to lose weight, but he enjoyed eating so much that he found it difficult to do so. He then reads about a product in the popular press, which guarantees that he can lose weight, as caloric intake due to starch ingestion will be reduced (a starch blocker). The over-the-counter product that he buys is claimed to inhibit which of the following enzymes?
(A) Pancreatic trypsinogen
(B) Pancreatic lipase
(C) Salivary amylase
(D) Gastric amylase
(E) Intestinal enteropeptidase

10 A 28-year-old male develops diabetes, as noted by constant, mildly elevated hyperglycemia. His father had similar symptoms at the same age as did his paternal grandmother. This patient is not obese, does not have hypertension, does not have dyslipidemia, and does not have antibodies directed against islet cells. This alteration in glucose homeostasis may be due to a mutation in which of the following enzymes?
(A) Pancreatic glucokinase
(B) Pancreatic hexokinase
(C) Liver glucokinase
(D) Muscle hexokinase
(E) Intestinal glucokinase

11 A 3-month-old girl with developing cataracts is shown to contain a reducing sugar in her urine, but the glucose oxidase test was negative. She has had no problems eating, and her growth curve is at the 60th percentile. Fasting blood glucose tests show normal levels of circulating glucose. A likely enzyme deficiency is which of the following?
(A) Fructokinase
(B) Hexokinase
(C) Galactokinase
(D) Galactose-1-phosphate uridylyltransferase
(E) Aldolase

12 The synthesis of one mole of glucose from two moles of lactate requires six moles of ATP. Which one of the following steps requires ATP in the gluconeogenic pathway?
(A) Pyruvate kinase
(B) Triosephosphate isomerase
(C) Glucose-6-phosphatase
(D) Fructose-1,6-bisphosphatase
(E) Phosphoglycerate kinase

13 An important product of the oxidation of the body's major energy source to provide energy for gluconeogenesis regulates which of the following key gluconeogenic enzymes?
(A) PEPCK
(B) Fructose-1,6-bisphosphatase
(C) Glucose-6-phosphatase
(D) Pyruvate carboxylase
(E) Pyruvate kinase

14 An individual with a BMI of 34 was advised by the physician to eat less and exercise more. The patient took this advice to an extreme, and has not eaten for 48 h. Which of the following best describes the patient's activity and phosphorylation state of the following key liver enzymes?

	Phosphofructokinase-1		Glucokinase		Pyruvate Kinase	
	Activity	**Phosphorylated?**	**Activity**	**Phosphorylated?**	**Activity**	**Phosphorylated?**
(A)	Low	Yes	Low	No	Low	Yes
(B)	Low	No	Low	No	Low	No
(C)	Low	No	Low	Yes	Low	Yes
(D)	Low	Yes	Low	No	Low	No
(E)	Low	No	Low	No	Low	Yes

15 Which of the following changes in enzyme activity will occur within 1 h of a type 1 diabetic taking an injection of insulin?

	Liver PFK-2	Liver PFK-1	Muscle Glucose Uptake
(A)	Active kinase	Active kinase	Increased
(B)	Inactive kinase	Active kinase	Increased
(C)	Active phosphatase	Active kinase	Increased
(D)	Inactive phosphatase	Active kinase	Decreased
(E)	Active kinase	Inactive kinase	Decreased

16 *Streptococcus mutans*, found in dental plaque, produces acids from the metabolism of carbohydrates. Topical fluoride treatment in the dental office can slow the production of acids, resulting in the accumulation of which metabolite?

(A) Glucose-6-phosphate
(B) Fructose-1,6-bisphosphate
(C) Glyceraldehyde-3-phosphate
(D) 2-phosphoglycerate
(E) Phosphoenolpyruvate

17 After eating a meal containing carbohydrates, the monosaccharides must be absorbed from the intestinal lumen. This transport is dependent on which of the following enzymes?

(A) Na^+/H^+ antiporter
(B) Glucose-6-phosphate dehydrogenase
(C) Hexokinase
(D) Chloride transporter
(E) Na^+, K^+ ATPase

18 Skeletal muscle PFK-2 is not regulated by phosphorylation, but heart muscle PFK-2 is. In the heart, phosphorylation of PFK-2 leads to what effect?

(A) Enhanced production of fructose-2,6-bisphosphate
(B) Reduced production of fructose-2,6-bisphosphate
(C) Degradation of fructose-1,6-bisphosphate
(D) Increased turnover of PFK-2
(E) Increased transcription of PFK-2

19 Your 20-year-old male patient received a medical discharge from the US Army. He has had multiple episodes of lightheadedness, sweating, fatigue, tremor, and intense hunger. He had one seizure. During two of these episodes, his blood glucose was 40 mg/dL. Which of the following tests could help you diagnose his problem?

(A) Fasting blood glucose
(B) HbA1c
(C) Noncontrast CT scan of the abdomen
(D) Blood glucose and insulin levels measured while he was symptomatic
(E) Determining the presence of islet cell antibodies

20 Under conditions of hypoglycemia, the liver is not utilizing glucose as an energy source due to which of the following?

(A) A low K_m for glucokinase
(B) A high K_m for glucokinase
(C) An inhibited, phosphorylated PFK-1
(D) An activated, phosphorylated PFK-1
(E) A reduction of glucose transporters in the membrane

ANSWERS

1 The answer is D: Providing substrate for glyceraldehyde-3-phosphate dehydrogenase. Under anaerobic conditions, the NADH generated by the glyceraldehyde-3-phosphate dehydrogenase step accumulates. Normally, the NADH would transfer its electrons to mitochondrial NAD^+, and the electrons would be donated to the electron transfer chain. However, in the absence of oxygen

NADH is generated by the glyceraldehyde 3-phosphate dehydrogenase reaction; in the absence of oxygen, NAD^+ is regenerated by the lactate dehydrogenase reaction. In the presence of oxygen, NADH donates its electrons to the electron transfer chain (regenerating NAD^+), which eventually donates the electrons to oxygen, forming water.

the electron transfer chain is not functioning. Thus, as NADH accumulates in the cytoplasm, the levels of NAD^+ decrease to the point that there would be insufficient NAD^+ available to allow the glyceraldehyde-3-phosphate dehydrogenase reaction to proceed, thereby inhibiting glycolysis. To prevent glycolytic inhibition, lactate dehydrogenase will convert pyruvate to lactate, regenerating NAD^+ for use in glycolysis, specifically as a substrate for the glyceraldehyde-3-phosphate dehydrogenase reaction. While hexokinase is inhibited by its product glucose-6-phosphate, this allosteric effect does not explain lactate formation under anaerobic conditions. Similarly, while phosphoglyceromutase does require 2,3-bisphosphoglycerate, anaerobiosis does not increase 2,3-bisphosphoglycerate levels, nor does it alleviate the lack of NAD^+ under these conditions. Pyruvate kinase is not inhibited by pyruvate (ATP and alanine are the allosteric inhibitors of this enzyme). AMP is an activator of phosphofructokinase-1; however, this activation does not relate to lactate formation under anaerobic conditions. The figure summarizes these key points outlined above.

2 The answer is C: Three moles of ATP. When glycogen produces glucose via the action of glycogen phosphorylase, glucose-1-phosphate is produced. As this is converted to two molecules of pyruvate, four moles of ATP are generated and one is utilized at the PFK-1 step for the net production of three moles of ATP. Two moles of NADH are also produced, but those are utilized by lactate dehydrogenase to reduce pyruvate to lactate (anaerobic conditions) such that NAD^+ can be regenerated for the glyceraldehyde-3-phosphate dehydrogenase step. A small amount of free glucose will be released from glycogen by the debranching enzyme (about 5% of the total); for that glucose, the net yield is two moles of ATP (since hexokinase has to phosphorylate the free glucose to glucose-6-phosphate), but since the majority of glucose released is in the form of glucose-1-phosphate, three moles of ATP is the better answer. These reactions are outlined below.

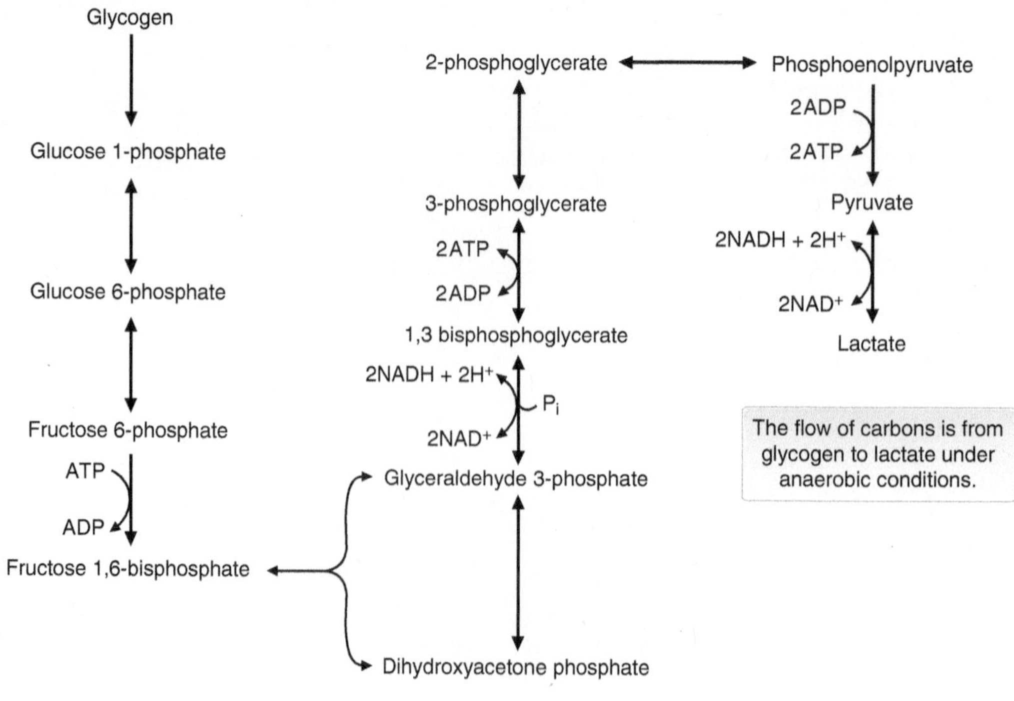

Answer 2

3 **The answer is B: Galactose-1-phosphate uridylyltransferase.** The child has classic galactosemia, a defect in galactose-1-phosphate uridylyltransferase. Due to the accumulation of galactose-1-phosphate, galactokinase is inhibited, and free galactose accumulates within the blood and tissues. The accumulation of galactose in the lens of the eye provides substrate for aldose reductase, converting galactose to its alcohol form (galactitol). The accumulation of galactitol leads to an osmotic imbalance across the lens, leading to cataract formation. Additionally, the increased galactose-1-phosphate, at very high levels in the liver, blocks phosphoglucomutase activity, resulting in ineffective glucose production from glycogen (phosphorylase degradation of glycogen will produce glucose-1-phosphate, but this cannot be converted to glucose-6-phosphate if phosphoglucomutase activity is inhibited). A defect in galactokinase will lead to nonclassical galactosemia, with cataract formation, but none of the feeding problems associated with classical galactosemia (associated with the accumulation of galactose-1-phosphate) are observed in nonclassical galactosemia. None of the other enzymes listed, if deficient, will give rise to the symptoms produced, particularly cataract formation. A defect in glycogen synthase would lead to reduced glycogen levels and fasting hypoglycemia. A defect in fructokinase leads to fructosuria (fructose in the urine), but no overt symptoms of disease. The figure below indicates the pathway for galactose metabolism and the defects in classical and nonclassical galactosemia.

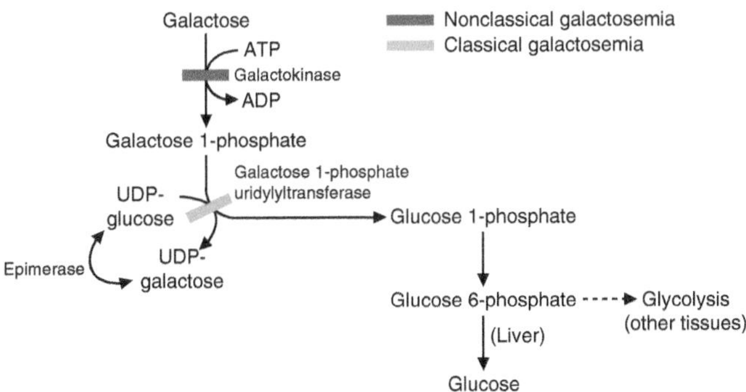

4 **The answer is B: Reduced effectiveness of carboxylation reactions, leading to reduced glucose production.** Raw eggs contain a potent binding partner to biotin, avidin, which, while bound to biotin, blocks biotin's participation in carboxylation reactions. This leads to reduced activity of pyruvate carboxylase, a necessary step in many gluconeogenic pathways, thereby leading to a reduced ability of the liver to properly maintain blood glucose levels. As oxaloacetate levels drop due to the need of oxaloacetate for gluconeogenesis, acetyl-CoA derived from fatty acid oxidation increases, leading to ketone body formation. Avidin does not affect NAD^+ or FAD levels, nor does it interfere with coenzyme A or vitamin C.

5 **The answer is E: Mechanical disruption of the intestinal epithelial cells, leading to loss of lactase from their surface.** Mechanical disruption of the intestinal epithelial cells (as brought about by acute viral gastroenteritis) leads to a loss of cell surface enzymes, but lactase is the most severely affected, as it is present at the lowest levels on these cells. While glucoamylase is also lost, its activity is in vast excess of what is required and its partial loss does not affect its ability to hydrolyze glucose–glucose linkages (it does not hydrolyze lactose). A lack of lactase means that the lactose in the diet passes undigested through the small intestine to the large intestine where the bacterial flora metabolize the lactose, producing gases and acids that disrupt the osmotic balance between the lumen of the bowel and the cells lining it. This leads to water secretion by the cells into the lumen of the bowel, resulting in diarrhea. Lactose is not directly transported by intestinal epithelial cells (its components, glucose and galactose, are, after hydrolysis of β-1,4 linkage between the two sugars), and a mechanical disruption of intestinal cells does not alter transcription of galactokinase and fructokinase.

6 **The answer is D: The high $NADH/NAD^+$ ratio impaired gluconeogenesis.** Ethanol oxidation to acetic acid (via acetaldehyde) generates large amounts of NADH. As liver glycogen stores have been depleted within 36 h of the fast, gluconeogenesis is required to maintain blood glucose levels. The major precursors for gluconeogenesis are glycerol, lactate, and amino acids (which give rise to pyruvate or TCA cycle precursors, which generate oxaloacetate). Because of the high $NADH/NAD^+$ ratio (due to the ethanol metabolism), pyruvate destined for gluconeogenesis is shunted to lactate in order to regenerate NAD^+ to allow alcohol metabolism to continue. Similarly, oxaloacetate is shunted to malate, also to regenerate NAD^+ for ethanol metabolism. Glycerol, which is converted to glycerol-3-phosphate, cannot go to dihydroxyacetone phosphate due to the high NADH levels in the liver. Thus, the high $NADH/NAD^+$ ratio diverts gluconeogenic precursors from entering gluconeogenesis, and the liver has trouble maintaining adequate blood glucose levels. Liver glycogen stores have been depleted within the first 36 h of the fast, but glycogen regulation is not affected by the $NADH/NAD^+$ ratio. Under conditions in which the liver is exporting glucose (glucagon administration, for example), liver glycolysis

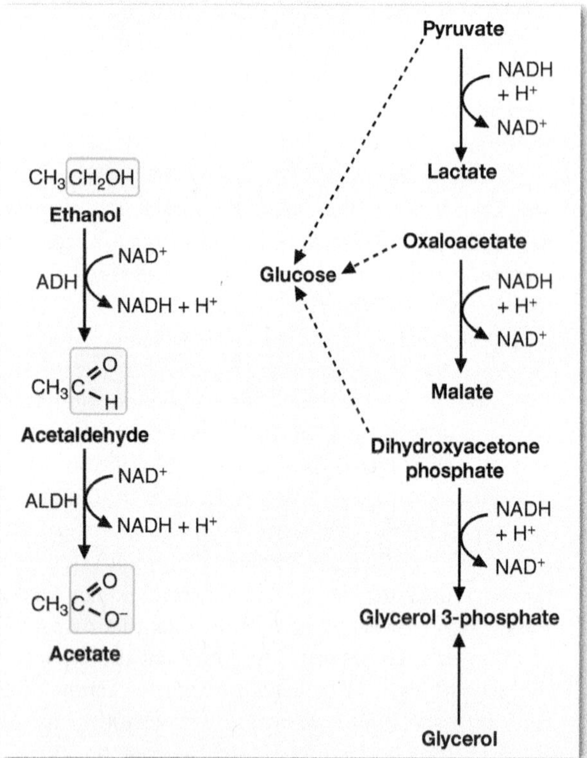

is inhibited by covalent modification of key regulatory enzymes, not the NADH/NAD^+ ratio. These pathways are indicated in the figure above.

7 **The answer is C: Aldolase.** The disorder is hereditary fructose intolerance, with a reduced ability to convert fructose-1-phosphate to dihydroxyacetone phosphate and glyceraldehyde. The specific defect is in aldolase B, with its activity reduced by as much as 85%. This problem is only evident when sucrose is introduced into the diet, and fructose enters the liver. The accumulation of fructose-1-phosphate, due to the reduced aldolase activity, leads to a constellation of physiological problems resulting in nausea, vomiting, and hypoglycemia. Elimination of fructose from the diet will reverse the symptoms. Galactokinase is needed for galactose metabolism; since the patient digests milk normally galactokinase activity is not altered. Similarly, glucose metabolism is not adversely affected (milk contains lactose, which is split into glucose and galactose), indicating that hexokinase and glucokinase activities are normal. The defect in aldolase B will hinder glycolysis, but the liver also contains aldolase C activity (this isozyme will not split fructose-1-phosphate), which enables glucose metabolism to be very close to normal. A deficiency in fructokinase will lead to an accumulation of fructose (not fructose-1-phosphate), which is released into the urine (fructosuria), but does not lead to the physiological symptoms exhibited by the patient. The fructose pathway (indicating the reaction catalyzed by aldolase B), and its relationship to glycolysis, is shown below.

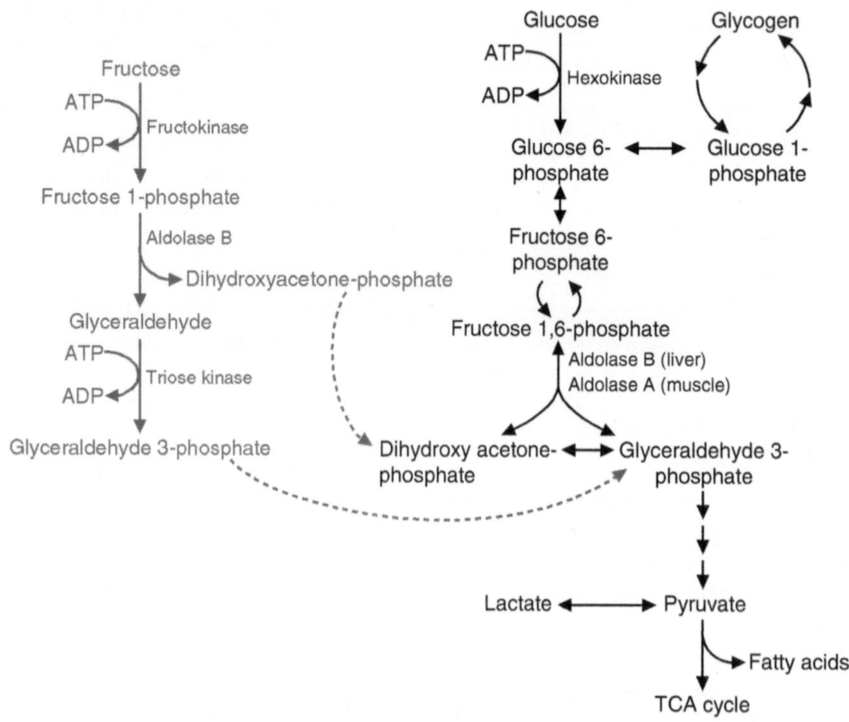

Answer 7

8 **The answer is C: Glycerol, lactate, and glutamine.** The woman has a BMI in the unhealthy range (15.7), indicating inadequate nutrient uptake. Since her nutrient uptake is poor, most of the glucose present in her blood is derived from gluconeogenesis, as her glycogen stores are most likely depleted. The substrates for gluconeogenesis are lactate (derived from red blood cell metabolism), glycerol (from triglyceride degradation), and amino acids derived from protein muscle degradation. Glutamine is a glucogenic amino acid, and is also used to transport nitrogen groups from the muscle to the liver for safe excretion via the urea cycle. Leucine is a strictly ketogenic amino acid (giving rise only to acetyl-CoA), and leucine carbons cannot be used to make glucose via gluconeogenesis. Fatty acids are also strictly ketogenic, and cannot be used for glucose production (fatty acids give rise to acetyl-CoA, which cannot be used to produce net glucose). Lysine is also a strictly ketogenic amino acid, and cannot be used for glucose production. Heme degradation gives rise to bilirubin, which cannot be further degraded, and none of the carbons of heme can be used for glucose production.

9 **The answer is C: Salivary amylase.** Starch blockers contain a natural inhibitor of salivary amylase, which will block starch digestion in the mouth. The other amylase that digests starch, pancreatic amylase, would only be inhibited by the starch blocker if the inhibitor would survive the conditions of the acidic stomach without becoming denatured. There is no gastric amylase. Intestinal enteropeptidase activates trypsinogen, which is required for protein digestion, not starch digestion. Pancreatic lipase is required for dietary triglyceride digestion, and is not active toward starch.

10 **The answer is A: Pancreatic glucokinase.** The boy has developed MODY (maturity onset diabetes of the young), and one variant of MODY is a mutated glucokinase (an inheritable disorder) such that the K_m for glucose has increased, and insulin release only occurs when hyperglycemia is present. Both an increase in ATP and NADPH are required for the pancreatic β-cell to release insulin. When pancreatic glucokinase has an increased K_m for glucose, ATP levels can only increase at greater than normal levels of glucose. Thus, moderate hyperglycemia is not sufficient to induce insulin release. As insulin release occurs from the pancreas, liver, muscle, or intestinal hexokinase will not affect the process. The pancreas does not express hexokinase, only glucokinase. MODY is a monogenetic autosomal dominant disease of insulin secretion. There are at least six amino acid substitutions known in a number of different proteins. MODY1 is a mutation in the transcription factor HNF4-α. MODY2 is a mutation in pancreatic glucokinase. MODY3 is a mutation in the transcription factor HNF1-α while MODY4 contains a mutation in insulin promoter factor 1. MODY5 is a mutation in another transcription factor, HNF1-β. MODY6 is a mutation in neurogenic differentiation factor 1. MODY is not insulin resistance. Therefore, all the other aspects of insulin resistance syndrome are not present (obesity, hypertension, and hypertriglyceridemia). Since MODY is autosomal dominant, it can be traced through the family tree. It was thought at one time that the patient had to be young to present with this disorder, but patients up to age 50 have been reported. It is not type 1 diabetes mellitus as no islet cell antibodies are present. Glucokinase is acting as a glucose sensor for the β-cell. A mutated, less sensitive sensor leads to mildly elevated blood glucose levels.

11 **The answer is C: Galactokinase.** The child has nonclassical galactosemia, a defect in galactokinase. With this disorder, galactose cannot be accumulated within cells, and so it accumulates in the blood, spilling over to the urine. Because of its high level, the galactose can enter the eye and be reduced to galactitol by aldose reductase, trapping the galactitol within the eye. As galactitol accumulates, an osmotic imbalance is created, leading to cataract formation. However, since galactose-1-phosphate is not accumulating (as occurs in classical galactosemia, a defect in galactose-1-phosphate uridylyl transferase), the other effects seen with classical galactosemia (hypoglycemia and neurological deficit) do not occur. The sugar that is accumulating in the urine is galactose, which contains an aldehyde, which generates a positive response in a reducing test. A defect in fructokinase leads to fructosuria, a benign condition (fructose is not a substrate for aldose reductase, as it is a ketose and not an aldose). A defect in hexokinase would lead to elevated glucose levels, and can lead to sorbitol production in the lens of the eye, but the urine reducing sugar test was negative for glucose. A defect in aldolase would lead to the intracellular accumulation of metabolites, but not a great increase in circulating galactose. Refer to the figure in the answer to question 3 of this chapter for the pathway of galactose metabolism and the enzyme defects in both classical and nonclassical galactosemia.

12 **The answer is E: Phosphoglycerate kinase.** In gluconeogenesis, phosphoglycerate kinase catalyzes the phosphorylation of 3-phosphoglycerate to 1,3-bisphosphoglycerate, a step which requires ATP. The other two steps requiring a high-energy phosphate bond in the conversion of pyruvate to glucose are pyruvate carboxylase and phosphoenolpyruvate carboxykinase. Fructose-1,6-bisphosphatase and glucose-6-phosphatase are

enzymes that remove phosphates from substrates, releasing the phosphates as inorganic phosphate. They do not require, nor generate, ATP. Pyruvate kinase is not utilized for gluconeogenesis, and triose phosphate isomerase catalyzes the conversion of dihydroxyacetone phosphate and glyceraldehyde-3-phosphate, without the involvement of a high-energy phosphate bond. These are shown in the pathway below.

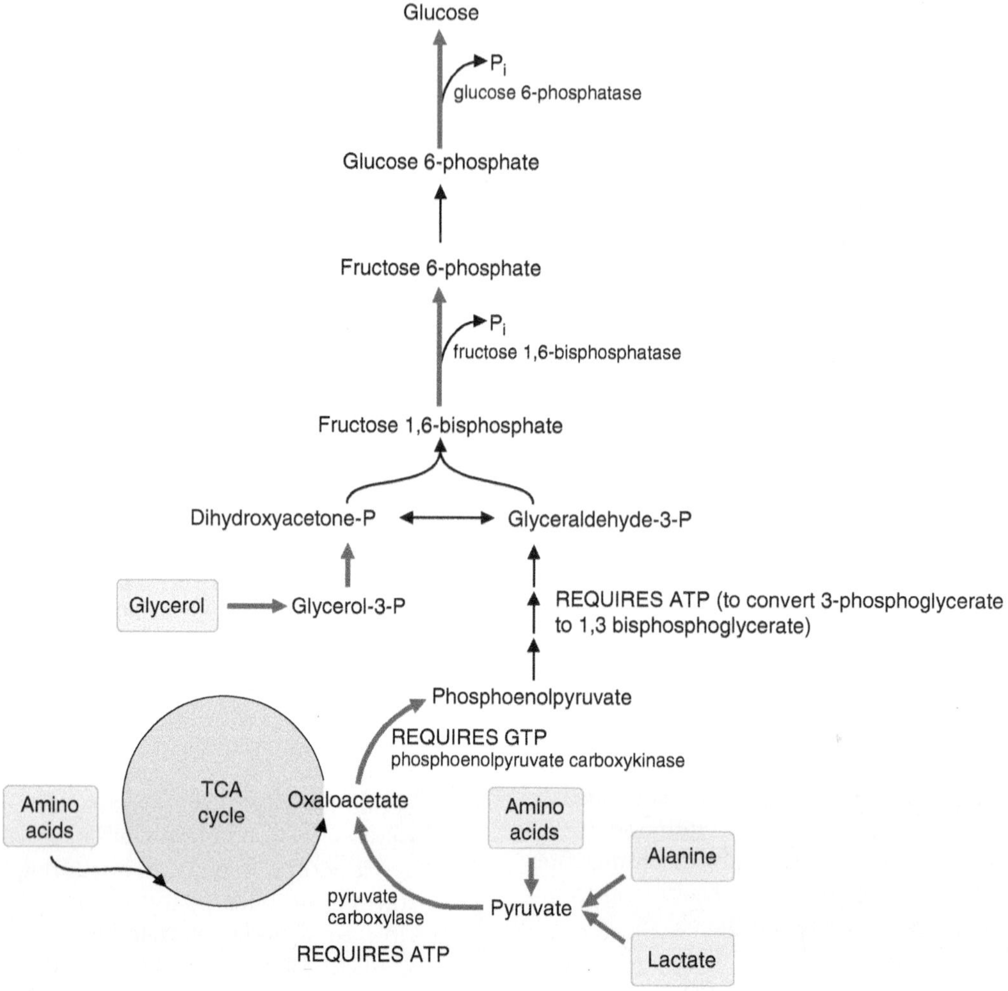

13 **The answer is D: Pyruvate carboxylase.** The body's major energy source for gluconeogenesis is fatty acids, which are oxidized to acetyl-CoA, at which point acetyl-CoA enters the TCA cycle to produce ATP. Acetyl-CoA activates pyruvate carboxylase (and inhibits pyruvate dehydrogenase), a key gluconeogenic enzyme. Acetyl-CoA does not regulate any of the other enzymes listed as potential answers (PEPCK is transcriptionally regulated by CREB; Fructose-1,6-bisphosphatase is inhibited by fructose-2,6-bisphosphate; glucose-6-phosphatase is regulated by a regulatory protein; and pyruvate kinase has both allosteric and covalent controls in the liver, but none involve acetyl-CoA).

14 **The answer is E.** Under the conditions of a 48-h fast, the liver is exporting glucose, and glycolysis will be inhibited. PFK-1 activity is reduced due to a reduction of fructose-2,6-bisphosphate levels, brought about by glucagon-induced phosphorylation of PFK-2, which activates PFK-2 phosphatase activity, which converts fructose-2,6-bisphosphate to fructose-6-phosphate. Pyruvate kinase activity, in the liver, is also reduced by phosphorylation by protein kinase A (which is activated by glucagon). As blood glucose levels have dropped during the fast, and the liver is exporting glucose, the concentration of glucose in the hepatocyte is not sufficient for glucokinase (which has a high K_m) to phosphorylate glucose. Glucokinase is not regulated by phosphorylation.

15 **The answer is A.** Upon insulin release, the cAMP phosphodiesterase is activated, reducing cAMP levels in the liver, thereby leading to inactivation of protein kinase A. In addition, protein phosphatase 1 has become active and dephosphorylates the enzymes that were phosphorylated by protein kinase A. Therefore, PFK-2 is not phosphorylated, which leads to an active kinase activity and an

inactive phosphatase activity (choices A, D, or E). The active kinase of PFK-2 produces more fructose-2,6-bisphosphate, leading to the activation of PFK-1 (answers A through D; combined with PFK-2 activity, now only choice A or D can be correct). Insulin stimulates preformed GLUT4 transporters in the muscle to fuse with the plasma membrane, thereby enhancing glucose transport into the muscle (choices A through C; combined with the other two columns, only choice A can be correct).

16 **The answer is D: 2-phosphoglycerate.** Fluoride inhibits the glycolytic enzyme enolase, which catalyzes the dehydration of 2-phosphoglycerate to phosphoenolpyruvate. Thus, 2-phosphoglycerate accumulates under these conditions.

17 **The answer is E: Na^+, K^+ ATPase.** Most monosaccharides are transported with sodium from the intestinal lumen into the enterocyte. The energy for active transport of the carbohydrate is derived from the sodium gradient that is established by the Na^+, K^+ ATPase, which pumps sodium out of the cell (three atoms of sodium) in exchange for potassium (two atoms of potassium). This creates both a sodium gradient (outside concentration higher) and a charge gradient (outside positive as compared to inside the cell) across the plasma membrane. Due to these gradients, the entry of sodium into the cell is energetically favorable, and the monosaccharide piggybacks with the sodium for transport into the cell. The Na /H^+ exchanger is not operative in intestinal epithelial cells, and none of the other enzymes (glucose-6-phosphate dehydrogenase, hexokinase, and chloride transporter) will create the necessary sodium gradient for monosaccharide transport. Carbohydrate transport into the enterocytes is outlined in the figure below.

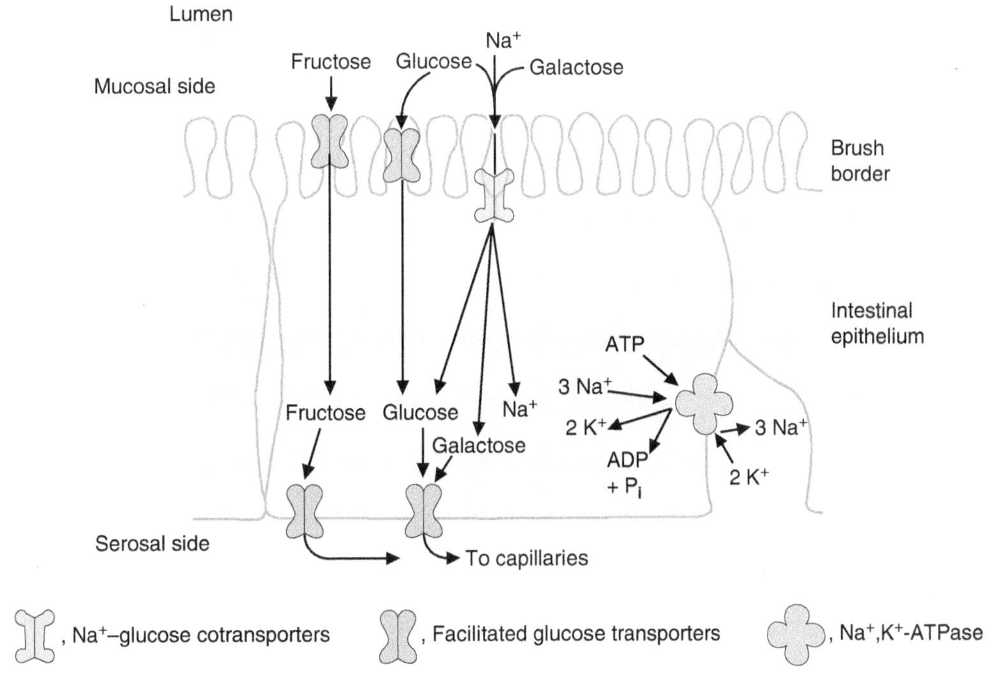

18 **The answer is A: Enhanced production of fructose-2, 6-bisphosphate.** When phosphorylated, heart PFK-2 is activated to produce more fructose-2,6-bisphosphate to stimulate heart PFK-1 and to increase the glycolytic rate of the heart. Phosphorylation of heart PFK-2 can be accomplished through the AMP-activated protein kinase (when the heart is having trouble generating energy) or in response to insulin (indicating that high levels of glucose are available for use). Phosphorylation of heart PFK-2 does not affect its transcription or turnover rate, and also does not affect the degradation of fructose-1, 6-bisphosphate.

19 **The answer is D: Blood glucose and insulin levels measured while he was symptomatic.** This patient probably has an insulinoma that releases insulin inappropriately at any blood glucose level, which would lead to hypoglycemia. The released insulin would stimulate glucose uptake into the peripheral tissues (muscle and fat), and if the patient had not eaten, blood glucose levels would rapidly fall. The insulin is also inhibiting the liver from producing glucose, either from glycogen degradation or gluconeogenesis, which only compounds the problem. The hypoglycemia and resultant epinephrine release account for all of his symptoms.

To diagnose an insulinoma, a low blood glucose level and an inappropriately high insulin level during symptoms must be documented. A fasting blood glucose and HbA1c could be perfectly normal and do not help in making the diagnosis, as insulinomas do not necessarily constantly secrete insulin; they do so episodically. The presence of islet cell antibodies helps diagnose type 1 diabetes mellitus, but not an insulinoma. A noncontrast CT scan might be used to locate the position of the insulinoma, but it is a very poor test even for location and would only be attempted once the diagnosis was confirmed.

20 **The answer is B: A high K_m for glucokinase.** The liver expresses glucokinase, which has a high K_m for glucose, particularly as compared to the K_m for hexokinase. This means that glucokinase will only phosphorylate glucose when the intrahepatic glucose concentrations are high, and the intrahepatic levels of glucose only reach these levels after a meal. Under normal, fasting conditions, the concentration of blood glucose is lower than the K_m for glucokinase, and very little phosphorylation of glucose will occur. PFK-1 is not a phosphorylated enzyme, and glucagon does not stimulate an increase in glucose transporters in the liver.

Chapter 11

TCA Cycle and Oxidative Phosphorylation

This chapter contains questions on the TCA cycle and oxidative phosphorylation, including questions integrated with other aspects of metabolism. Metabolic diseases affecting aspects of the TCA cycle and oxidative phosphorylation are also covered in this chapter.

QUESTIONS

Select the single best answer.

1 A chronic alcoholic, while out on a binge, became very confused and forgetful. The police found the man and brought him to the emergency department. Upon examination, he displayed nystagmus and ataxia. Which enzyme is displaying reduced activity in his brain under these conditions?

(A) Glyceraldehyde-3-phosphate dehydrogenase
(B) Isocitrate dehydrogenase
(C) α-ketoglutarate dehydrogenase
(D) Succinate dehydrogenase
(E) Malate dehydrogenase

2 The energy yield from the complete oxidation of acetyl-CoA to carbon dioxide is which of the following in terms of high-energy bonds formed?

(A) 6
(B) 8
(C) 10
(D) 12
(E) 14

3 Ethanol ingestion is incapable of supplying carbons for gluconeogenesis. This is due to which of the following?

(A) Ethanol is converted to acetone, and the carbons are lost during exhalation
(B) Ethanol is lost directly in the urine
(C) Ethanol cannot enter the liver, where gluconeogenesis predominantly occurs
(D) Ethanol's carbons are lost as carbon dioxide before a gluconeogenic precursor can be generated
(E) Ethanol is converted to lysine, which is strictly a ketogenic amino acid

4 A family that had previously had a newborn boy die of a metabolic disease has just given birth to another boy, small for gestational age, and with low Apgar scores. The child displayed spasms a few hours after birth. Blood analysis indicated extremely high levels of lactic acid. Analysis of cerebrospinal fluid showed elevated lactate and pyruvate. Hyperalaninemia was also observed. The child died within 5 days of birth. The biochemical defect in this child is most likely which of the following?

(A) The E1 subunit of pyruvate dehydrogenase
(B) The E2 subunit of pyruvate dehydrogenase
(C) The E3 subunit of pyruvate dehydrogenase
(D) Citrate synthase
(E) Malate dehydrogenase

5 A 3-month-old girl developed lactic acidemia. Blood analysis also indicated elevated levels of pyruvate, α-ketoglutarate, and branched-chain amino acids. A urinalysis showed elevated levels of lactate, pyruvate, α-hydroxyisovalerate, α-ketoglutarate, and α-hydroxybutyrate. A likely mutation in which of the following proteins would lead to this clinical finding?

(A) The E1 subunit of pyruvate dehydrogenase
(B) The E2 subunit of pyruvate dehydrogenase
(C) The E3 subunit of pyruvate dehydrogenase
(D) Citrate synthase
(E) Malate dehydrogenase

6 A human geneticist is studying two different families. In one family, all of the children of a mildly affected mother display myoclonic epilepsy, developmental display, and abnormal muscle biopsy (ragged red fibers). In the other family, the three children of an affected woman endure strokelike episodes and a mitochondrial myopathy. The common link between these two diseases is which of the following?

(A) Mutations in pyruvate dehydrogenase complex
(B) Mutations in cytoplasmic tRNA
(C) Mutations in mitochondrial tRNA
(D) Mutations in malate dehydrogenase
(E) Mutations in pyruvate carboxylase

7 A toddler has been diagnosed with a mild case of Leigh syndrome. One possible treatment is which of the following?

(A) Increased carbohydrate diet
(B) Additional B_6 in the diet
(C) Decreased lipoamide in the diet
(D) Additional thiamine in the diet
(E) Decreased fat diet

8 A patient was diagnosed with a mitochondrial DNA mutation that led to reduced complex I activity. This patient would have difficulties in which of the following electron transfers?

(A) Succinate to complex III
(B) Cytochrome c to complex IV
(C) Coenzyme Q to complex III
(D) Malate to coenzyme Q
(E) Coenzyme Q to oxygen

9 A pair of farm workers in Mexico was spraying pesticide on crops when they both developed the following severe symptoms: heavy, labored breathing, significantly elevated temperature, and loss of consciousness. The pesticide contained an agent that interfered with oxidative phosphorylation, which most closely resembled which of the following known inhibitors?

(A) Oligomycin
(B) Atractyloside
(C) Cyanide
(D) Rotenone
(E) Dinitrophenol

10 A crazed friend of yours has gone on an orange juice, fish, and vitamin pill diet. He tells you that the citric acid, since it is a component of the TCA cycle, is always recycled and does not count toward his caloric total each day. You disagree, and inform him that citrate can, in addition to having its carbons stored as glycogen or fat for later use, produce energy for his daily metabolic needs. The energy yield for the complete oxidation of citrate to six carbon dioxides and water is which of the following?

(A) 15.0 moles of ATP per mole of citrate
(B) 17.5 moles of ATP per mole of citrate
(C) 20.0 moles of ATP per mole of citrate
(D) 22.5 moles of ATP per mole of citrate
(E) 25.0 moles of ATP per mole of citrate

11 You have been following a patient for several years, who has recently become clinically depressed, and is eating very little and drinking alcohol very heavily. He presents to you one day with noticeable swelling of the lower legs, increased heart rate, lung congestion, and complaints of shortness of breath with virtually any activity. These symptoms have come about due to which of the following?

(A) Lack of energy to the nervous system due to niacin deficiency
(B) Heart has trouble generating energy due to niacin deficiency
(C) Lack of energy to the nervous system due to B_1 deficiency
(D) Lack of energy to the heart due to B_1 deficiency
(E) Lack of TCA cycle activity in the kidneys, leading to excessive water retention

12 An 8-month-old girl was taken to the emergency department due to the onset of sudden seizures. The child had brittle hair, with some bald spots, and skin rashes. An ophthalmologist noted optic atrophy. Urinalysis showed slightly elevated ketones and the presence of other organic acids (such as propionate and lactate). Treatment of this child with which of the following can successfully alleviate the problems?

(A) Thiamine
(B) Niacin
(C) Riboflavin
(D) Carnitine
(E) Biotin

13 The refilling of TCA cycle intermediates is frequently dependant upon which of the following cofactors?

(A) Niacin
(B) Riboflavin
(C) Carnitine
(D) Pyridoxal phosphate
(E) Lipoate

14 The concentration of TCA cycle intermediates can be reduced under certain conditions. Consider a patient who initiates taking barbiturates. During the initial phase of his taking this drug, which TCA cycle intermediate is reduced in concentration?

(A) Citrate
(B) α-ketoglutarate
(C) Succinyl-CoA
(D) Fumarate
(E) Oxaloacetate

Questions 15 and 16 are based on the following graph of oxygen consumption by carefully washed mitochondria as a function of time. ATP, ADP, inorganic phosphate, and oxygen are present, but no oxidizable substrates. Once a compound is added to the mixture, it is not removed, nor is the length of the experiment sufficient to use up all of the compounds added to the mitochondrion.

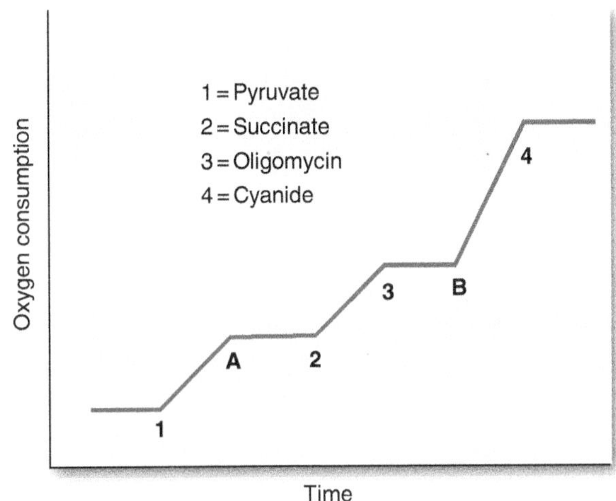

15 What compound was added at the point indicated as A?
(A) Antimycin A
(B) Atractyloside
(C) Rotenone
(D) Dinitrophenol
(E) Lactate

16 What compound was added at the point indicated as B?
(A) Antimycin A
(B) Atractyloside
(C) Rotenone
(D) Dinitrophenol
(E) Lactate

17 An inactivating mutation in which of the following enzymes would lead to lactic acid accumulation in the liver?
(A) Glucokinase
(B) Phosphofructokinase-1
(C) Cytoplasmic malate dehydrogenase
(D) Pyruvate kinase
(E) Glycerol-3-phosphate dehydrogenase

18 A researcher was studying oxidative phosphorylation in a suspension of carefully washed and isolated mitochondria. ATP, ADP, inorganic phosphate, lactate, lactate dehydrogenase, and oxygen were introduced to the suspension, and he was able to demonstrate ATP production within the mitochondria. The researcher then added oligomycin to the mixture, which stopped oxygen uptake. This occurred due to which of the following?
(A) Inhibition of complex I
(B) Inhibition of complex II
(C) Inhibition of complex III
(D) Inhibition of complex IV
(E) Inhibition of the proton translocating ATPase

19 A newborn displays lethargy and crying episodes. Blood analysis indicates lactic acidosis and hyperalaninemia. In order to distinguish between a pyruvate dehydrogenase complex deficiency and a pyruvate carboxylase deficiency, one can measure which of the following in the blood?
(A) Fasting blood glucose
(B) Alanine aminotransferase activity
(C) Free fatty acids levels when fasting
(D) Insulin levels when fasting
(E) Glucagon levels when fasting

20 Your obese patient has type 2 diabetes mellitus and you have started him on metformin. One of the possible complications of metformin therapy is lactic acidosis. Why is this a concern with metformin therapy?
(A) Metformin reduces insulin resistance
(B) Metformin blocks hepatic gluconeogenesis
(C) Metformin blocks the TCA cycle
(D) Metformin inhibits glycolysis
(E) Metformin inhibits dietary protein absorption

ANSWERS

1 **The answer is C: α-ketoglutarate dehydrogenase.** The alcoholic has become deficient in vitamin B_1, thiamine, which is converted to thiamine pyrophosphate for use as a coenzyme. One of the symptoms of B_1 deficiency is neurological, due to insufficient energy generation within the nervous system. B_1 is required for a small number of enzymes, including transketolase, pyruvate dehydrogenase, and α-ketoglutarate dehydrogenase. By reducing the activity of the latter two enzymes, glucose oxidation to generate energy is impaired, and the nervous system suffers because of it.

2 **The answer is C: 10.** When acetyl-CoA enters the TCA cycle, and is converted to two molecules of carbon dioxide, and oxaloacetate is regenerated, three molecules of NADH are produced, along with one molecule of $FADH_2$ and one substrate-level phosphorylation resulting in the generation of GTP. As each NADH can give rise to 2.5 ATP, and each $FADH_2$ to 1.5 ATP via oxidative phosphorylation, the net yield of high-energy bonds from one acetyl-CoA being oxidized by the cycle is 10 (7.5 from NADH, 1.5 from $FADH_2$, and 1 from GTP). This is shown in the figure below.

3 **The answer is D: Ethanol's carbons are lost as carbon dioxide before a gluconeogenic precursor can be generated.** Ethanol is converted to acetaldehyde, which is further oxidized to acetic acid and is then activated to acetyl-CoA. The acetyl-CoA enters the TCA cycle to generate energy, and two carbons are lost for each turn of the cycle as CO_2. Thus, ethanol cannot provide carbons for the net synthesis of glucose. Ethanol is not converted

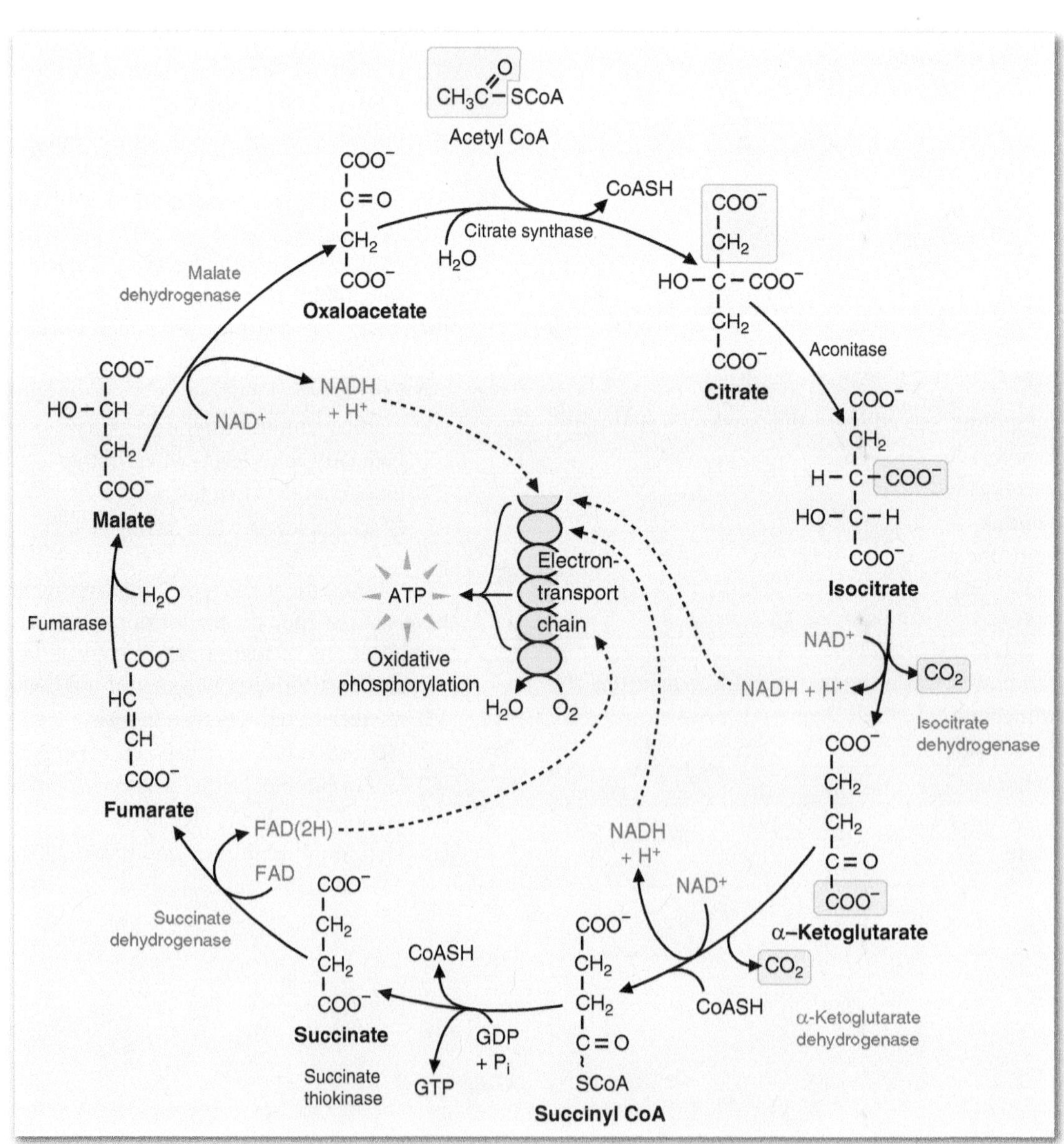

Answer 2: The Krebs tricarboxylic acid cycle.

to acetone, nor is it directly lost in the urine. Ethanol is primarily oxidized in the liver, and its carbons cannot be used for the biosynthesis of lysine, which is an essential amino acid for humans. Ethanol oxidation is outlined in the figure below.

CH_3CH_2OH
Ethanol
ADH (NAD^+ → $NADH + H^+$)
CH_3CHO
Acetaldehyde
ALDH (NAD^+ → $NADH + H^+$)
CH_3COO^-
Acetate

Ethanol metabolism.

4 **The answer is A: The E1 subunit of pyruvate dehydrogenase.** Lactic acidosis can result from a defect in an enzyme that metabolizes pyruvate (primarily pyruvate dehydrogenase and pyruvate carboxylase). The pyruvate dehydrogenase complex consists of three major catalytic subunits, designated E1, E2, and E3. The E1 subunit is the one that binds thiamine pyrophosphate and catalyzes the decarboxylation of pyruvate. The gene for the E1 subunit is on the X chromosome, so defects in this subunit are inherited as X-linked diseases, which primarily affects males. Since this is the second male child to have these symptoms, it is likely that the mother is a carrier for this disease. The pattern of inheritance distinguishes this diagnosis from that of an E2 or E3 deficiency. In addition, an E3 deficiency would affect more than pyruvate metabolism, as this subunit is shared with other enzymes that catalyze oxidative decarboxylation reactions, and other metabolites would also be accumulating. Defects in citrate synthase and malate dehydrogenase would not lead to severe lactic acidosis and would not be male-specific disorders. As an example, the three subunits of α-ketoglutarate dehydrogenase are shown below.

5 **The answer is C: The E3 subunit of pyruvate dehydrogenase.** The child is defective in a variety of oxidative decarboxylation reactions (pyruvate dehydrogenase, leading to a buildup of lactate and pyruvate; α-ketoglutarate dehydrogenase, leading to the buildup of α-ketoglutarate; and branched-chain α-ketoacid dehydrogenase, leading to a buildup of many of the other metabolites). Enzymes, which catalyze oxidative decarboxylation reactions, contain three catalytic subunits, E1, E2, and E3 (see the figure in the answer to the previous question). E3 subunit, which contains the dihydrolipoyl dehydrogenase activity, is common among these enzymes. Thus, a mutation in E3 would render all of these enzymes inoperable, leading to a buildup of the α-ketoacid precursors. Defects in citrate synthase or malate dehydrogenase would not lead to the buildup of these α-ketoacids.

6 **The answer is C: Mutations in mitochondrial tRNA.** Both families are suffering from mitochondrial diseases. Family 1 has MERRF (myoclonic epilepsy with ragged red fibers) while family 2 has MELAS (mitochondrial myopathy, encephalopathy, lactic acidosis, and stroke). Both disorders are due to mutations in a mitochondrially encoded tRNA. MERRF is a mutation in $tRNA^{lys}$, whereas MELAS has a mutation in a $tRNA^{leu}$ gene. In both cases, the tRNA mutations interfere with protein synthesis within the mitochondria, leading to a reduction of functional proteins necessary

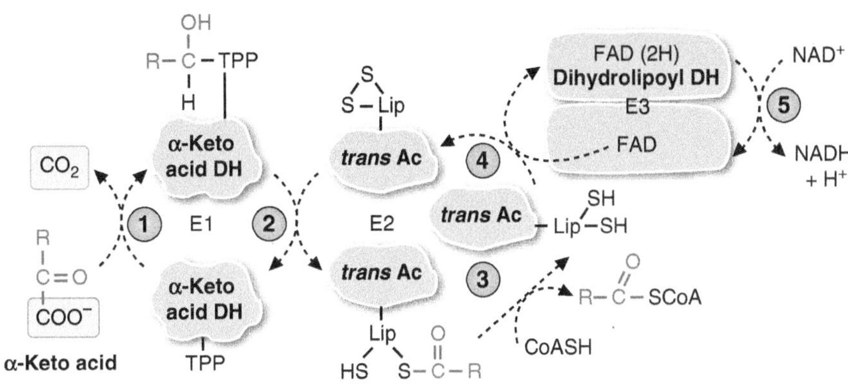

Answer 4: Mechanism of α-keto acid dehydrogenase complexes. R represents the portion of the α-keto acid that begins with the β carbon. Three different subunits are required for the reaction, E1 (α-keto acid decarboxylase), E2 (transacylase), and E3 (dihydrolipoyl dehydrogenase). TPP refers to the cofactor thiamine pyrophosphate. Lip refers to the cofactor lipoic acid.

for various aspects of oxidative phosphorylation. These disorders are not due to mutations in nuclear encoded genes (which eliminates all of the other answers).

7 The answer is D: Additional thiamine in the diet. Leigh syndrome can result from a deficiency of pyruvate dehydrogenase (PDH) activity, leading to lactic acidosis. In some cases, the enzyme has a reduced affinity for thiamine pyrophosphate, a required cofactor for the enzyme. Adding thiamine to the diet may overcome this deficiency by raising the concentration of thiamine pyrophosphate such that it will bind to the altered enzyme. Increasing the carbohydrate in the diet will make the disease worse, as more pyruvate would be generated due to the increase in the glycolytic rate. Vitamin B_6 does not play a role in glycolysis or the PDH reaction. Lipoamide is a required cofactor for the PDH reaction, so reducing lipoamide would have an adverse effect on the activity of PDH. Decreasing the fat content of the diet may be harmful, particularly if the calories are replaced as carbohydrate.

8 The answer is D: Malate to coenzyme Q. Complex I accepts electrons from NADH, and will transfer them to coenzyme Q. Malate dehydrogenase will convert malate to oxaloacetate, generating NADH in the process. The NADH will then donate electrons to complex I to initiate electron transfer. Succinate donates electrons at complex II (via succinate dehydrogenase, a component of complex II), which donates to coenzyme Q, thereby bypassing complex I. Cytochrome c transfers electrons from complex III to complex IV. Once electrons are carried by coenzyme Q, complex I is no longer required for electron transfer to oxygen. These transfers are outlined in the figure below.

9 The answer is E: Dinitrophenol. The key is the elevation in temperature. Dinitrophenol is an uncoupler of oxidation and phosphorylation in that uncouplers destroy the proton gradient across the membrane (thereby inhibiting the synthesis of ATP) without blocking the transfer of electrons through the electron transfer chain to oxygen. The energy that should have been generated in the form of a proton gradient is lost as heat, which elevates the body temperature of the affected workers. Electron flow is also enhanced in the presence of an uncoupler, so additional oxygen is required to allow the chain to continue (hence the heavy breathing). The other agents added would have stopped electron transfer totally, which would not allow for an increase in temperature, and would actually decrease the rate of breathing (since oxygen is no longer required for the nonfunctioning electron transfer chain). Atractyloside inhibits the ATP/ADP exchanger, and once there is no ADP in the mitochondrial matrix, electron flow will stop due to the inability to synthesize ATP (normal coupling). Oligomycin works in a similar mechanism in that it blocks the ATP synthase, preventing ATP synthesis, and, due to coupling, electron transfer through the chain. Rotenone blocks complex I transfer to coenzyme Q, which significantly reduces electron flow, and will not lead to an increase in temperature.

10 The answer is D: 22.5 moles of ATP per mole of citrate. The following steps (see the figure on page 95) are required for the complete oxidation of citrate to carbon dioxide and water. First, citrate goes to isocitrate, which goes to α-ketoglutarate (this last step generates carbon dioxide and NADH, which can give rise to 2.5 ATP). The α-ketoglutarate is further oxidized to succinyl-CoA, plus carbon dioxide and NADH (this is the second carbon released as CO_2, and another 2.5 ATP). Succinyl-CoA is converted to succinate, generating a GTP (at this point, five high-energy bonds have been created, plus two carbons lost as carbon dioxide).

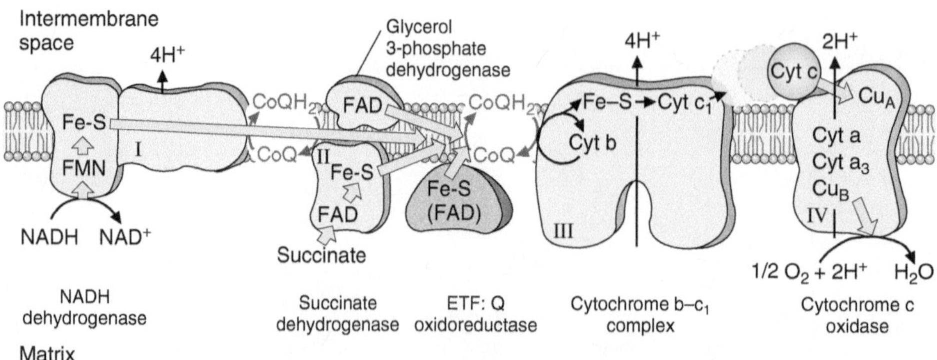

Answer 8: Electron flow through the electron-transport chain.

Succinate goes to fumarate, with the generation of $FADH_2$ (another 1.5 ATP), fumarate is converted to malate, and malate leaves the mitochondria (via the malate/aspartate shuttle) for further reactions. Once in the cytoplasm, the malate is oxidized to oxaloacetate, generating NADH (another 2.5 ATP if the malate/aspartate shuttle is used). At this point, citrate has been converted to cytoplasmic oxaloacetate, with the generation of ten high-energy bonds and the loss of two carbons as carbon dioxide. The oxaloacetate is then converted to phosphoenolpyruvate and carbon dioxide at the expense of a high-energy bond (GTP, the phosphoenolpyruvate carboxykinase reaction). The high-energy bond is recovered in the next step, however, as PEP is converted to pyruvate, generating an ATP. Thus, at this point in our conversion, citrate has gone to pyruvate, plus three CO_2, with a net yield of ten ATP (or high-energy bonds). The pyruvate re-enters the mitochondria and is oxidized to acetyl-CoA and carbon dioxide, also generating NADH (another 2.5 ATP). When this acetyl-CoA goes around the TCA cycle, two carbon dioxide molecules are produced, along with another ten high-energy bonds. The net total is therefore six carbon dioxide molecules and 22.5 high energy bonds for the complete oxidation of citrate.

11 **The answer is D: Lack of energy to the heart due to B_1 deficiency.** The patient has thiamine deficiency, and because of this, his heart is having trouble generating sufficient energy to effectively pump his blood (due to a reduction in the rate of both pyruvate oxidation and TCA oxidative steps). The resultant congestive heart failure leads to edema in the lower extremities, pulmonary edema, and inability to participate in even mild exercise. The thiamine deficiency has resulted from the patient's poor diet and the effect of ethanol blocking thiamine absorption from the diet. The nervous system also suffers from thiamine deficiency, in which case, neurological signs of the deficiency would be evident. These are not yet observed in this patient. The symptoms observed are not due to niacin deficiency (which are dementia, dermatitis, and diarrhea). The problem is also not due to insufficient energy for the kidney to appropriately filter the blood.

12 **The answer is E: Biotin.** The child has biotinidase deficiency, which results in a functional biotin deficiency. Biotinidase is required to remove covalently linked biotin from proteins in our diet and from proteins that have turned over within the body. An inability to do this leads to a biotin deficiency (as most ingested biotin is

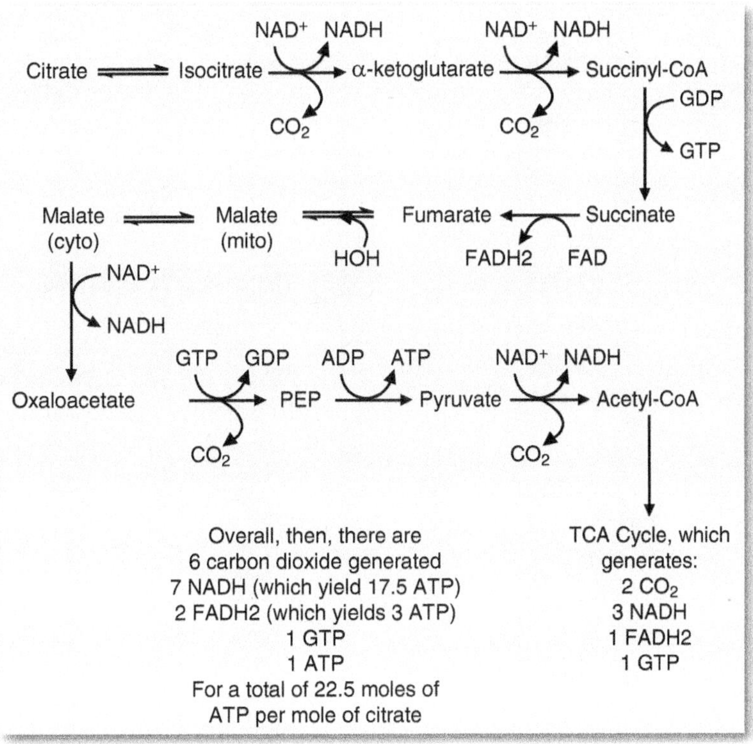

Answer 10: The pathway required for the complete oxidation of citrate to carbon dioxide and water.

linked to proteins). The hair and scalp problems have been attributed to an inability to synthesize fatty acids (as acetyl-CoA carboxylase is missing biotin). Since pyruvate carboxylase is also inoperative (due to the lack of biotin), gluconeogenesis is impaired, and ketone bodies will be synthesized by the liver to compensate for reduced glucose production. Priopionyl-CoA carboxylase is also impaired, leading to the elevated levels of propionic acid. Since gluconeogenesis is impaired, excess pyruvate will be converted to lactate since it cannot be converted to oxaloacetate. The optic atrophy may be due to an inability to synthesize fatty acids within the neurons or a lack of energy due to reduced gluconeogenesis.

13 **The answer is D: Pyridoxal phosphate.** Pyridoxal phosphate is required for the transamination of aspartate to oxaloacetate and glutamic acid to α-ketoglutarate. Both the α-keto acids are TCA cycle components, and when their levels decrease, they can be replenished through such a reaction. Niacin, riboflavin, and lipoate are required for oxidative decarboxylation reactions, but that reaction type does not lead to a refilling of TCA cycle intermediates. Carnitine is required to transport acyl groups into the mitochondria and is not used to transport TCA cycle intermediates from the cytoplasm to the mitochondria. Biotin would be a correct answer (for the pyruvate carboxylase reaction, to regenerate oxaloacetate from pyruvate), but it was not offered as a choice. A typical transamination reaction is shown below.

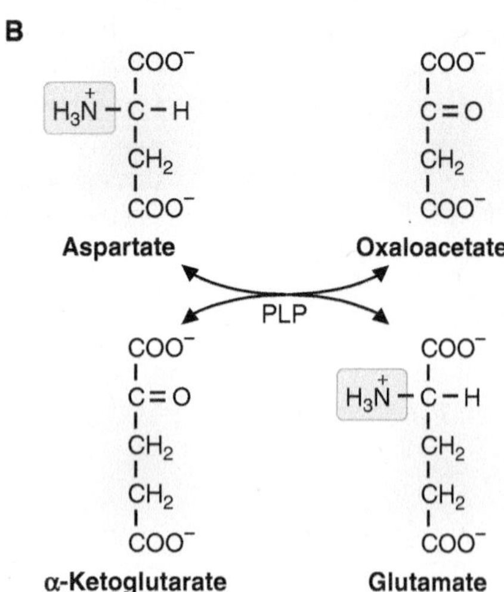

Panel **A** indicates the general reaction for a transamination reaction whereas Panel **B** shows the transamination between aspartic acid and α-ketoglutarate.

14 **The answer is C: Succinyl-CoA.** Barbiturates are metabolized via cytochrome P450 enzymes, which are induced by their substrates. The induction of synthesis requires that heme be synthesized, and the first step in heme synthesis requires succinyl-CoA and glycine and occurs within the mitochondrial matrix (see the figure below). Thus, succinyl-CoA levels can drop in the matrix during heme synthesis, and anaplerotic reactions are required to keep the cycle going.

Succinyl CoA

\+

Glycine

δ-ALA synthase

PLP

$CoAS^-$

CO_2

δ-Aminolevulinic acid (δ-ALA)

The first step in heme biosynthesis.

15 **The answer is C: Rotenone.** At point 1, an oxidizable substrate was added to the mixture as indicated in the figure (pyruvate), which is oxidized to form NADH. The NADH can add electrons to complex I to initiate electron flow across the chain. Since at point 2 the addition of succinate allows electron flow to reoccur, after being inhibited, it suggests that the inhibitor added at point A blocks electron flow from complex I to complex III (recall, succinate will add electrons at complex II, bypassing complex I). The only inhibitor in the list that does this is rotenone. Antimycin A blocks electron flow from complex III to complex IV. Atractyloside blocks ATP/ADP exchange across the inner mitochondrial membrane and will stop electron flow due to an inhibition of phosphorylation. The addition of succinate would not be able to overcome an inhibition of ATP synthesis due to lack of substrate (ADP). Dinitrophenol is an uncoupler, but would not allow electron flow from complex 1 in the presence of rotenone. Lactate is another oxidizable substrate, which would not overcome the block of electron transfer from complex I as lactate oxidation will generate NADH, which adds electrons to complex I.

16 **The answer is D: Dinitrophenol.** The increase in oxygen uptake stimulated by succinate (which is allowing electron flow from complex II to oxygen) is being blocked by oligomycin, which inhibits ATP synthesis. The block in ATP synthesis leads to the cessation of oxygen consumption due to the coupling of oxidation and phosphorylation. The only drug that can allow electron flow, in the absence of ATP synthesis, is an uncoupler, which uncouples the link between oxygen consumption and ATP production. Dinitrophenol is the only uncoupler on the list of answers. Note also that the rate of oxygen consumption has increased as compared to that when either NADH or succinate was donating electrons. This is due to the lack of a proton gradient in the presence of an uncoupler, so there is no "back pressure" to oxygen consumption, and the electron flow is faster than in the absence of the uncoupler.

17 **The answer is C: Cytoplasmic malate dehydrogenase.** The cytoplasmic malate dehydrogenase is required in liver as part of the malate/aspartate shuttle in transferring reducing equivalents across the inner mitochondrial membrane. In the absence of such an activity, NADH levels will build up in the cytoplasm (since the electrons cannot be transferred to the mitochondrial matrix) and will lead to the reduction of pyruvate to lactate to regenerate NAD^+ for other cytoplasmic reactions. A defect in glucokinase will block glycolysis, with no pyruvate or lactate formation from glucose. The same is true for an inactivating mutation in PFK-1. If pyruvate kinase were defective, PEP would accumulate, which cannot be converted to lactate without forming pyruvate first. A defect in glycerol-3-phosphate dehydrogenase will prevent the glycerol-3-phosphate shuttle from transferring electrons to the mitochondrial matrix, but the liver uses primarily the malate/aspartate shuttle for this activity. See the figure below for an overview of the malate/aspartate shuttle system.

18 **The answer is E: Inhibition of the proton translocating ATPase.** Oligomycin blocks the F_0 component of the proton-translocating ATPase, thereby blocking proton flow through the enzyme and ATP synthesis. Oligomycin does not affect any other complex of oxidative phosphorylation.

19 **The answer is A: Fasting blood glucose.** A pyruvate carboxylase deficiency will impair gluconeogenesis from lactate and pyruvate, thereby leading to fasting hypoglycemia more easily than a pyruvate dehydrogenase deficiency (which will primarily affect the ability to generate energy from carbohydrates). Alanine amino transferase activity in the blood is a measure of liver damage, which would not distinguish between the two possibilities. Free fatty acid levels would be the same under both conditions, during fasting conditions, as would insulin and glucagon levels.

20 **The answer is B: Metformin blocks hepatic gluconeogenesis.** Metformin leads to a reduction of hepatic gluconeogenesis. This is accomplished through the activation of the AMP-activated protein kinase, which phosphorylates and sequesters within the cytoplasm TORC2, which is a coactivator of CREB activity (a transcription factor needed for expression of two gluconeogenic enzymes, PEP carboxykinase and glucose-6-phosphatase). Thus, when TORC2 is absent from the nucleus, gluconeogenesis is impaired as the synthesis of two key enzymes is greatly reduced. One of the major gluconeogenic precursors is lactate, generated from the red blood cells and exercising muscle. In the Cori cycle, two lactates are converted to one glucose, which is then exported. If gluconeogenesis is blocked, lactate is not utilized and its levels can increase, and potentially lead to lactic acidosis. However, in the absence of congestive heart failure or renal insufficiency, this does not occur. The heart, with its massive amount of muscle and mitochondria, can utilize the lactate for energy unless the heart is dysfunctional or has lost muscle mass. Good, functional kidneys can also overcome

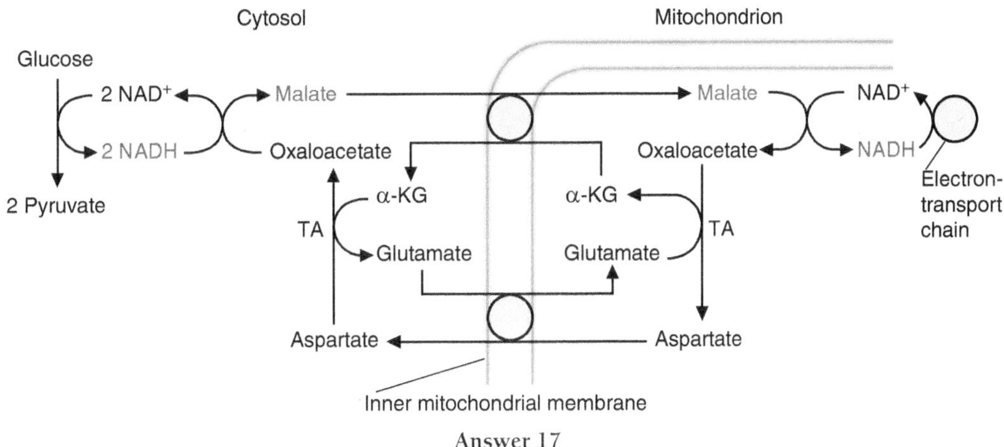

Answer 17

the lactate imbalance caused by metformin treatment. Metformin does decrease the insulin resistance, but this does not increase lactate in the aerobic state. Metformin does not inhibit the TCA cycle, glycolysis, or dietary protein absorption. These interactions are outlined in the figure below.

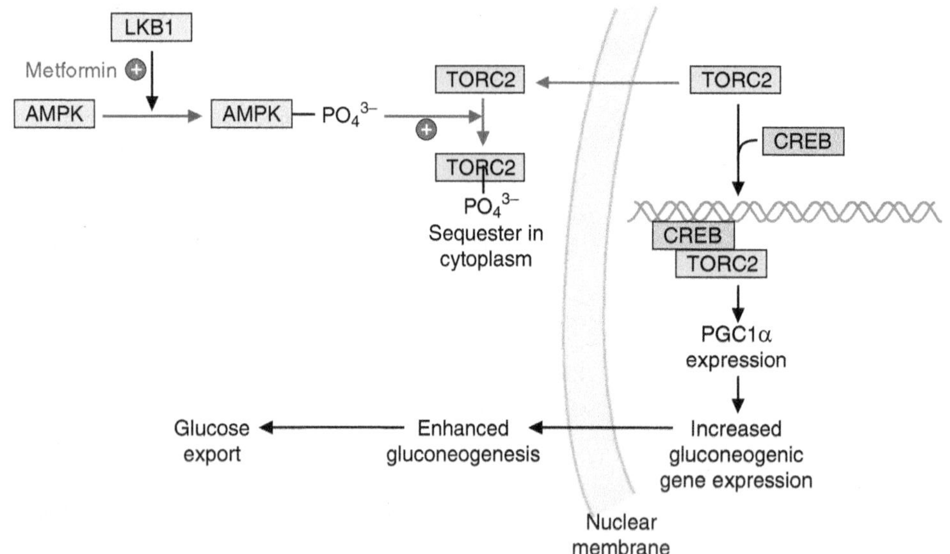

TORC2 sequestration in the cytoplasm after phosphorylation by the AMP-activated protein kinase, which is activated by metformin treatment. This leads to reduced synthesis of key gluconeogenic enzymes, thereby reducing gluconeogenesis in the liver.

Chapter 12

Glycogen Metabolism

This chapter quizzes the student on various aspects of the synthesis and degradation of the major carbohydrate storage molecule in the body. Regulation of these processes is also key as is the understanding of the multitude of diseases that alter glycogen metabolism.

QUESTIONS

Select the single best answer.

1 A 3-month-old infant was brought to the pediatrician due to muscle weakness (myopathy) and poor muscle tone (hypotonia). Physical exam revealed an enlarged liver and heart, and heart failure. The infant had always fed poorly, had failure to thrive, and had breathing problems. He also had trouble holding up his head. Blood work indicated early liver failure. A liver biopsy indicated that glycogen was present and of normal structure. A potential defect in this child is which of the following?

(A) Liver glycogen phosphorylase
(B) Liver glycogen synthase
(C) Liver α-glucosidase
(D) Liver debranching enzyme
(E) Liver branching enzyme

2 A 7-year-old boy is brought to the pediatrician due to severe exercise intolerance. In gym class, the boy has trouble with anaerobic activities. Laboratory tests showed a lack of lactate production under such conditions. The boy was eventually found to have a mutation in which one of the following enzymes?

(A) Liver glycogen phosphorylase
(B) Liver PFK-1
(C) Muscle PFK-1
(D) Muscle glucose-6-phosphatase
(E) Liver glucose-6-phosphatase

3 A 3-month-old infant, when switched to a formula diet plus fruit juices, begins to vomit and displays severe hypoglycemia after eating. Removal of the fruit juices from the diet seemed to reduce the severity of the symptoms. At the pediatrician's office, an inborn error of metabolism was considered, which could explain the hypoglycemia. Which explanation is most likely?

(A) Fructose inhibition of the debranching enzyme
(B) Galactose-1-phosphate inhibition of glycogen phosphorylase
(C) Fructose-1-phosphate inhibition of glycogen phosphorylase
(D) Fructose-6-phosphate inhibition of glycogen phosphorylase
(E) Galactose inhibition of aldolase

4 A 6-month-old infant was brought to the pediatrician due to fussiness and a tender abdomen. The child seemed to do well until the time between feeding was increased to more than 3 h. The baby always seemed hungry and irritable if not fed frequently. Upon examination, hepatomegaly and enlarged kidneys were noted, and blood work showed fasting hypoglycemia. Subsequent laboratory analysis demonstrated that in response to a glucagon challenge, only about 10% of the normal amount of glucose was released into circulation, which significantly contributed to the fasting hypoglycemia. Which enzyme defect in the patient is the most likely?

(A) Glycogen synthase
(B) Branching enzyme
(C) Debranching enzyme
(D) Glucose-6-phosphatase
(E) Fructose-1,6-bisphosphatase

5 A 4-month-old infant is seen by the pediatrician for failure to thrive. Examination shows distinct hepatosplenomegaly. Lab results show elevated transaminases and bilirubin, suggestive of liver failure. The boy dies shortly thereafter, and upon autopsy, precipitated carbohydrate was found throughout the liver. The boy most likely had a mutation in which of the following enzymes?

(A) Glycogen phosphorylase
(B) Debranching enzyme
(C) Glycogen synthase
(D) β-glucosidase
(E) Branching enzyme

6 An inactivating mutation in which of the following proteins can lead to fasting hypoglycemia?
(A) Liver PFK-1
(B) Liver glucokinase
(C) Adenylate cyclase
(D) Galactokinase
(E) Fructokinase

7 If the turnover number of all enzymes involved in glycogen metabolic regulation and activity is 100 reactions per second, how many glucose molecules could be removed from glycogen in 1 s upon activation of one molecule of protein kinase A (PKA)?
(A) 100
(B) 1,000
(C) 10,000
(D) 100,000
(E) 1,000,000

8 An individual is taking a serene walk in the park when he spots an escaped alligator from the zoo. The individual runs away as fast as he can. Glycogen degradation is occurring to supply glycolysis with a substrate even before epinephrine has reached the muscle. This is due to which of the following?
(A) Sudden decrease in blood glucose levels
(B) Increase in sarcoplasmic calcium levels
(C) Insulin binding to muscle cell receptors
(D) Decline in ATP levels
(E) Lactate production

9 As the individual in the previous question continues to run from the alligator, the muscle begins to import glucose from the circulation. This occurs due to which of the following?
(A) Insulin binding to muscle cells
(B) Epinephrine binding to muscle cells
(C) Glucagon binding to muscle cells
(D) Increase in intracellular AMP levels
(E) Increase in intracellular calcium levels

10 An 18-year-old man visits the doctor due to exercise intolerance. His muscles become stiff or weak during exercise, and he sometimes cramps up. At times, his urine appears reddish-brown after exercise. An ischemic forearm exercise test indicates very low lactate production. A potential enzyme defect in this man is which of the following?
(A) Muscle glycogen phosphorylase
(B) Liver glycogen phosphorylase
(C) Liver PFK-1
(D) Muscle glucose-6-phosphatase
(E) Muscle GLUT4 transporters

11 Patients with von Gierke disease display hepatomegaly. Glycogen content in the liver is increased, relative to normal, due to which of the following effects of glucose-6-phosphate in these patients?
(A) Inhibition of phosphorylase a
(B) Stimulation of phosphorylase b
(C) Inhibition of glycogen synthase I
(D) Stimulation of glycogen synthase D
(E) Inhibition of glycogen phosphorylase kinase

12 The hyperuricemia observed in patients with von Gierke disease comes about due to which of the following?
(A) Glucose-6-phosphate inhibition of kidney tubule absorption of urate
(B) Lactate inhibition of kidney tubule absorption of urate
(C) Glucose-6-phosphate inhibition of glucose-6-phosphate dehydrogenase activity
(D) Glucose-6-phosphate stimulation of glycogen synthase D
(E) Glucose-6-phosphate activation of amidophosphoribosyl transferase activity

13 Consider the case of an athlete who has just completed a work out. At this point, the athlete consumes a sports drink, which contains a large amount of glucose, which enters the circulation. Glycogen degradation is inhibited in the liver under these conditions, prior to insulin release, due to allosteric inhibition of which of the following enzymes?
(A) Glycogen synthase I
(B) Phosphorylase kinase a
(C) Phosphorylase a
(D) Protein phosphatase 1
(E) Adenylate kinase

14 A muscle cell line has been developed with a nonfunctional adenylate cyclase gene. Glycogen degradation can be induced in this cell line via which of the following mechanisms?
(A) Addition of glucagon
(B) Addition of epinephrine
(C) Increase in intracellular magnesium
(D) Increase in intracellular AMP
(E) Increase in intracellular ADP

15 A researcher created a liver cell line that displayed very low levels of glycogen. The glycogen that was synthesized was of normal structure, but the overall levels of glycogen were about 5% of normal. Which of the following is a potential alteration in the cell line that would lead to these results?

(A) An altered glycogen synthase with a reduced K_m for UDPglucose
(B) An altered phosphorylase kinase with an increased K_m for glycogen
(C) An altered UTPglucose-1-phosphate uridyl transferase with a decreased K_m for glucose-1-phosphate
(D) An altered glycogenin with an increased K_m for UDPglucose
(E) An altered phosphorylase kinase with an increased K_m for glycogen synthase

16 Ten hours into a fast, in a normal individual, which of the following best represents the activity and phosphorylation state of a number of key enzymes within the liver?

	PFK-1		Glycogen Synthase		Phosphorylase Kinase		Pyruvate Dehydrogenase	
	Active?	**Phosphorylated?**	**Active?**	**Phosphorylated?**	**Active?**	**Phosphorylated?**	**Active?**	**Phosphorylated?**
(A)	No	Yes	No	Yes	Yes	Yes	No	Yes
(B)	No	No	No	No	Yes	Yes	No	Yes
(C)	No	No	No	Yes	Yes	Yes	No	No
(D)	No	No	No	Yes	Yes	No	No	Yes
(E)	No	No	No	Yes	Yes	Yes	No	Yes

17 A woman with nonclassical galactosemia is considering becoming pregnant and is concerned that she will be unable to synthesize lactose in order to breast-feed her child. Her physician, who recalls her biochemistry, tells her this should not be a problem, and that she will be able to synthesize lactose at the appropriate time. This is true due to the presence of which of the following?
(A) Galactose-1-phosphate uridyl transferase
(B) Phosphoglucomutase
(C) Fructokinase
(D) Aldolase
(E) Phosphohexose isomerase

18 The energy required to store one molecule of glucose-6-phosphate as a portion of glycogen is which of the following?
(A) One high-energy bond
(B) Two high-energy bonds
(C) Three high-energy bonds
(D) Four high-energy bonds
(E) No high-energy bonds

19 An individual has been eating a large number of oranges during the winter months to protect against getting a cold. The excess carbons of citrate can be used to produce glycogen in the liver. Which one of the following liver enzymes is required for this conversion to occur?
(A) α-ketoglutarate dehydrogenase
(B) Pyruvate carboxylase
(C) Pyruvate kinase
(D) PFK-1
(E) Glucose-6-phosphatase

20 Your patient is a marathon runner and has visited your office to ask you about carbohydrate loading to increase his performance during a race. For a full week prior to a race, he eats three meals a day of pancakes, potatoes, brown rice, and pasta and does not exercise at all. He has not noticed any success with this regimen. Which of the following answers best explains why he is getting no benefit from his "carb loading"?
(A) Carbohydrate loading is a myth
(B) He is not depleting glycogen stores prior to loading
(C) He is not on the carbohydrate loading diet long enough prior to the race
(D) He is eating the incorrect foods for carbohydrate loading
(E) He is too highly trained as an athlete for anything to increase his performance

ANSWERS

1 **The answer is C: Liver α-glucosidase.** The infant has Pompe disease, a loss of liver α-glucosidase activity. This is glycogen storage disease II. The finding of normal glycogen structure eliminates liver debranching and branching activities as being deficient. The missing enzyme is a lysosomal enzyme, and nondegraded glycogen accumulates in the lysosome, interfering with lysosomal function (hence, a lysosomal storage disease). The malfunctioning of the lysosomes is what leads to the muscle and liver problems. A defect in glycogen phosphorylase (liver) would lead to fasting hypoglycemia, and an enlarged liver, but not the muscle problems exhibited by

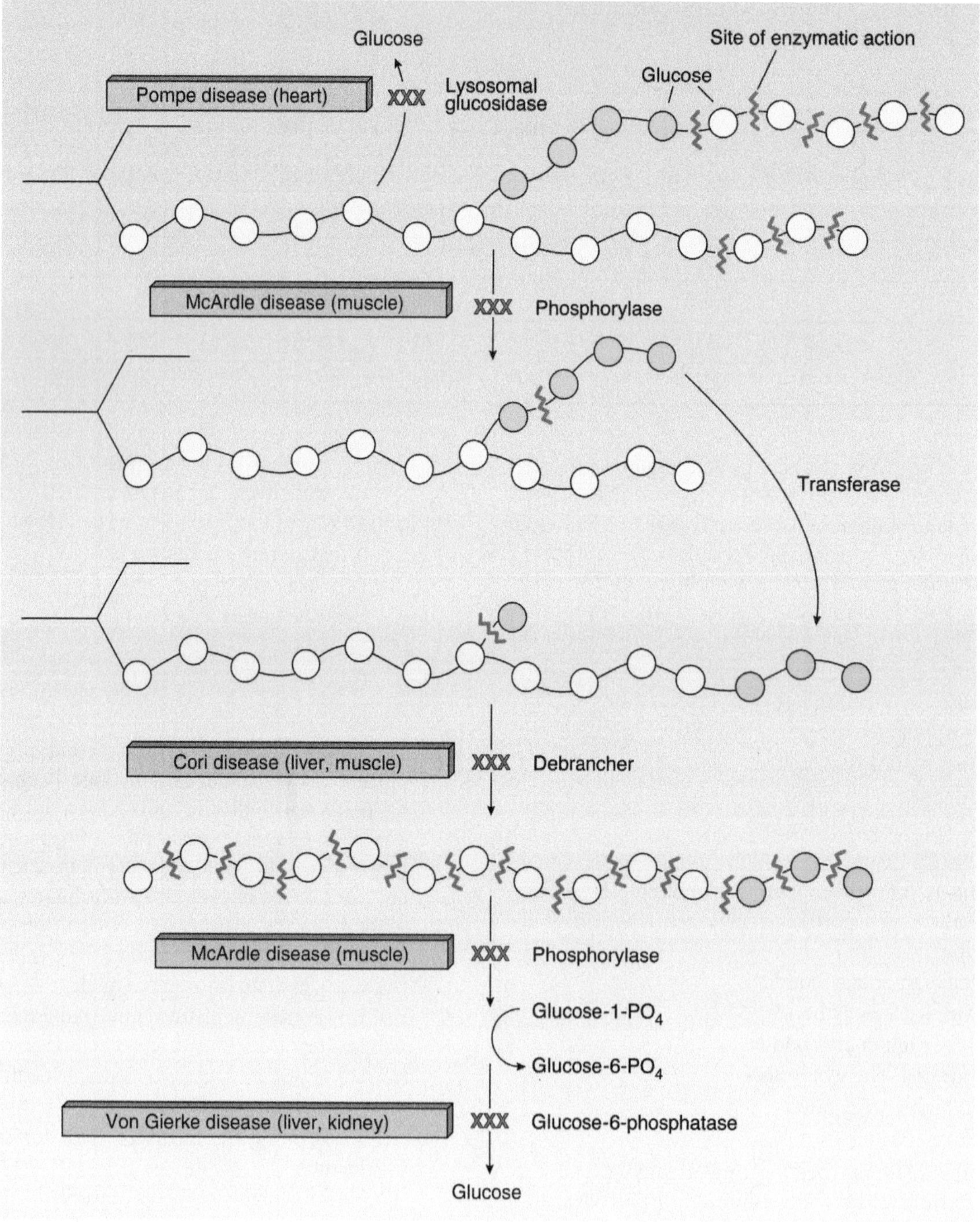

The catabolism of glycogen and an indication of some of the enzymes that are deficient in various glycogen storage diseases. Glycogen phosphorylase hydrolyzes the α-1,4 linkages in glycogen, releasing glucose-1-phosphate. The debranching enzyme transfers a small number of glucose residues from branch points and adds them to a longer chain of sugars (reaction 1). The debranching enzyme also removes the α-1,6-linked sugar at the original branch point (reaction 2). Once glucose-1-phosphate is converted to glucose-6-phosphate, glucose is released by the action of glucose-6-phosphatase. A small proportion of glycogen is totally degraded within lysosomes by acid α-glucosidase.

the child. A defect in glycogen synthase would also lead to fasting hypoglycemia, but would not lead to severe muscle and liver disease. Additionally, in an individual with a defect in glycogen synthase, glycogen would not be found in the liver biopsy since it could not be formed. The figure on page 102 summarizes steps involved in glycogen degradation, and the glycogen storage disease that results if an enzyme is defective.

2 **The answer is C: Muscle PFK-1.** The child has a form of glycogen storage disease known as type VII, Tarui disease, which is a lack of muscle phosphofructokinase 1 (PFK-1) activity. The lack of muscle PFK-1 means that glycolysis is impaired, so anaerobic activities are significantly curtailed in such individuals. Slow, aerobic activities, which can be powered by fatty acid oxidation, are normal in such children. Strenuous activity will lead to muscle damage and weakness due to this block in glycolysis. Glucose-6-phosphatase is only found in the liver (and to a small extent, the kidney), and a lack of such activity would lead to fasting hypoglycemia, but would not affect muscle glycolytic activity. A defect in liver PFK-1 activity would not affect muscle glycolysis. A defect in liver glycogen phosphorylase would also lead to fasting hypoglycemia, but would not alter the rate of muscle glycolysis, or lactate formation from that pathway.

3 **The answer is C: Fructose-1-phosphate inhibition of glycogen phosphorylase.** The child has hereditary fructose intolerance, a defect in aldolase B activity in the liver. This leads to an accumulation of fructose-1-phosphate in the liver (and, as fructokinase has a high V_{max}, a large amount of fructose-1-phosphate accumulates). At high levels, fructose-1-phosphate, through similarity in structure to glucose-1-phosphate, inhibits glycogen phosphorylase activity, leading to hypoglycemia (glycogen degradation is inhibited when blood glucose levels drop). The fructose is derived from the fruit juices introduced to the child's diet. Fructose does not inhibit debranching enzyme, and fructose-6-phosphate has no effect on glycogen phosphorylase (recall, one of the products of the glycogen phosphorylase reaction is glucose-1-phosphate, not glucose-6-phosphate). Galactose is found in lactose, which, while present in milk, is not found in fruit juice.

4 **The answer is D: Glucose-6-phosphatase.** The child has Von Gierke disease, glycogen storage disease type I, a lack of glucose-6-phosphatase. In such a disorder, glucose-6-phosphate, whether produced from glycogen degradation or gluconeogenesis, cannot be dephosphorylated for glucose export, and the liver cannot maintain blood glucose levels. The small amount of glucose which is exported (10% of the expected) is derived from the activity of debranching enzyme, which hydrolyzes an α-1,6-glucose linkage, which produces free glucose. The hepatomegaly arises due to excess glycogen in the liver (glucose-6-phosphate will activate glycogen synthase D), as does the increase in kidney size. A picture of a 25-month-old untreated child with this disorder is shown below. A lack of glycogen synthase would not lead to hepatomegaly, while a lack of branching enzyme leads to a different glycogen storage disease, with very different symptoms. A lack of debranching activity would not lead to hepatomegaly and would allow more glucose release than is observed through the normal action of glycogen phosphorylase. A defect in fructose-1,6-bisphosphatase would impair gluconeogenesis, but should not affect the ability of glycogen to be degraded to raise blood glucose levels.

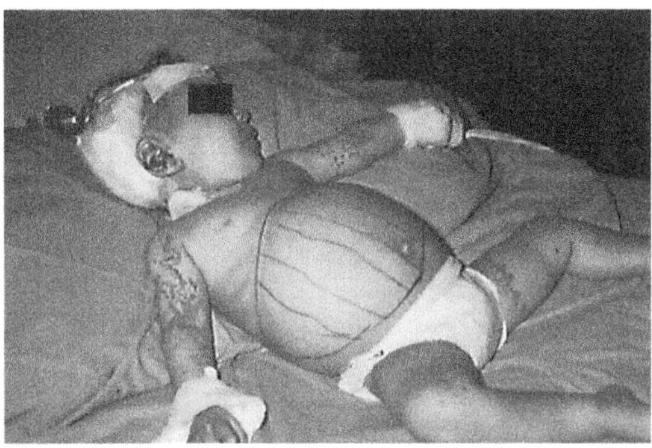

A 25-month-old child with von Gierke disease. Note the hepatomegaly and eruptive xanthomas on the arms and legs. The child is in the third percentile for height and weight, indicating a failure to thrive.

5 **The answer is E: Branching enzyme.** The child has a lack of branching enzyme activity, another glycogen storage disease, type IV (Andersen disease). In this case, the glycogen produced is a long, straight chain amylopectin, which has limited solubility, and precipitates in the liver (recall, the liver has the highest concentration of glycogen of all tissues). This leads to early liver failure (thus, the high bilirubin and transaminases in the serum) and death if a liver transplant is not performed. Defects in any of the other enzymes listed would lead to a different clinical scenario. Lack of glycogen phosphorylase or synthase, within the liver, would lead to fasting hypoglycemia, but not liver failure. Lack of these enzymes in the muscle would lead to exercise intolerance but would not affect blood glucose levels. Lack of α-glucosidase is Pompe disease, which also leads to an early death, but is due to the lack of a lysosomal enzyme, and there is no glycogen precipitation within the body of the liver. A lack of debranching activity is glycogen storage disease III, but would also lead to fasting hypoglycemia, without glycogen precipitation within the liver. A number of the glycogen storage diseases are summarized in the figure on page 104.

Types of Glycogenoses

Type	Glycogenosis	Deficient enzyme	Biochemical diagnosis	Clinical symptoms
1	Hepatorenal g., Gierke disease	glucose-6-phosphatase	Normal glycogen; excessive amounts in liver and kidneys	Hypoglycemia, hyperlipemia, ketosis, hyperuricemia, hepatomegaly, dwarfism
2	Generalized, malignant g.; Pompe disease; cardiomegalia glycogenica	α-1,4-glucosidase	Normal glycogen, excessive in all organs	Muscle hypotonia, heart failure, neurologic symptoms, infant death
3	Hepatomuscular, benign g.; Cori disease, Forbes disease (with subvariants 3b through f)	Amylo-1,6-glucosidase	Abnormal glycogen, with short outer chains, in liver and (more rarely) in muscles	Hepatomegaly, hypoglycemia; mild course of disease
4	Liver, cirrhotic, reticuloendothelial g.; Anderson disease; amylopectinosis	α-1,4-glucan: α-1,4-glucan-6-glycosyltransferase	Abnormal glycogen, with long outer chains, in liver, spleen, and lymph nodes	Cirrhosis of the liver; hepatosplenomegaly
5	Muscular g., Mcardle-Schmid-Pearson disease	α-glucanphosphorylase of the muscle	Normal glycogen, excessive amounts in muscle	Generalized myasthenia and myalgia, myoglobinuria
6	Hepatic g., Hers disease	α-glucanphosphorylase I of the liver	Normal glycogen, excessive amounts in liver	Hepatomegaly, relatively benign
7	Muscular g.; Tarui disease	Phosphofructokinase of the muscle	Normal glycogen, in the skeletal muscle	Muscle cramping, myoglobinuria
8	Hepatic g.; X-chromosome inheritance	Phosphorylase-b kinase of the liver	Normal glycogen, in the liver	Clinically mild manifestation, hepatomegaly, hypoglycemia

Answer 5: A summary of the glycogen storage diseases.

6 **The answer is C: Adenylate cyclase.** If adenylate cyclase is defective, glucagon cannot initiate the activation of glycogenolysis and inhibition of glycolysis in the liver (cAMP levels will not increase, and PKA will stay inactive). Under such conditions, only the allosteric effectors in liver will be active, and there is no activator of glycogen phosphorylase b. When the hypoglycemia is severe enough, epinephrine release, working through its α-receptors, will activate phospholipase C, leading to calcium release. The increased calcium can activate phosphorylase kinase, which will activate phosphorylase, but fasting hypoglycemia will still occur. Defects in liver PFK-1 or glucokinase will not affect glycogenolysis or gluconeogenesis. Defects in liver galactokinase or fructokinase will not allow for metabolism of galactose or fructose, but do not affect the ability of the liver to degrade glycogen, or perform gluconeogenesis from other precursors.

7 **The answer is E: 1,000,000.** One active PKA can activate in 1 s 100 molecules of phosphorylase kinase. Each phosphorylase kinase can, in 1 s activate 100 molecules of glycogen phosphorylase (so at this point we have 100 times 100 active molecules of phosphorylase, or 10,000 active phosphorylase molecules). Each active phosphorylase molecule can release 100 glucose residues per second from glycogen, and since there are 10,000 active phosphorylase molecules, 1,000,000 molecules of glucose are released per second once a single molecule of PKA has been activated. This is an example of cascade amplification, in which an increase in activity of just one molecule at the top of the cascade can result in a large response further down the cascade.

8 **The answer is B: Increase in sarcoplasmic calcium levels.** When the individual begins to run away from the alligator, muscle contraction leads to calcium release from the sarcoplasmic reticulum to the sarcoplasm. This increase in sarcoplasmic calcium binds to the calmodulin subunit of phosphorylase kinase and activates the enzyme in an allosteric manner, in the absence of any covalent modification. The activated phosphorylase kinase will phosphorylate and activate glycogen phosphorylase, which will initiate glycogen degradation. When epinephrine reaches the muscle, phosphorylase kinase will be fully activated via phosphorylation by PKA. The activation of glycogen degradation under these conditions is not due to a decrease in blood glucose levels, insulin binding (insulin would not be released under these conditions), a decline in ATP levels (the AMP-activated

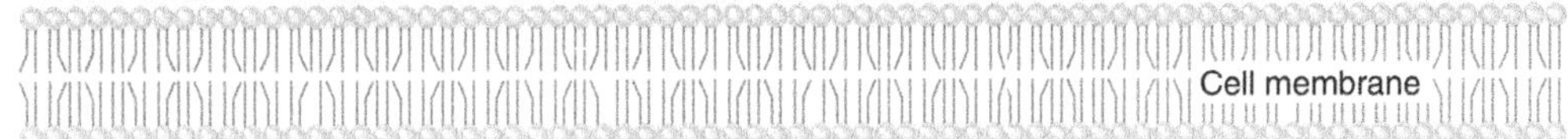

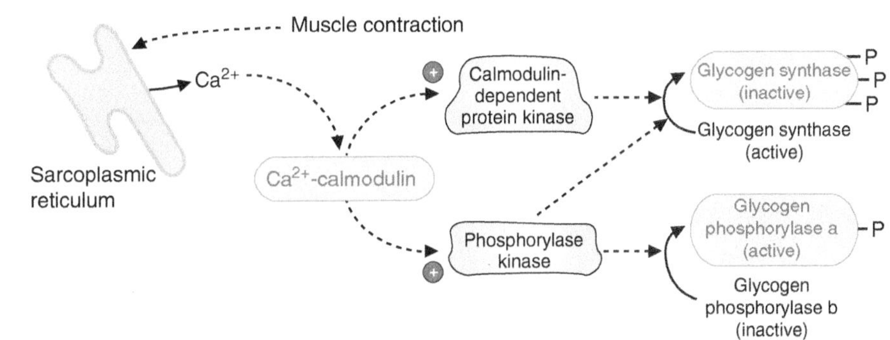

Answer 8: Regulation of glycogen synthesis and degradation by calcium in the muscle. Muscle contraction leads to calcium release from the sarcoplasmic reticulum, which binds to calmodulin, activating phosphorylase kinase, and leading to the inhibition of glycogen synthesis and the activation of glycogen degradation.

protein kinase does not activate glycogen degradation), or lactate production, the end product of anaerobic metabolism. The figure above shows the stimulation of glycogen degradation, working through calcium activation of the calmodulin subunit of phosphorylase kinase.

9 **The answer is D: Increase in intracellular AMP levels.** As AMP levels increase in the muscle due to the need for ATP for muscle contraction, and the activity of the adenylate kinase reaction, the AMP-activated protein kinase is turned on. One of the effects of the AMP-activated protein kinase is to increase the number of GLUT4 transporters in the muscle membrane, in a process similar to the action of insulin. This enables muscle to take up glucose efficiently from the circulation when internal energy levels are low. The ability of the muscle to take up glucose under these conditions is not due to an increase in epinephrine levels, an increase in sarcoplasmic calcium levels, or insulin binding to muscle cells. Under conditions as described in the question, insulin will not be present in the circulation to bind to the muscle cells. As the muscle does not contain glucagon receptors, there is no effect on muscle when glucagon is present in the circulation.

10 **The answer is A: Muscle glycogen phosphorylase.** The patient is lacking muscle glycogen phosphorylase and cannot utilize muscle glycogen for energy. This is another glycogen storage disease, type V, McArdle disease. The lack of muscle glycogen phosphorylase is why lactate production during exercise is very low. As shown in the figure below, there are many glycogen particles present in the muscle cells just below the sarcolemma, as the glycogen is not able to be degraded. Muscle damage also results from vigorous exercise, releasing myoglobin into the circulation, which is what leads to the reddish-brown urine after exercise. Alterations in liver enzymes (phosphorylase or PFK-1) would not affect exercise tolerance in the muscle. Muscle does not contain glucose-6-phosphatase, and this problem is not due to a lack of muscle GLUT4 transporters, as the muscle cannot utilize stored, internal glucose supplies.

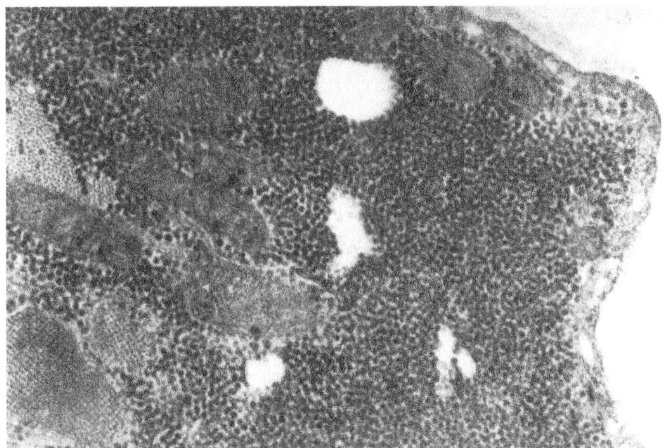

The electron micrograph demonstrates an abnormal mass of glycogen (not surrounded by a membrane) particles just beneath the sarcolemma, which distinguishes this disorder from Pompe disease (a lysosomal disorder in which glycogen within the lysosomes cannot be degraded).

11 **The answer is D: Stimulation of glycogen synthase D.** Glycogen synthase D (the inactive, phosphorylated form) can be allosterically activated by glucose-6-phosphate binding to the enzyme. Glucose-6-phosphate will inhibit the AMP-stimulation of muscle phosphorylase b, but does not have any allosteric effect on the other enzymes listed (PFK-1, glucose-6-phosphatase, or GLUT4 transporters) as answer choices for this problem.

12 **The answer is B: Lactate inhibition of kidney tubule absorption of urate.** Patients with von Gierke disease display elevated levels of lactate, which interferes with the kidney's ability to remove uric acid from the blood and place it in the urine. This leads to hyperuricemia. The reason lactate levels are elevated is that the high glucose-6-phosphate in the cell (recall, the defect in this disorder is a lack of glucose-6-phosphatase activity) forces glycolysis forward, producing pyruvate, which is converted to lactate in order to regenerate NAD^+ to allow glycolysis to continue. Glucose-6-phosphate does not inhibit glucose-6-phosphate dehydrogenase (that enzyme is regulated by the $NADP^+$ levels), nor does it regulate a committed step of de novo purine synthesis, amidophosphoribosyl transferase (which is regulated by adenine and guanine nucleotides). Glucose-6-phosphate does stimulate glycogen synthase D, but that activation does not play a role in elevated urate levels. Glucose-6-phosphate does not affect urate absorption within the kidney.

13 **The answer is C: Phosphorylase a.** The glucose in the sports drink will bind to liver glycogen phosphorylase a and inhibit its activity allosterically. Once the insulin signal reaches the liver, phosphorylase a will be converted to the dephosphorylated phosphorylase b by activated phosphatases. There is no allosteric inhibitor for glycogen synthase I, or protein phosphatase 1 (which is regulated by protein inhibitor 1). Adenylate kinase is not regulated allosterically, and there is no allosteric inhibitor of phosphorylase kinase a (the nonphosphorylated form can be activated by calcium).

14 **The answer is D: Increase in intracellular AMP.** AMP will activate muscle glycogen phosphorylase b allosterically, allowing glycogen degradation to begin before any hormonal signal has reached the muscle. The addition of epinephrine to the muscle requires activation of adenylate cyclase to initiate glycogen degradation, and adenylate cyclase has been inactivated in this cell line. Muscle lacks glucagon receptors, so cannot respond to this hormone. An increase in intracellular calcium would lead to glycogen degradation (via activation of phosphorylase kinase b), but magnesium does not have the same effect as calcium. Increases in ADP levels will not activate glycogen phosphorylase b; the allosteric activator is specific for AMP. The table below summarizes the allosteric interactions involved in glycogen metabolism.

Form of enzyme	Tissue	Activator	Inhibitor
Phosphorylase a	Liver	Already active	Glucose
	Muscle	Already active	Creatine-phosphate
Phosphorylase b	Liver	None	None
	Muscle	AMP	ATP, G6P
Phosphorylase kinase b	Liver and Muscle	Ca^{2+}	None
Glycogen synthase D	Liver and Muscle	Glucose-6-phosphate	None

15 **The answer is D: An altered glycogenin with an increased K_m for UDPglucose.** A reduction in overall glycogen synthesis suggests that the biosynthetic pathway is defective in some step. All glycogen molecules have, at their core, a glycogenin protein molecule, which autocatalyzes the addition of six glucose residues, using UDPglucose as the carbohydrate donor. This structure then provides the initial primer required by glycogen synthase. If the K_m for UDPglucose is increased, the rate of formation of glycogen primers will be decreased, as the levels of UDP-glucose may not be sufficient to allow glycogenin to self-prime. This would result in an overall reduction of glycogen levels within the cell. If a glycogen synthase had a reduced K_m for UDPglucose, then the enzyme would be active at lower UDPglucose levels, and one would expect greater than normal glycogen synthesis. Phosphorylase kinase has as its substrate phosphorylase, not glycogen, so answer B is not correct. If the uridyl transferase had a reduced K_m for a substrate, it would proceed at low substrate levels and would not give the resultant phenotype. And, if phosphorylase kinase had an increased K_m for glycogen synthase, then glycogen synthase would not be inactivated as rapidly, and glycogen synthesis would be expected to continue under conditions where it should not, leading to enhanced glycogen synthesis.

16 **The answer is E.** Under fasting conditions, the liver is exporting glucose, so the pathways of glycogenolysis and gluconeogenesis will be active, while glycolysis will be inhibited (all due to the effects of glucagon and activation of PKA). In glycolysis, PFK-2 is phosphorylated, activating its phosphatase activity, which leads to a reduction in fructose-2,6-bisphosphate levels. This

results in a reduction of PFK-1 activity (thus, PFK-1 is not active, but is not phosphorylated). Glycogen degradation has been activated, and synthesis inhibited, via the phosphorylation of glycogen synthase, inactivating the enzyme (thus, glycogen synthase is not active, but is phosphorylated). Phosphorylase kinase has been activated, and phosphorylated, by PKA (so phosphorylase kinase is active, and phosphorylated). Pyruvate dehydrogenase is inactive under these conditions (due to fatty acid oxidation in the mitochondria acetyl-CoA levels and NADH levels are high, which slows down the TCA cycle and inhibits pyruvate dehydrogenase), and it is also phosphorylated by the PDH-kinase, which is activated by NADH.

17 **The answer is B: Phosphoglucomutase.** For this woman to synthesize lactose, she needs to synthesize the precursors UDPgalactose and glucose, both of which are available from glucose. Glucose is converted to glucose-6-phosphate by hexokinase in the breast, and then phosphoglucomutase will convert this to glucose-1-phosphate (G1P). The G1P will react with UTP in the glucose-1-phosphate uridyl transferase reaction, producing UDPglucose. The C4 epimerase will then produce UDPgalactose from UDPglucose. The UDPgalactose then condenses with free glucose (using lactose synthase) to produce lactose and UDP. The other enzymes listed as answers are not required to produce lactose from the single precursor glucose. Fructokinase is unique for fructose metabolism. Aldolase is a glycolytic enzyme, which is deficient in hereditary fructose intolerance. Phosphohexose isomerase coverts glucose-6-phosphate to fructose-6-phosphate, which is not required for lactose synthesis. Classical galactosemia (severe, type 1) is a deficit of galactose-1-phosphate uridyl transferase. Patients cannot metabolize galactose, and the accumulating galactose-1-phosphate interferes with glycogen degradation. Nonclassical galactosemia (type 2) is a deficit in galactokinase, such that galactose cannot be phosphorylated. The complications in type 1 galactosemia due to the accumulation of galactose-1-phosphate are not seen in type 2 galactosemia. In either case, the missing enzymes are not required for the synthesis of lactose. See the figure below for both the pathway of lactose synthesis, and the defects in classical and nonclassical galactosemia.

18 **The answer is A: One high-energy bond.** For a molecule of glucose-6-phosphate (G6P) to be incorporated into glycogen, the following pathway must be utilized: G6P is converted to glucose-1-phosphate (G1P) via phosphoglucomutase, the G1P reacts with UTP to form UDPglucose via glucose-1-phosphate uridyl transferase, releasing pyrophosphate. The resultant pyrophosphate is hydrolyzed to two inorganic phosphates, with the loss of one high-energy bond. The UDPglucose then reacts with glycogen to produce a glycogen chain with one additional sugar, and UDP is released. The overall equation for these steps is: G6P + UTP + glycogen$_n$ yields UDP + 2Pi + (glycogen)$_{n+1}$. These steps are outlined below:

Gluose-6-phosphate → Glucose-1-phosphate
Glucose-1-phosphate + UTP → UDPglucose + PPi
PPi + H_2O → 2 Pi
UDPglucose + glycogen$_n$ → Glycogen$_{n+1}$ + UDP
UDP + ATP → UTP + ADP
Sum: Glucose-6-phosphate + ATP
+ glycogen$_n$ + H_2O → glycogen$_{n+1}$ + ADP + 2Pi

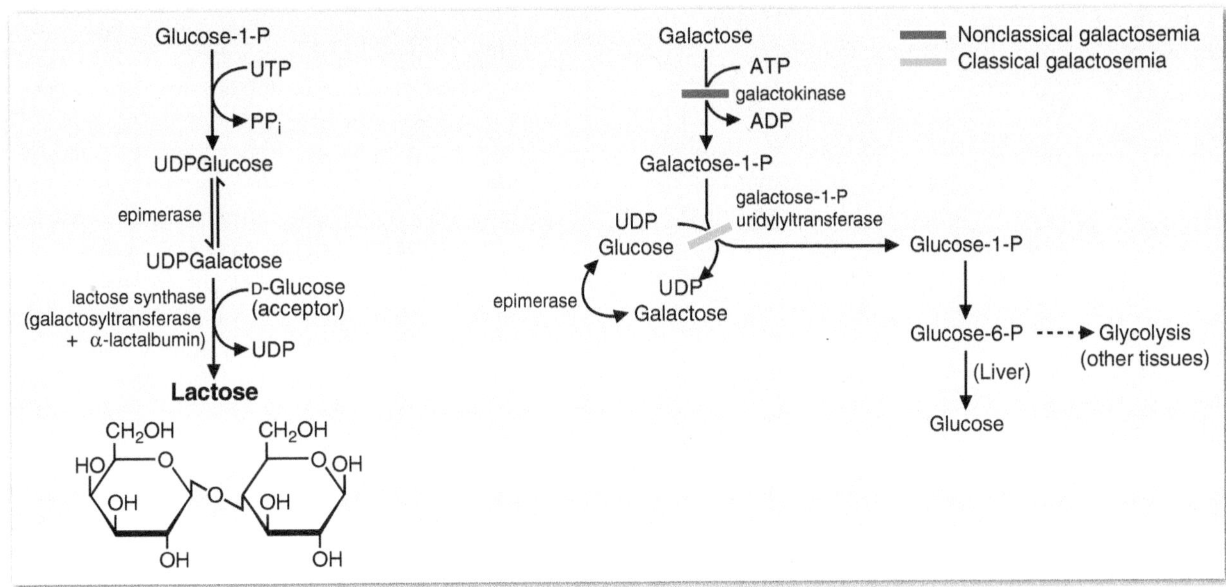

Answer 17

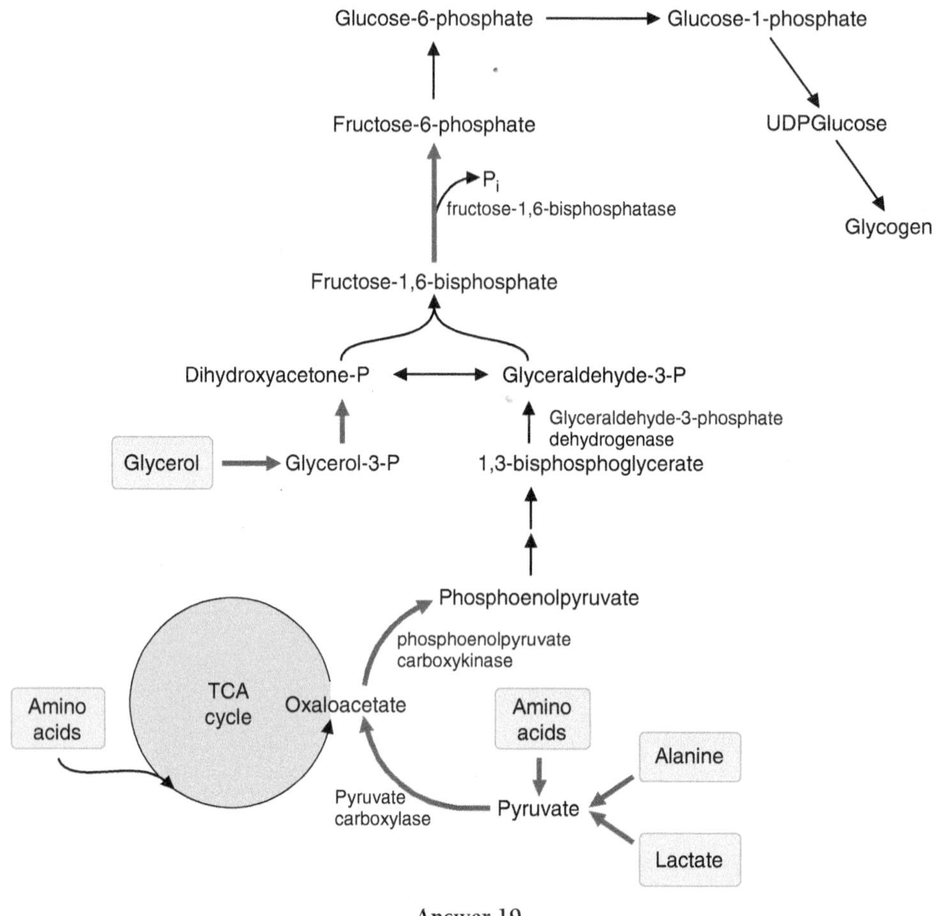

Answer 19

19 **The answer is A: α-ketoglutarate dehydrogenase.** In order for citrate to be converted to glycogen, the citrate must first be converted to oxaloacetate in the TCA cycle (which requires the participation of α-ketoglutarate dehydrogenase). From oxaloacetate, PEP carboxykinase will convert this to PEP, which will go through the gluconeogenic pathway up to glucose-6-phosphate. From there, G1P is produced, then UDPglucose, and finally incorporation of the glucose into glycogen. Pyruvate carboxylase, while being a gluconeogenic enzyme, converts pyruvate to OAA, which is not required in this series of reactions. PFK-1 and pyruvate kinase are irreversible enzymes of glycolysis and are not used in the gluconeogenic pathway. Glucose-6-phosphatase removes the phosphate from G6P, which is not required when glycogen is being synthesized. See the figure above for the pathways.

20 **The answer is B: He is not depleting glycogen stores prior to loading.** Marathon runners deplete their stores of glycogen during a race and need to catabolize other sources for energy to continue running. In the vernacular of the sport, when all the glycogen stores are exhausted, the runner "hits the wall." This is usually somewhere around mile 20. Research has shown that proper "carb loading" prior to a race can increase body stores of glycogen and increase performance. Though it is a small increase (1% to 2%), it has been documented repeatedly in research studies even in highly trained athletes. Therefore, it is not a myth. To properly carbohydrate load, one must deplete glycogen stores with very vigorous exercise about 2 to 3 days prior to a race. This stimulates glycogen synthase which increases glycogen stores over the next 2 to 3 days before it returns to baseline levels. This is a critical step in the process of "overbuilding" glycogen stores. This is the step the patient is not doing properly. Vigorous exercise cannot then be continued during the 2 to 3 days of glycogen building or the glycogen stores will be utilized. Pancakes, potatoes, brown rice, and pasta are excellent sources of simple carbohydrates.

Chapter 13

Fatty Acid Metabolism

This chapter examines the students' ability to integrate their knowledge of fatty acid metabolism with clinical problems and carbohydrate metabolism.

QUESTIONS

Select the single best answer.

1 You prescribe ibuprofen to help reduce your patient's inflammation. Which of the following pathways is blocked as an anti-inflammatory mechanism of action of nonsteroidal anti-inflammatory drugs?
(A) Prostaglandin synthesis
(B) Thromboxane synthesis
(C) Leukotriene synthesis
(D) All eicosanoid synthesis
(E) Arachidonic acid release from the membrane

2 You have an asthmatic patient who is already on an inhaled steroid and albuterol, but is still having difficulty. You add montelukast to her regimen. Montelukast (Singulair) specifically blocks the product of which of the following metabolic pathways?
(A) Cyclooxygenase
(B) Lipoxygenase
(C) P450
(D) Cori cycle
(E) TCA cycle

3 Coconut palm tress cannot survive growing outdoors in Kansas. Which of the following is the best explanation for this finding?
(A) Coconut/palm oil is a saturated fat
(B) Coconut/palm oil is a monounsaturated fat
(C) Coconut/palm oil is a polyunsaturated fat
(D) Kansas soil is not sandy enough to support growth
(E) Kansas soil is too rocky to support growth

4 An inactivating mutation in the ETF:CoQ oxidoreductase will lead to an initial inhibition of which of the following enzymes in fatty acid oxidation?
(A) Carnitine acyltransferase I
(B) Carnitine acyltransferase II
(C) Acyl-CoA dehydrogenase
(D) Enoyl-CoA dehydrogenase
(E) β-keto thiolase

5 A 3-month-old child had her first ear infection and was feeding poorly due to the ear pain. One morning the parents found the child in a nonresponsive state and rushed her to the emergency department. A blood glucose level was 45 mg/dL, and upon receiving intravenous glucose the child became responsive. Further blood analysis displayed the absence of ketone bodies, normal levels of acyl-carnitine, and the presence of the following unusual carboxylic acids shown below. The enzymatic defect in this child is most likely in which of the following enzymes?

$$^{-}O(O{=})C-CH_2-CH_2-CH_2-CH_2-C({=}O)O^{-}$$

$$^{-}O(O{=})C-CH_2-CH_2-CH_2-CH_2-CH_2-CH_2-C({=}O)O^{-}$$

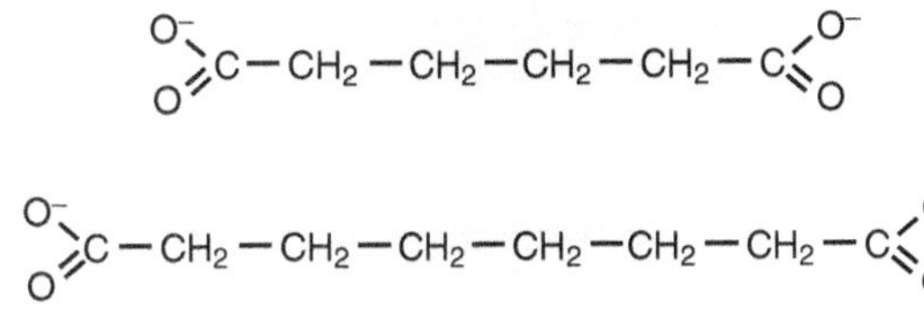

(A) Fatty acyl-CoA synthetase
(B) Carnitine translocase
(C) Carnitine acyltransferase I
(D) Carnitine acyltransferase II
(E) Medium chain acyl-CoA dehydrogenase

6 Regarding the child described in question 5, why were fasting blood glucose levels so low?
(A) Acyl-carnitine inhibition of gluconeogenesis
(B) Dicarboxylic acid inhibition of gluconeogenesis
(C) Insufficient energy for gluconeogenesis
(D) Dicarboxylic acid inhibition of glycogen phosphorylase
(E) Reduction of red blood cell production of lactate for gluconeogenesis

7 A 6-month-old child presents to the physician in a hypotonic state. The child has previously had a number of hypoglycemic episodes, at which times blood glucose

levels were between 25 and 50 mg/dl. Blood work shows normal levels of ketone bodies (not elevated) during hypoglycemic episodes. Carnitine levels in the blood were, however, below normal. Free fatty acid levels were elevated in the blood, however acyl-carnitine levels were normal. Dicarboxylic acid levels were non-detectable in the blood. A liver biopsy shows elevated levels of triglyceride. A likely enzymatic defect is which of the following?
(A) Carnitine acyltransferase I
(B) Carnitine acyltransferase II
(C) Medium chain acyl-CoA dehydrogenase
(D) Hormone sensitive lipase
(E) Carnitine transporter

8 Carnitine deficiency can occur in a number of ways. Secondary carnitine deficiency can be distinguished from primary carnitine deficiency by measuring which of the following in the blood?
(A) Fatty acids
(B) Acyl-carnitine
(C) Lactic acid
(D) Glucose
(E) Ketone bodies

9 Which one of the following fatty acids will generate the largest amount of ATP upon complete oxidation to carbon dioxide and water?
(A) C16:0
(B) cisΔ9 C16:1
(C) cisΔ9 C18:1
(D) cisΔ6 C18:1
(E) cisΔ9, Δ12 C18:2

10 An individual contains an inactivating mutation in a particular muscle protein, which leads to weight loss due to unregulated muscle fatty acid oxidation. Such an inactivated protein could be which of the following?
(A) Malonyl-CoA decarboxylase
(B) Carnitine acyl transferase I
(C) Carnitine acyl transferase II
(D) Medium chain acyl-CoA dehydrogenase
(E) Acetyl-CoA carboxylase 2

11 The net energy yield obtained (moles of ATP per mole of substrate oxidized) when acetoacetate is utilized by the nervous system as an alternative energy source is which of the following? Consider that acetoacetate must be oxidized to four molecules of carbon dioxide during the reaction sequence.
(A) 17
(B) 18
(C) 19
(D) 20
(E) 21

12 A mouse model has been generated as an in vivo system for studying fatty acid synthesis. An inactivating mutation was created which led to the cessation of fatty acid synthesis and death to the mice. This mutation is most likely in which of the following proteins?
(A) Carnitine acyl transferase I
(B) Carnitine acyl transferase II
(C) Citrate translocase
(D) Glucose-6-phosphate dehydrogenase
(E) Medium chain acyl-CoA dehydrogenase

13 α-oxidation would be required for the complete oxidation of which of the following fatty acids?

A $CH_3-(CH_2)_n-CH(CH_3)-CH_2-CH_2-COO^-$

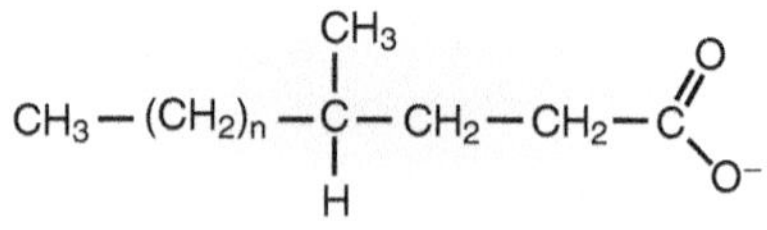

B $CH_3-(CH_2)_n-CH_2-CH(CH_3)-CH_2-COO^-$

C $CH_3-(CH_2)_n-CH_2-CH_2-CH(CH_3)-COO^-$

D $CH_3-(CH_2)_n-CH(CH_2CH_3)-CH_2-CH_2-COO^-$

E $CH_3-(CH_2)_n-CH(CH_3)-CH_2-CH(CH_3)-COO^-$

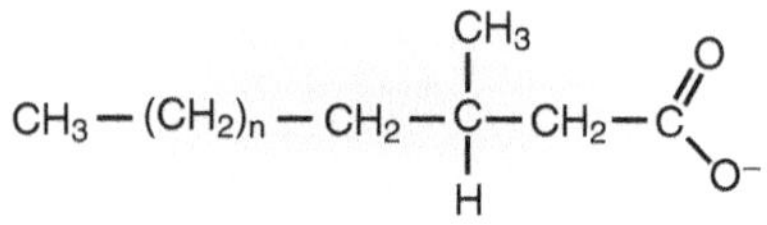

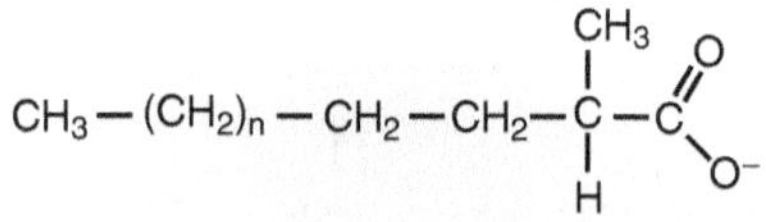

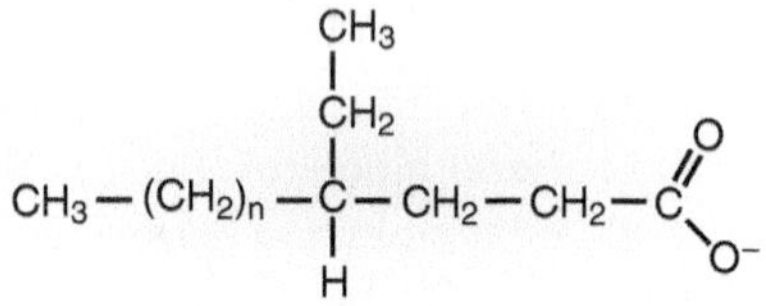

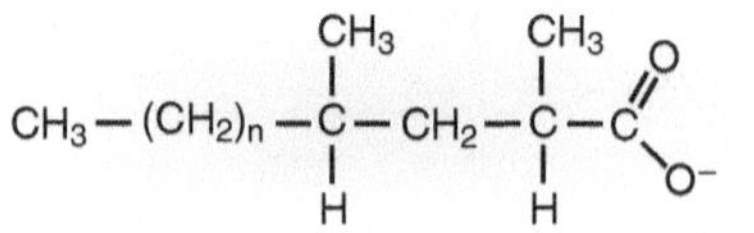

14 A 2-month-old infant with failure to thrive displays hepatomegaly, high levels of iron and copper in the blood, and vision problems. This child has difficulty in carrying out which of the following types of reactions?
(A) Oxidation of very long chain fatty acids
(B) Synthesis of unsaturated fatty acids
(C) Oxidation of acetyl-CoA
(D) Oxidation of glucose
(E) Synthesis of triacylgycerol

15 A 55-year-old man had been advised by his physician to take 81 mg of aspirin per day to reduce the risk of blood clots leading to a heart attack. The rationale for this treatment is which of the following?

(A) To reduce prostaglandin synthesis
(B) To reduce leukotriene synthesis
(C) To reduce thromboxane synthesis
(D) To increase prostacyclin synthesis
(E) To increase Lipoxin synthesis

16 You are examining a patient who exhibits fasting hypoglycemia and need to decide between a carnitine deficiency and a carnitine acyltransferase 2 deficiency as the possible cause. You order a blood test to specifically examine the levels of which one of the following?

(A) Glucose
(B) Ketone bodies
(C) Insulin
(D) Acyl-carnitine
(E) Carnitine

17 Inhibitors specific for cyclooxygenase 2 (COX-2) were deemed more efficacious for certain conditions than inhibitors which blocked both COX-1 and COX-2 activities. This is due to which of the following?

(A) Inhibiting COX-1 increased the frequency of heart attacks
(B) Inhibiting COX-2 did not alter prostaglandin production
(C) COX-2 is specifically induced during inflammation
(D) Specifically inhibiting COX-2 reduces the rate of heart attacks
(E) COX-1 is inducible and only expressed during wound repair, while COX-2 is expressed constitutively

18 An individual with a biotinidase deficiency was shown to produce fatty acids at a greatly reduced rate (in the absence of supplements) as compared to someone who did not have the deficiency. This is due to which of the following?

(A) Low activity of citrate lyase
(B) Reduced activity of malic enzyme
(C) Reduced activity of acetyl transacylase
(D) Defective acyl carrier protein
(E) Reduced ability to form malonyl-CoA

19 Liver fatty acid oxidation leads to an enhancement of gluconeogenesis via which of the following?

(A) Generation of precursors for glucose synthesis
(B) Activation of pyruvate carboxylase
(C) Activation of phosphoenolpyruvate carboxykinase
(D) Inhibition of pyruvate kinase
(E) Inhibition of PFK-2

20 A 35-year-old man in New York city, originally from Jamaica, purchased an illegally imported fruit from a street vendor and, within 4 h of eating the fruit, began vomiting severely. When brought to the emergency department the man was severely dehydrated and exhibited several seizures. The toxic effects of the fruit were interfering with which of the following?

(A) Fatty acid release from the adipocyte
(B) Fatty acid entry into the liver cell
(C) Fatty acid activation
(D) Fatty acid transport into the mitochondria
(E) Oxidative phosphorylation

ANSWERS

1 **The answer is A: Prostaglandin synthesis.** Eicosanoids are potent regulators of cellular function. They are derived from arachidonic acid and are metabolized by three pathways: the cyclooxygenase pathway (prostaglandins and thromboxanes), lipoxygenase pathway (leukotrienes), and the cytochrome P450 pathway (epoxides) (see the figure below). Nonsteroidal anti-inflammatory drugs (NSAIDs) do not block arachidonic acid release from the membrane (which would block all eicosanoid synthesis); however, they do interfere with the cyclooxygenase pathway. Prostaglandins affect inflammation, thromboxanes affect formation of blood clots, and leukotrienes affect bronchoconstriction and bronchodilatation. NSAIDs block prostaglandins as one of their anti-inflammatory mechanisms. Thus, while NSAIDS will block both prostaglandin and thromboxane synthesis, it is the blockage of prostaglandin synthesis which will block the inflammatory symptoms.

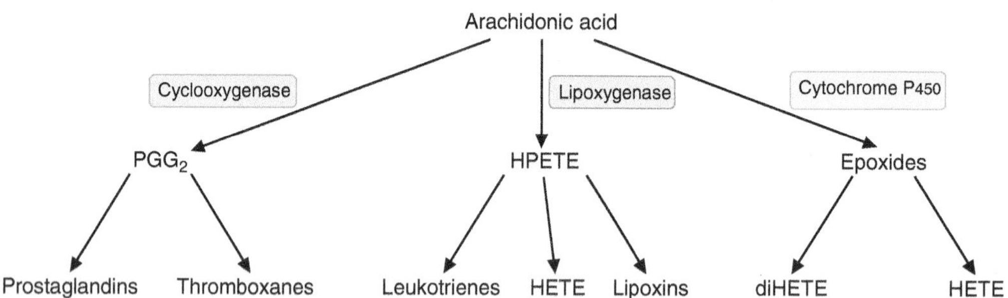

2 **The answer is B: Lipoxygenase.** Montelukast is a leukotriene blocker. Leukotrienes are formed through the lipoxygenase pathway and affect bronchoconstriction and allergy pathways (see the figure in answer to question 1). The cyclooxygenase pathway produces prostaglandins and thromboxanes. The P450 pathway produces epoxides. The Cori cycle is related to gluconeogenesis (lactate transfer from the muscle to the liver), while the TCA cycle is utilized to oxidize acetyl-CoA to CO_2 and H_2O.

3 **The answer is A: Coconut/palm oil is a saturated fat.** Saturated fats do not liquefy until a much higher temperature than that at which monounsaturated or polyunsaturated fats do (the melting temperature for saturated fats is greater than that for unsaturated fats). Conversely, saturated fats are solids at a higher temperature than unsaturated fats and cannot exist in a liquid form at a lower temperature. Since the oil of a plant is its "lifeblood," at a lower temperature, a saturated oil would solidify and the plant would die. Saturated oil plants cannot survive in a temperate climate (Kansas) and need a tropical climate of warm temperatures all year round. Only polyunsaturated oil plants can survive in a temperate climate (corn, flax, wheat, and canola). Monounsaturated oils need a warmer climate, but not as warm as the tropics (olive, peanut). Knowing where a plant grows gives a large clue as to whether the oil will be saturated, monounsaturated, or polyunsaturated. The difference in oil content between plants appears to be an evolutionary process. Kansas soil is very rich and supports growth of most plants.

4 **The answer is C: acyl-CoA dehydrogenase.** The acyl-CoA dehydrogenases catalyze the first step of the fatty acid oxidation spiral in that these enzymes create a carbon–carbon double bond between carbons 2 and 3 of the fatty acyl-CoA, generating an FADH2 in the process. The FADH2 then donates its electrons to the electron transfer flavoprotein (ETF), which then transfers the electrons to coenzyme Q (via the ETF:CoQ oxidoreductase). A lack of the oxidoreductase activity will lead to an accumulation of mitochondrial FADH2, depleting FAD levels, and reducing the activity of the acyl-CoA dehydrogenases. The lack of FAD does not directly inhibit the β-ketothiolase or enoyl-CoA dehydrogenase steps, nor does it affect the activity of the carnitine acyltransferases. The figure below shows the normal transport of electrons from FADH2 to coenzyme Q when the FADH2 is generated by the acyl-CoA dehydrogenases.

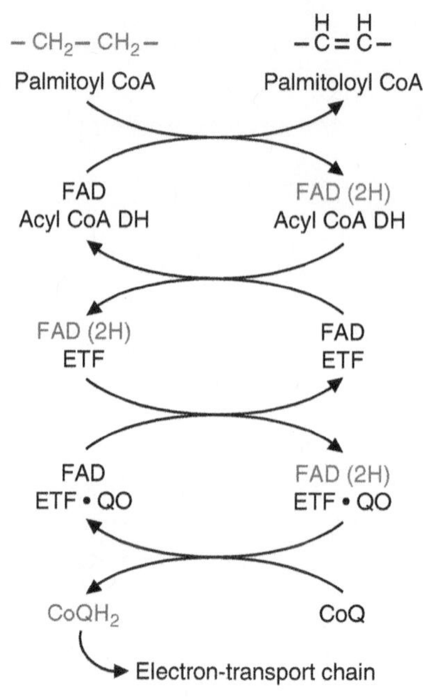

5 **The answer is E: Medium chain acyl-CoA dehydrogenase.** The child has MCAD (medium-chain acyl-CoA dehydrogenase) deficiency, an inability to completely oxidize fatty acids to carbon dioxide and water. With an MCAD deficiency, gluconeogenesis is impaired due to a lack of energy from fatty acid oxidation, and an inability to fully activate pyruvate carboxylase, as acetyl-CoA activates pyruvate carboxylase, and acetyl-CoA production from fatty acid oxidation is greatly reduced. In an attempt to generate more energy, medium-chain fatty acids are oxidized at the ω ends to generate the dicarboxylic acids seen in the question (see the figure below for an overview of ω oxidation). The finding of such metabolites (dicarboxylic acids) in the blood is diagnostic for MCAD deficiency. If there were mutations in any aspect of carnitine metabolism, there would be no oxidation of fatty acids (the fatty acids would not be able to enter the mitochondria), and the dicarboxylic acids (which are byproducts of fatty acid metabolism) would not be observed. Similarly, a mutation in the fatty acyl-CoA synthetase (the activating enzyme, converting a free fatty acid to an acyl-CoA) would also result in a lack of fatty acid oxidation, as fatty acids are not able to enter the mitochondria in their free (nonactivated) form.

$$\underset{\omega}{CH_3} - (CH_2)_n - \overset{O}{\overset{\|}{C}} - O^-$$

$$\downarrow$$

$$HO - CH_2 - (CH_2)_n - \overset{O}{\overset{\|}{C}} - O^-$$

$$\downarrow$$

$$\downarrow$$

$$^-O - \overset{O}{\overset{\|}{C}} - (CH_2)_n - \overset{O}{\overset{\|}{C}} - O^-$$

6 **The answer is C: Insufficient energy for gluconeogenesis.** Defects in fatty acid oxidation deprive the liver of energy when fatty acids are the major energy source (such as during exercise, or a fast). Because of this, there is insufficient energy to synthesize glucose from gluconeogenic precursors (it requires 6 moles of ATP to convert 2 moles of pyruvate to 1 mole of glucose). Acyl-carnitines and dicarboxylic acids have no effect on the enzymes of gluconeogenesis, nor do they hinder the ability of the red blood cell to utilize glucose through the glycolytic pathway. Additionally, acetyl-CoA levels are low due to the lack of complete fatty acid oxidation and pyruvate carboxylase, a key gluconeogenic enzyme, is not fully activated. This also contributes to the reduced gluconeogenesis observed in patients with MCAD defective.

7 **The answer is E: Carnitine transporter.** The child has a mutation in the enzyme which transports carnitine into liver and muscle cells, leading to a primary carnitine deficiency. The carnitine stays in the blood and is eventually lost in the urine (the same carnitine transporter is required to recover the carnitine from the urine in the kidney). Since the liver is carnitine deficient, ketone body production is minimal at all times, even during a fast (thus, the lack of baseline ketone bodies in the circulation under these conditions). Fatty acids will rise in circulation, as they cannot be stored in the cells as acyl-CoA. The liver shows evidence of triglyceride formation as the acyl-CoA cannot be degraded, and acyl-CoA accumulates within the cytoplasm, leading to triglyceride formation. A defect in carnitine acyl transferase 1 would lead to elevated levels of carnitine in the circulation. A defect in carnitine acyltransferase II would lead to elevated levels of acyl-carnitine in the circulation (since the acyl group cannot be removed from the carnitine). The lack of circulating dicarboxylic acids indicates that the defect is not in MCAD (medium-chain acyl-CoA dehydrogenase). A defect in hormone sensitive lipase would show a decrease in free fatty acid levels, rather than the increase observed in the patient.

8 **The answer is B: acyl-carnitine.** Primary carnitine deficiency is a lack of carnitine within the cell (such as a mutation in the carnitine transporter); secondary carnitine deficiency occurs when the carnitine is sequestered in the form of acyl-carnitine (the carnitine cannot be removed from the acyl group, such as a defect in carnitine acyl transferase 2). Thus, elevated levels of acyl-carnitine would be expected in a secondary carnitine deficiency, but not in a primary carnitine deficiency. In both types of carnitine deficiencies, fatty acid oxidation is significantly reduced, so the levels of ketone bodies, glucose, lactate, and fatty acids would be similar under both conditions.

9 **The answer is C: cisΔ9 C18:1.** An 18-carbon fatty acid will generate an additional acetyl-CoA, one NADH, and one FADH2 as compared to a 16-carbon fatty acid. Thus, the addition of two carbons will add 14 additional ATP to the overall energy yield (10 ATP per acetyl-CoA, 2.5 for NADH, and 1.5 for FADH2). An unsaturation at an odd carbon position will require the use of an isomerase during oxidation, and this will result in the loss of generation of 1 FADH2; an unsaturation at an even carbon position will require the use of the 2,4 dienoyl-CoA reductase, and this will result in the loss of generation of 1 NADPH. Thus, an unsaturation at an odd position results in the loss of 1.5 ATP, while an unsaturation at an even position results in the loss of 2.5 ATP. Thus, in comparing two 18-carbon fatty acids, one with an unsaturation at position 9, and the other at position 6, the fatty acid with the double bond at position 9 will

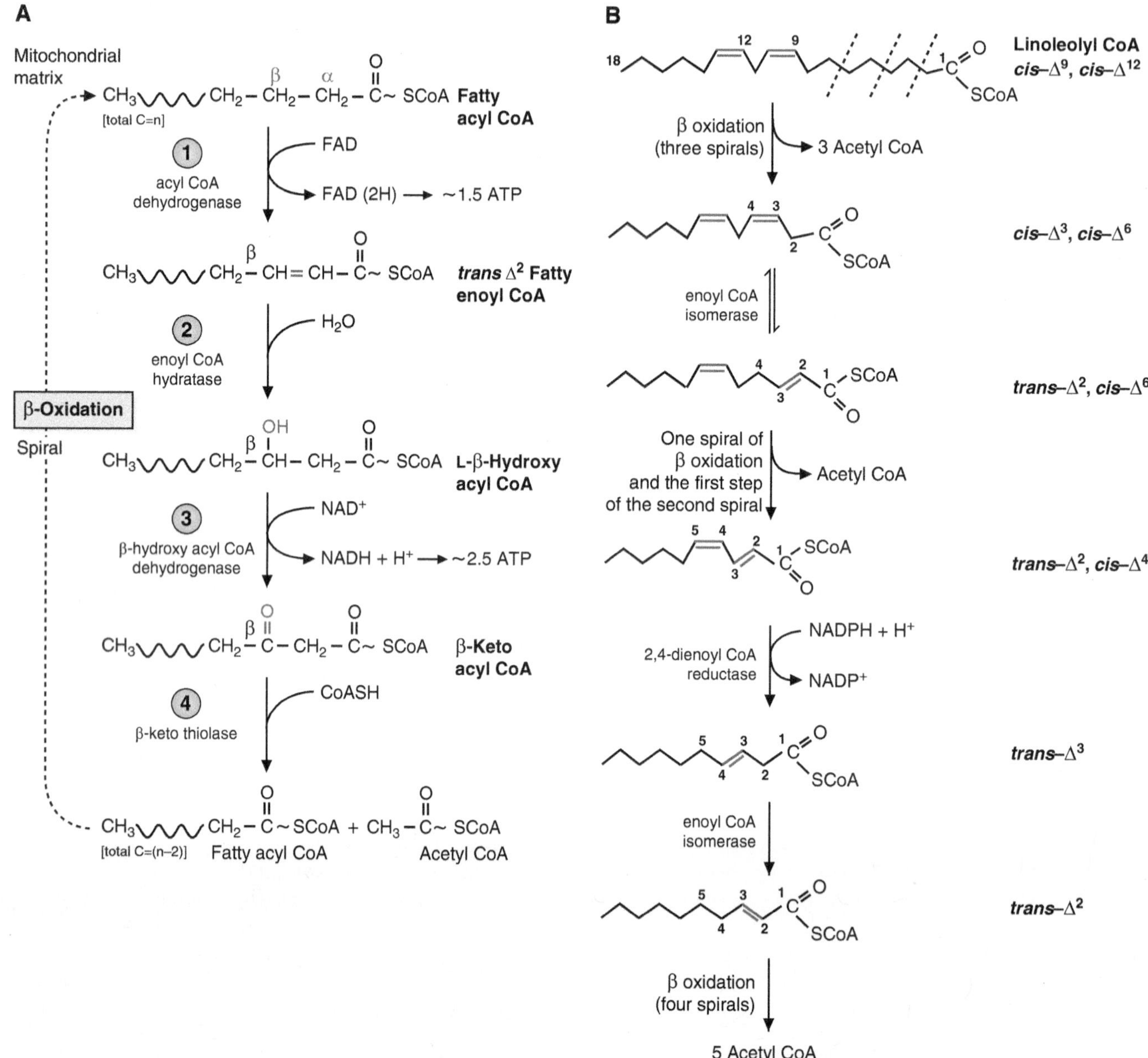

Answer 9: Panel A: The steps of β-oxidation. The four steps are repeated until an even-chain fatty acid is completely converted to acetyl-CoA. The FAD(2H) and NADH are reoxidized by the electron-transport chain, producing ATP. **Panel B**: The additional reactions required for the oxidation of unsaturated fatty acids. The two new enzymes required are the enoyl-CoA isomerase and the 2,4 dienoyl-CoA reductase.

yield one more ATP than the fatty acid with the unsaturation at position 6. An overview of the fatty acid oxidation spiral is shown above, along with the reactions required for the oxidation of unsaturated fatty acids.

10 The answer is E: acetyl-CoA carboxylase 2. An inactivating mutation in acetyl-CoA carboxylase would lead to an inability to produce malonyl-CoA, which regulates fatty acid oxidation through an inhibition of carnitine acyl transferase 1. As malonyl-CoA levels increase, fatty acid oxidation is reduced, and as the levels decrease, fatty acid oxidation will increase. If malonyl-CoA decarboxylase were inactivated, malonyl-CoA levels would remain elevated, and fatty acid oxidation would be inhibited. Inactivating mutations in either carnitine acyltransferase 1 or 2 would lead to an inability to oxidize fatty acids, as they would not enter the mitochondria. A defect in medium-chain acyl-CoA dehydrogenase (MCAD) would also result in reduced fatty acid oxidation, as the initial step of the oxidation spiral would be inhibited once the fatty acid had been reduced to about 10 carbons in length. The reactions catalyzed by malonyl-CoA decarboxylase and acetyl-CoA carboxylase are shown below.

$CH_3-\overset{O}{\overset{\|}{C}}\sim SCoA$

Acetyl CoA

CO_2 (Malonyl CoA decarboxylase)

CO_2, Biotin, acetyl CoA carboxylase; ATP → ADP + P_i

$^{-}O-\overset{O}{\overset{\|}{C}}-CH_2-\overset{O}{\overset{\|}{C}}\sim SCoA$

Malonyl CoA

11 **The answer is C: 19.** Acetoacetate will react with succinyl-CoA to produce acetoacetyl-CoA and succinate (this costs 1 GTP, as the succinate thiokinase step is skipped). The acetoacetyl-CoA is converted to two acetyl-CoA, each of which can generate 10 ATP when completely oxidized (each acetyl-CoA generates 1 GTP, 3 NADH, and 1 FADH2). The sum, then, is 20 minus the 1 lost in the CoA transferase step, for a net yield of 19 ATP.

12 **The answer is C: Citrate translocase.** Citrate translocase is required for citrate to exit the mitochondria and enter the cytoplasm in order to deliver acetyl-CoA for fatty acid biosynthesis (see the figure below). Acetyl-CoA, which is produced exclusively in the mitochondria, has no direct path through the inner mitochondrial membrane. However, under conditions conducive to fatty acid biosynthesis (high energy levels, and allosteric inhibition of the TCA cycle), citrate will accumulate and leave the mitochondria (see the figure below). Once in the cytoplasm, citrate lyase will cleave the citrate to

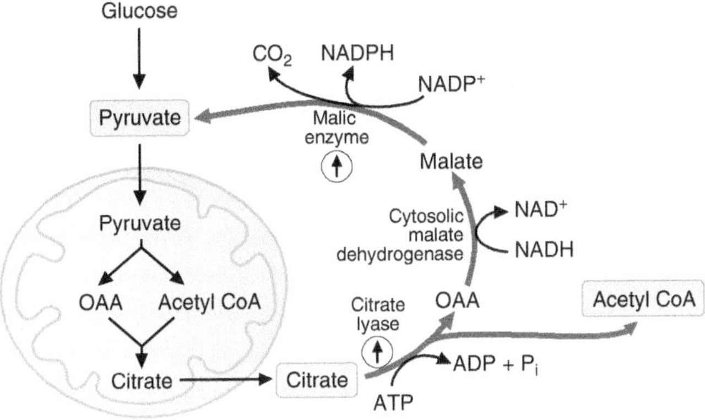

Citrate leaving the mitochondria and delivering acetyl-CoA to the cytoplasm for fatty acid synthesis.

produce acetyl-CoA and oxaloacetate. The oxaloacetate is recycled to pyruvate, producing NADPH in the process, which is also required for fatty acid biosynthesis. A defect in either carnitine acyl transferase will not affect fatty acid biosynthesis, as those enzymes are required to transport the fatty acid into the mitochondria for its oxidation. A lack of glucose-6-phosphate dehydrogenase will not interfere with fatty acid synthesis, as malic enzyme can provide sufficient NADPH for the pathway. MCAD is involved in fatty acid oxidation and does not affect fatty acid synthesis.

13 **The answer is B.** α-oxidation leads to the oxidation of the α-carbon of a branched chain fatty acid to generate an α-keto acid, which undergoes oxidative decarboxylation. This reorients the methyl groups on the branched chain fatty acid such that they are on the α-carbon, rather than the β-carbon. In this manner, the methyl groups do not interfere with the β-oxidation spiral (if the methyl group were on the β-carbon, a carbonyl group would be unable to form on that carbon, which would block further oxidation of the fatty acid). Answer choices A, C, D, and E are eliminated as requiring α-oxidation because, after one round of normal β-oxidation, the methyl group (or butyl group) will be on the α-carbon and would not interfere with the β-oxidation spiral. An overview of α-oxidation is shown below.

β-Oxidation

CH_3 CH_3 CH_3 CH_3 COO^-

CH_3

α-Oxidation

The figure depicts the oxidation of phytanic acid. A peroxisomal α-hydroxylase oxidizes the α-carbon, and its subsequent oxidation to a carboxyl group releases the carboxyl group as carbon dioxide. Subsequent spirals of peroxisomal β-oxidation alternately release propionyl and acetyl-CoA.

14 **The answer is A: Oxidation of very long chain fatty acids.** The child has Zellweger's syndrome, an absence of peroxisomal enzyme activity. Of the pathways listed as answers, only the oxidation of very long chain fatty acids is a peroxisomal function. Fatty acid synthesis occurs in the cytoplasm. Acetyl-CoA oxidation takes place in the mitochondria. Glucose oxidation is a combination of glycolysis (cytoplasm) and the TCA cycle (mitochondria). Triglyceride synthesis occurs in the cytoplasm.

15 **The answer is C: To reduce thromboxane synthesis.** Thromboxane A2 release from platelets is an essential element of forming blood clots, and aspirin will block prostaglandin, prostacyclin, and thromboxane synthesis. It is the thromboxane inhibition which reduces the risk of blood clots. Leukotrienes and lipoxins require the enzyme lipoxygenase, which is not inhibited by aspirin. These pathways are outlined below.

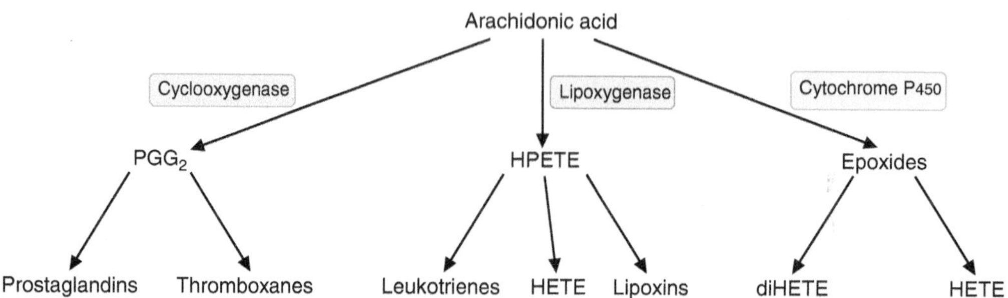

16 **The answer is D: acyl-carnitine.** With a carnitine deficiency, fatty acids cannot be added to carnitine, and acyl-carnitine would not be synthesized. With a carnitine acyl-transferase 2 deficiency, the fatty acids are added to carnitine, but the acyl-carnitine cannot release the acyl group within the mitochondria. This will lead to an accumulation of acylcarnitine, which will lead to an accumulation in the circulation. The end result of either deficiency is a lack of fatty acid oxidation, such that ketone body levels would be minimal under both conditions, and blood glucose levels would also be similar in either condition. Insulin release is not affected by either deficiency, and carnitine levels, normally low, would not be significantly modified in either deficiency.

17 **The answer is C: COX-2 is specifically induced during inflammation.** COX-2 is induced during inflammatory conditions, while COX-1 is constitutively expressed. Thus, when an injury occurs, and an immune response is mounted at the site of injury, COX-2 is induced in those cells to produce second messengers that play a role in mediating the pain response. Specifically inhibiting the COX-2 isozyme will block the production of those second messengers, without affecting the normal function of COX-1. Inhibiting COX-1 may reduce the frequency of heart attacks, and inhibiting COX-2 will block prostaglandin production via the cylco-oxygenase. Recent data suggests that certain drugs that specifically block COX-2 have unwanted side effects, such as an increase in heart attacks.

18 **The answer is E: Reduced ability to form malonyl-CoA.** Biotinidase is required to remove covalently-bound biotin from proteins, which is how most of the biotin in our diet is received. In the absence of biotinidase, individuals can become functionally biotin-deficient, due to the lack of free biotin in the body (as compared to being covalently bound to proteins). The formation of malonyl-CoA, via acetyl-CoA carboxylase, requires biotin as a required cofactor (see the figure below). Citrate lyase, malic enzyme, acetyl transacylase (an activity of fatty acid synthase) and acyl carrier protein (another component of fatty acid synthase) do not require biotin for their activity.

$CH_3-\overset{O}{\overset{\|}{C}}\sim SCoA$

Acetyl CoA

CO_2, Biotin, ATP → ADP + P_i (Acetyl CoA carboxylase)

$^{-}O-\overset{O}{\overset{\|}{C}}-CH_2-\overset{O}{\overset{\|}{C}}\sim SCoA$

Malonyl CoA

19 **The answer is B: Activation of pyruvate carboxylase.** Fatty acid oxidation increases the levels of acetyl-CoA within the mitochondrial matrix, and acetyl-CoA is a potent activator of pyruvate carboxylase, a key gluconeogenic enzyme (it will convert pyruvate to oxaloacetate, a necessary first step to bypass the irreversible pyruvate kinase reaction). Acetyl-CoA cannot be used to synthesize net glucose, so it is not an effective precursor of glucose production. Acetyl-CoA does not activate PEP carboxykinase (that enzyme is transcriptionally controlled), nor does it affect pyruvate kinase (a cytoplasmic enzyme). PFK-2 is not regulated by acetyl-CoA (phosphorylation by protein kinase A is the key regulator effect for PFK-2 in the liver).

20 **The answer is D: Fatty acid transport into the mitochondria.** The man had eaten the unripe fruit of the ackee tree (from Jamaica). The unripened fruit contains the toxin hypoglycin A, which will interfere with carnitine's ability to transport acyl-carnitine groups across the inner mitochondrial membrane. This leads to a complete shutdown of fatty acid oxidation in all tissues in the affected individual, leading to severe hypoglycemia. Hypoglycin has no effect on fatty acid release from the adipocyte, or fatty acid entry into liver cells. Fatty acid oxidation is not directly inhibited, nor does this toxin directly inhibit the complexes of the electron transport chain and the proton-translocating ATPase.

Chapter 14

HMP Shunt and Oxidative Reactions

This chapter covers questions related to the pentose phosphate shunt pathway and reactions that generate and protect against radical oxygen species. Interactions of this pathway with other metabolic pathways are also emphasized.

QUESTIONS

Select the single best answer.

1 A 52-year-old man has had bouts of alcohol abuse in his past. During his binges, he takes acetaminophen to help control some muscle pain. He then gets very ill (nausea, vomiting, and right upper quadrant pain), and is rushed to the emergency department. A potential treatment for this patient's symptoms is to take which of the following?

(A) Aspirin
(B) A mercaptan
(C) Rifampin
(D) Iron
(E) Vitamin C

2 A 34-year-old man was prescribed barbiturates 6 months ago for a seizure disorder. However, with time, the physician has had to increase his daily dosage to maintain the same therapeutic drug level. This is due to which of the following?

(A) Downregulation of drug receptors on the cell surface
(B) Decreased absorption of the drug from the stomach
(C) Increased synthesis of opposing neurotransmitters
(D) Induction of drug-metabolizing enzymes
(E) Induction of targeted enzyme synthesis

3 Considering the patient in question 2, one night, the patient consumes a large amount of alcohol. He continues to take his usual dose of seizure medication. He dies that night in his sleep. This is due to which of the following?

(A) Ethanol stimulating barbiturate absorption by the stomach
(B) Ethanol inhibition of a cytochrome P450 system
(C) Acetaldehyde reacting with the drug, creating a toxic compound
(D) Acetyl-CoA production leads to enhanced energy production, which synergizes with barbiturate action
(E) Ethanol's dehydration effect leads to toxic concentrations of the seizure medication in the blood

4 A chronic alcoholic presents to the emergency department with nystagmus, peripheral edema, pulmonary edema, ataxia, and mental confusion. The physician orders a test to determine if there is a vitamin deficiency. An enzyme used for such a test can be which of the following?

(A) Transaldolase
(B) Aldolase
(C) Transketolase
(D) β-ketothiolase
(E) Acetylcholine synthase

5 A researcher is studying the HMP shunt pathway in extracts of red blood cells, in the absence of $NADP^+$, and in which PFK-1 has been chemically inactivated. Which carbon substrates are required to generate ribose-5-phosphate in this system?

(A) Glucose-6-phosphate and sedoheptulose-7-phosphate
(B) Glucose-6-phosphate and glyceraldehyde-3-phosphate
(C) Fructose-6-phosphate and glyceraldehyde-3-phosphate
(D) Fructose-6-phosphate and pyruvate
(E) Glucose-6-phosphate and pyruvate

6 Which one of the following is an obligatory intermediate in the conversion of ribose-5-phosphate to glucose-6-phosphate?
(A) Pyruvate
(B) 1,3-bisphosphoglycerate
(C) Oxaloacetate
(D) Xylulose-5-phosphate
(E) 6-phosphogluconate

7 A 23-year-old man of Mediterranean descent was recently prescribed ciprofloxacin to treat a urinary tract infection. After 2 days on the drug, the patient was feeling worse, and weak, and went to the emergency department. He was found to have hemolytic anemia. This most likely resulted due to which of the following?
(A) Induction of red blood cell cytochrome P450s, leading to membrane damage
(B) Oxidative damage to red blood cell membranes
(C) Drug induced ion pores in the red blood cell membrane
(D) Drug induced inhibition of the HMP shunt pathway
(E) Oxidative damage to bone marrow, interfering with red blood cell production

8 You are seeing a male patient of African American descent, whose grandparents live in a chloroquine resistant malaria belt in Africa. He wants to visit his grandparents, and you want to give him primaquine as a malaria prophylaxis, but before you do so, you should test the patient for which of the following nonsymptomatic enzymatic deficiencies?
(A) Transketolase
(B) Pyruvate dehydrogenase
(C) α-Ketoglutarate dehydrogenase
(D) Glucose-6-phosphate dehydrogenase
(E) Glyceraldehyde-3-phosphate dehydrogenase

9 A patient has an insidious and steadily progressing neurologic disorder that, after several years, results in wasting and paralysis of the muscles of the limbs and trunk, loss of ability to speak, and swallowing difficulties. His paternal uncle had the same disease. A mutation in which enzyme may lead to these symptoms?
(A) Superoxide dismutase
(B) Catalase
(C) Myeloperoxidase
(D) NO synthase
(E) Tyrosine hydroxylase

10 A researcher has generated a cell line in which the γ-glutamyl cycle is defective, and glutathione cannot be synthesized. Which radical species might you initially expect to accumulate in this cell?
(A) Superoxide
(B) Nitrogen dioxide
(C) Nitrous oxide
(D) Hydrogen peroxide
(E) Peroxynitrate

11 A 25-year-old African American male, in good health, had read about fava beans in "Silence of the Lambs." For dinner one night, the man had liver with fava beans and a nice Chianti. About 8 h after eating the beans, the man was tired and weak. Blood work showed hemolytic anemia. This patient most likely has a defect in regenerating which of the following?
(A) NADH
(B) NAD^+
(C) Reduced glutathione
(D) Oxidized glutathione
(E) ATP

12 A 52-year-old male complained of sudden onset of left-sided chest pain radiating down his left arm. Rapid breathing, sweating, and a feeling of doom accompanied this. He was rushed to the emergency department. An angiogram revealed 90% occlusion of the left anterior descending artery (LAD) and no occlusions in any other artery. The LAD was opened by angioplasty. However, shortly after this procedure, with normal blood flow through the LAD, the patient's condition worsened. This was most likely due to which of the following?
(A) Disruption of the HMP shunt in cardiac cells
(B) Damage to healthy cells by loss of essential enzymes from cells due to membrane damage
(C) Development of intimal narrowing in another artery
(D) Radical-induced damage once blood flow was reinitiated
(E) Lack of glycogen for ATP synthesis in the heart

13 Consider an intestinal epithelial cell in S phase, and for which the major, active biosynthetic pathway is nucleotide synthesis. Which one of the following best represents the activity state of a series of key enzymes under these conditions?

	Glucose-6-phosphate dehydrogenase	Transketolase	PFK-1
(A)	Active	Active	Active
(B)	Active	Inactive	Inactive
(C)	Inactive	Active	Inactive
(D)	Inactive	Inactive	Active
(E)	Inactive	Active	Active

14 A researcher is studying cultured human hepatocytes and is examining the specific condition in which fatty acid synthesis is activated, but the cell remains in the G_0 phase of the cell cycle. Under such conditions, what would be the activity state of the following enzymes?

	Glucose-6-phosphate dehydrogenase	Transketolase	Transaldolase	Fructose-1, 6-bisphosphatase
(A)	Active	Active	Inactive	Inactive
(B)	Active	Active	Active	Active
(C)	Active	Inactive	Active	Inactive
(D)	Inactive	Active	Inactive	Active
(E)	Inactive	Inactive	Active	Inactive

15 Individuals with a superactive glutathione reductase will develop gout. This occurs due to which of the following?
(A) Activation of glucose-6-phosphate dehydrogenase
(B) Inhibition of glucose-6-phosphate dehydrogenase
(C) Activation of transketolase
(D) Activation of transaldolase
(E) Inhibition of transketolase

16 Glucose-6-phosphate labeled in carbon 6 with ^{14}C was added to a test tube with the enzymes phosphohexose isomerase, PFK-1, aldolase, transketolase, and transaldolase. ATP was also added to the test tube. At equilibrium, in which position would the radioactive label be found in the newly produced ribose-5-phosphate?
(A) 1
(B) 2
(C) 3
(D) 4
(E) 5

17 Which one of the following disorders would lead to increased activity of the HMP shunt pathway?
(A) Glycogen phosphorylase deficiency
(B) Glucose-6-phosphatase deficiency
(C) Fructose-1,6-bisphosphatase deficiency
(D) Pyruvate kinase deficiency
(E) Pyruvate dehydrogenase deficiency

18 A 45-year-old man was diagnosed with hypercholesterolemia, for which he was prescribed a statin. After a month on medications, the patient decided to adopt a healthier life style and replaced eggs and coffee for breakfast with fruit juices and whole-wheat toast. Within 2 weeks of changing his diet, the man developed severe muscle pain in his arms and shoulders. The muscle pain could be the result of which of the following?
(A) Induction of a detoxifying cytochrome P450 system
(B) Inhibition of a detoxifying cytochrome P450 system
(C) Increased mevalonate inhibiting actin/myosin interactions
(D) Increased mevalonate stabilizing actin/myosin interactions
(E) HMG-CoA stimulation of calcium efflux from the sarcoplasmic reticulum

19 A patient is recovering from acute respiratory distress syndrome (ARDS). Which of the following is a major antioxidant found in the fluid lining the bronchial epithelium needed in high concentration for recovery from ARDS?
(A) Glucuronic acid
(B) Pyruvate
(C) Sorbitol
(D) Glycogen
(E) Glutathione

20 Which of the following biochemical pathways produces the antioxidant referred to in the previous question?
(A) TCA cycle
(B) Glycolysis
(C) γ-Glutamyl cycle
(D) HMP shunt
(E) Polyol pathway

ANSWERS

1 **The answer is B: A mercaptan.** The man is suffering from acetaminophen poisoning. As shown below, MEOS (the microsomal ethanol oxidizing system, also named CYP2E1) will convert acetaminophen into a toxic intermediate. In a chronic alcoholic, the MEOS has been induced and is very active. The toxic intermediate (NAPQI) can be rendered inactive by adding glutathione to the compound for safe excretion, and glutathione is a mercaptan (a compound with a free sulfhydryl group). Individuals with acetaminophen poisoning are given N-acetyl cysteine as a mechanism to increase glutathione production. Iron and vitamin C will not aid in detoxifying the toxic intermediate. Rifampin blocks RNA polymerase in bacteria. Aspirin will block cyclooxygenase, but will not stimulate NAPQI excretion.

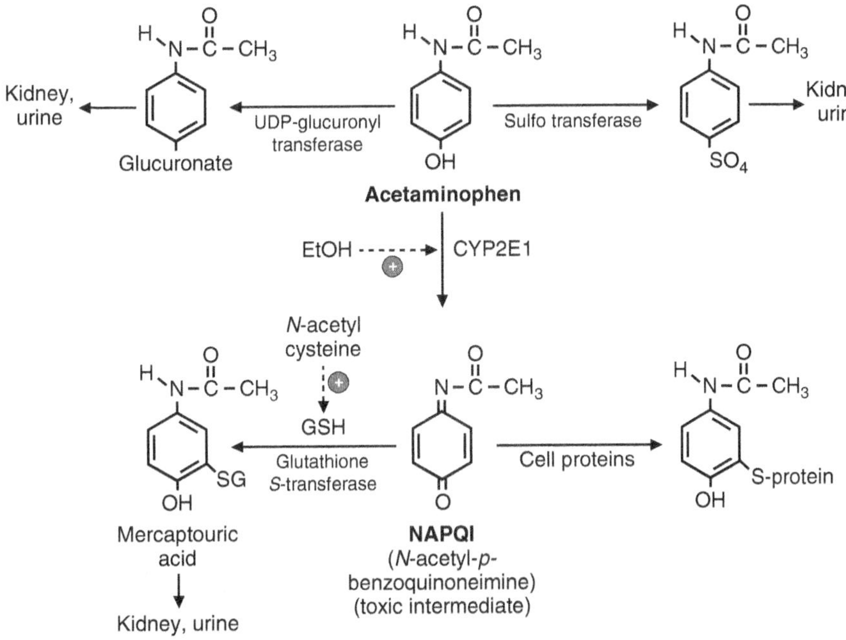

2 **The answer is D: Induction of drug-metabolizing enzymes.** Barbiturates are xenobiotics, and the body induces specific cytochrome P450 systems to help detoxify and excrete the barbiturates. When the man first begins taking the drug, a low concentration of drug is sufficient to exert a physiological effect, as the drug detoxifying system has not yet been induced. As the detoxifying system is induced, however, higher concentrations of drug are required to have the same effect, as the rate of excretion of the drug is increased as the detoxification system is induced. The "tolerance" to drugs, in this case, is not due to downregulation of drug receptors or decreased absorption of the drug from the stomach. There is no induction of target gene expression, leading to enhanced drug action, nor are opposing neurotransmitters expressed. The tolerance comes about due to enhanced inactivation of the drug due to the induction of drug-metabolizing enzymes.

3 **The answer is B: Ethanol inhibition of a cytochrome P450 system.** Ethanol inhibits the drug detoxifying system for barbiturates; thus, in the presence of ethanol, the high levels of barbiturates being taken (due to the tolerance) are now toxic (the system that breaks down the drug has been inhibited). Ethanol does not increase absorption of the drug from the digestive tract, nor does acetaldehyde, ethanol's oxidation product, react with barbiturates. Barbiturate action is not affected by energy production (acetyl-CoA). The ethanol inhibition of cytochrome P450 systems is also not due to ethanol's dehydration effect.

4 **The answer is C: Transketolase.** The patient is experiencing the symptoms of vitamin B_1 (thiamine) deficiency. Ethanol blocks thiamine absorption from the gut, so in the United States, one will usually only see a B_1 deficiency in chronic alcoholics. One assay for B_1 deficiency is to measure transketolase activity (which requires B_1 as an essential cofactor) in the presence and absence of added B_1. If the activity level increases when B_1 is added, a vitamin deficiency is assumed. None of the other enzymes listed (transaldolase, aldolase, β-ketothiolase, and acetylcholine synthase) require B_1 as a cofactor,

and, thus, could not be used as a measure of B_1 levels. A reaction catalyzed by transketolase is shown below (note the breakage of a carbon–carbon bond, and then the synthesis of a carbon–carbon bond to generate the product of the reaction).

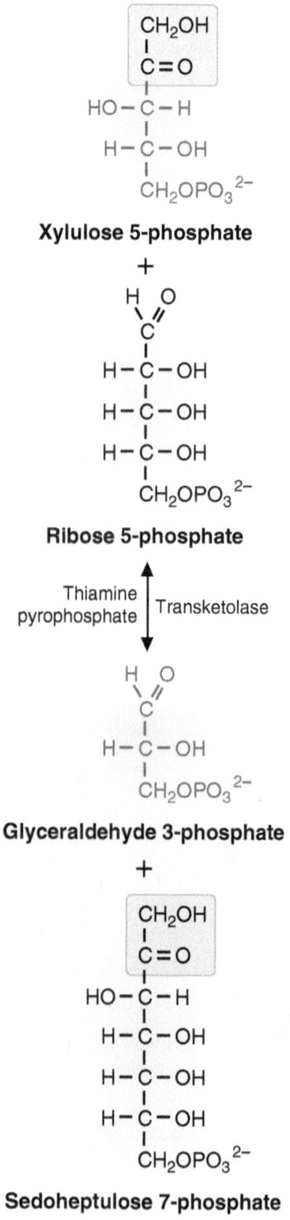

CH_2OH – C=O – HO–C–H – H–C–OH – $CH_2OPO_3^{2-}$

Xylulose 5-phosphate

+

HC=O – H–C–OH – H–C–OH – H–C–OH – $CH_2OPO_3^{2-}$

Ribose 5-phosphate

Thiamine pyrophosphate ⇅ Transketolase

HC=O – H–C–OH – $CH_2OPO_3^{2-}$

Glyceraldehyde 3-phosphate

+

CH_2OH – C=O – HO–C–H – H–C–OH – H–C–OH – H–C–OH – $CH_2OPO_3^{2-}$

Sedoheptulose 7-phosphate

5 **The answer is C: Fructose-6-phosphate and glyceraldehyde-3-phosphate.** In the absence of $NADP^+$, the oxidative steps of the HMP shunt pathway are nonfunctional, so only the nonoxidative steps will occur. In addition, PFK-1 has been made nonfunctional, such that glyceraldehyde-3-phosphate (G3P) cannot be produced from either fructose-6-phosphate (F6P) or glucose-6-phosphate (G6P). In order to generate ribose-5-phosphate (R5P) under these conditions, both F6P and G3P need to be provided. These two substrates will react, using transketolase as a substrate, to generate erythrose-4-phosphate (E4P) and xylulose-5-phosphate (X5P, step 1 in the figure below). The X5P will be epimerized to ribulose-5-phosphate (Ru5P, step 2 in the figure below), and then isomerized to R5P (step 3 in the figure below). Glucose-6-phosphate cannot be used as a substrate because it cannot be converted to G3P (due to the block in PFK-1). Pyruvate cannot be used as a substrate in extracts of red blood cells because such cells do not have pyruvate carboxylase, so the pyruvate cannot be converted to either F6P or G3P.

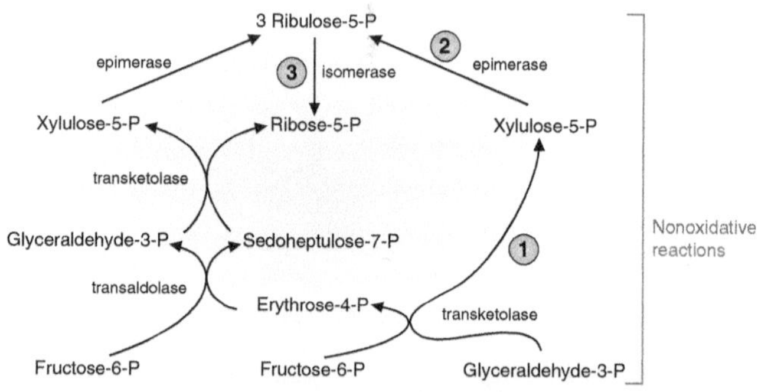

6 **The answer is D: Xylulose-5-phosphate.** In order for ribose-5-phosphate to be converted to glucose-6-phosphate, the nonoxidative reactions of the HMP shunt pathway must be used (the oxidative steps are not reversible reactions). In order for this to occur, the ribose-5-phosphate is isomerized to ribulose-5-phosphate, which is then epimerized to xylulose-5-phosphate (steps 1 and 2 in the figure on page 123). R5P and X5P then initiate a series of reactions utilizing transketolase (step 3 in the figure on page 123) and transaldolase (step 4 in the figure on page 123) to generate fructose-6-phosphate, which can be isomerized to glucose-6-phosphate (step 5 in the figure on page 123). Glyceraldehyde-3-phosphate is also formed during this series of reactions, which then goes back to fructose-6-phosphate production. Pyruvate, oxaloacetate, 1,3-bisphosphoglycerate, and 6-phosphogluconoate are not obligatory intermediates in this conversion.

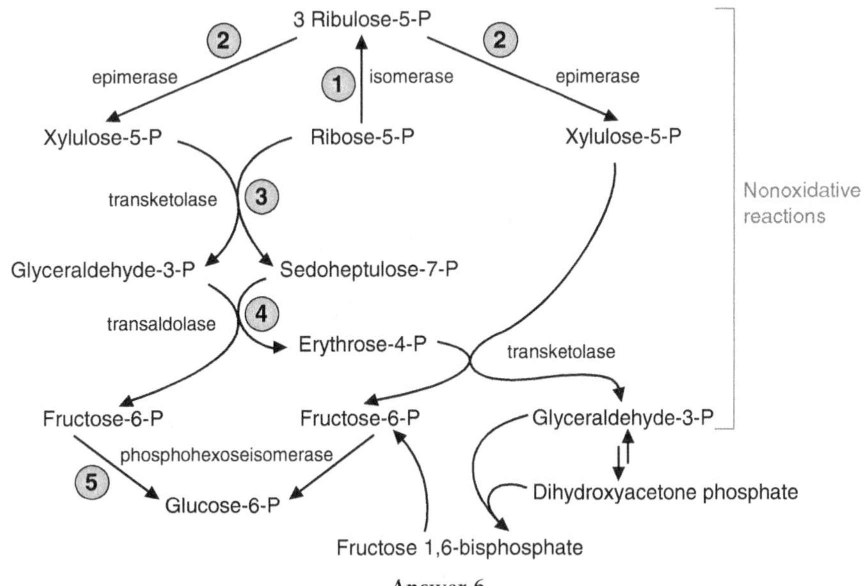

Answer 6

7 **The answer is B: Oxidative damage to red blood cell membranes.** The man has glucose-6-phosphate dehydrogenase deficiency and is incapable of regenerating reduced glutathione to protect red blood cell membranes from oxidative damage. In the presence of a strong oxidizing agent (the new drug the patient was taking), the red cell membranes undergo oxidative damage and the red cell bursts, leading to hemolytic anemia. This is all due to a lack of protective glutathione in the membrane. As the red cell lacks a nucleus, the cell cannot induce new gene synthesis. The drug the patient was taking does not induce ion pores in red cell membranes or inhibit the HMP shunt pathway. It also does not cause oxidative damage to bone marrow. The drugs to avoid while prescribing for a patient with a G6PDH deficiency include primaquine, dapsone, nitrofurantoin, and sulfonylurea. The reduced (Panel A) and oxidized (Panel B) forms of glutathione are indicated to the side.

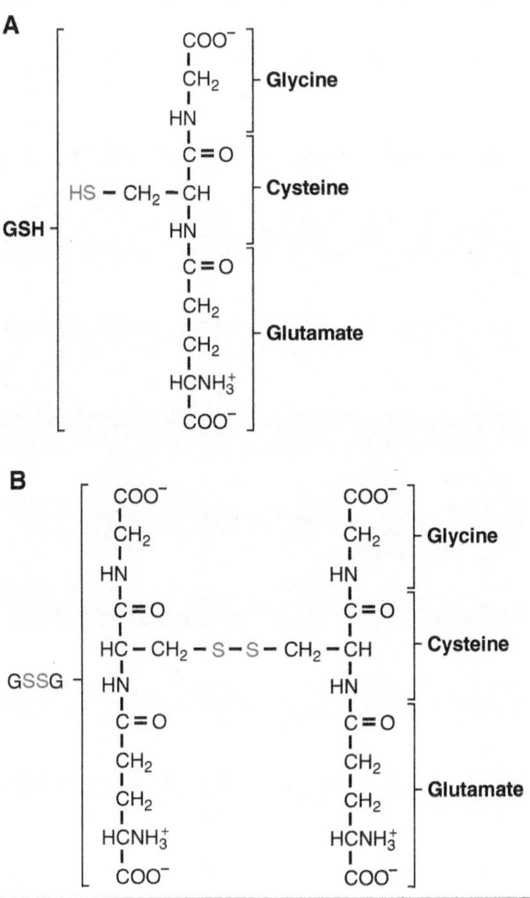

Answer 7: **Panel A** indicates reduced glutathione (GSH) while **Panel B** indicates oxidized glutathione (GSSG).

8 **The answer is D: Glucose-6-phosphate dehydrogenase.** Given the demographics of the patient's ancestry (and the need for obtaining an accurate history), and the fact that the patient is a male, the patient may have glucose-6-phosphate dehydrogenase deficiency (an X-linked disorder). If a person with this enzyme deficiency is given primaquine, which is a strong oxidizing agent, hemolytic anemia is likely to develop. If a physician suspects that a patient may have such an enzymatic deficiency, it is imperative to check before prescribing strong oxidizing agents to the patient, or prescribe another antimalarial prophylaxis that is not a strong oxidizing agent (such as tetracycline). If individuals were deficient in transketolase, pyruvate dehydrogenase, α-ketoglutarate dehydrogenase, or glyceraldehyde-3-phosphate dehydrogenase, red cell lysis would not occur. One should also recall that the red cells lack mitochondria, so these cells do not contain pyruvate dehydrogenase or α-ketoglutarate dehydrogenase.

9 **The answer is A: Superoxide dismutase.** The patient is experiencing the symptoms of familial ALS. A mutation in superoxide dismutase 1 (SOD1) in humans has been linked to the development of familial ALS through an unknown mechanism. Familial ALS only constitutes between 5% and 10% of all ALS cases diagnosed. The disease process, when SOD1 is mutated, is not linked to a loss of enzymatic activity, although the SOD1 may have been mutated such that it will produce other radical species and is no longer specific for superoxide. A second model proposes a misfolding problem similar to prion disease. For more information on such models see Nature Med. 2000;6:1320–1321 and Ann Neurol. 2007 Dec;62(6):553–559. None of the other enzymes listed (catalase, myeloperoxidase, NO synthase, and tyrosine hydroxylase) have been linked to the development of ALS, or an ALSlike disease. The reaction catalyzed by SOD1 is shown below.

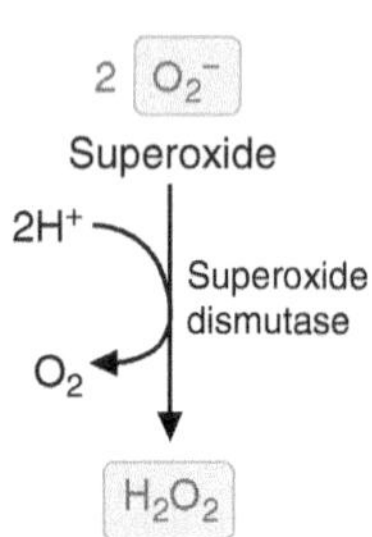

10 **The answer is D: Hydrogen peroxide.** In the absence of glutathione, the enzyme glutathione peroxidase will be less active due to the lowered concentration of glutathione. Glutathione peroxidase catalyzes the oxidation of two reduced glutathione molecules by hydrogen peroxide, generating oxidized glutathione and two molecules of water. As glutathione peroxidase is one mechanism whereby hydrogen peroxide levels are reduced, hydrogen peroxide would be expected to accumulate, and can then lead to radical damage of membrane proteins and lipids. Glutathione peroxidase does not require, or react with, superoxide, nitrogen dioxide, nitrous oxide, and peroxynitrate. It is possible that under these conditions, superoxide would also accumulate, due to the increase in concentration of one of the reaction products of superoxide dismutase, hydrogen peroxide. However, there is no evidence that hydrogen peroxide accumulation will inhibit the reaction catalyzed by superoxide dismutase.

11 **The answer is C: Reduced glutathione.** The patient has glucose-6-phosphate dehydrogenase deficiency, and his red blood cells cannot convert oxidized glutathione to reduced glutathione due to a lack of NADPH. Fava beans contain a potent oxidizing agent that will, in some patients (but not all), lead to hemolytic anemia in individuals with glucose-6-phosphate dehydrogenase deficiency; in individuals with a normal G6PDH, the oxidizing agent is handled by glutathione. The red blood cells, under these conditions, do not have a problem in regenerating NADH, NAD^+, or ATP.

12 **The answer is D: Radical induced damage once blood flow was reinitiated.** The patient is experiencing ischemic reperfusion injury. When oxygen delivery to cardiac cells was compromised, the electron transfer chain in the mitochondria was fully reduced, as the terminal oxygen acceptor was missing. When oxygen is reintroduced to the cell, at a high concentration, the likelihood of electron transfer from reduced coenzyme Q to oxygen is increased, such that the possibility of superoxide generation is increased. The superoxide produced reacts with lipids and proteins and can lead to cell death above that originally occurring from the initial heart attack. Radicals do not form during the ischemic event since oxygen is missing from the tissues. There is no effect on glycogen stores or the HMP shunt pathway under these conditions. Intimal narrowing occurs over a long time period, not over the short time period covered in this case. Injured cells do leak enzymes into the bloodstream, but these enzymes do not cause the death of other, healthy cells.

13 **The answer is E.** Under the conditions described, DNA synthesis is occurring without any requirement for NADPH (such as fatty acid synthesis). Under these conditions, NADPH levels are high and glucose-6-phosphate dehydrogenase is inactive. The cell requires ribose-5-phosphate, however, for nucleotide biosynthesis, and this is synthesized from fructose-6-phosphate and glyceraldehyde-3-phosphate using the nonoxidative reactions of the pathway. Thus, both transketolase and transaldolase will be active under these conditions. PFK-1 is active as well, as the only way to generate glyceraldehyde-3-phosphate from a sugar precursor is via enzymes of the glycolytic pathway.

14 **The answer is B.** The conditions of the cell indicate that NADPH is required for fatty acid synthesis, but there is no need for ribose-5-phosphate, as the cells are in G_0 phase and are not undergoing DNA synthesis (so nucleotides are not required). The HMP shunt will utilize the oxidative reactions to generate NADPH, and then the ribulose-5-phosphate produced will use the nonoxidative reactions to regenerate glucose-6 -phosphate. For this to occur, transketolase, transaldolase, glucose-6-phosphate dehydrogenase (as the major oxidative enzyme of the pathway), and fructose-1,6-bisphosphatase all have to be active. These nonoxidative reactions are indicated in the figure on page 125.

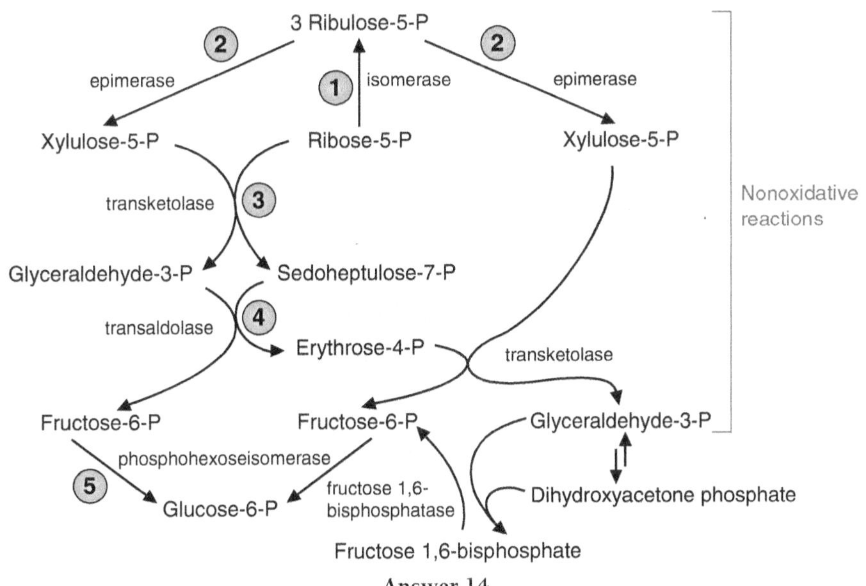

Answer 14

15 **The answer is A: Activation of glucose-6-phosphate dehydrogenase.** Glutathione reductase will utilize NADPH and reduce oxidized glutathione to reduced glutathione, generating $NADP^+$. If Glutathione reductase is superactive, $NADP^+$ levels accumulate, which activates glucose-6-phosphate dehydrogenase. This will lead to NADPH production via the oxidative reactions of the HMP shunt, along with ribulose-5-phosphate (Ru5P). The Ru5P will lead to increased ribose-5-phosphate production, increased 5′-phosphoribosyl 1′-pyrophosphate (PRPP) production, and increased 5′-phosphoribosyl 1′-amine levels. This eventually leads to increased purine production, in excess of what is required. The excess purines are converted to uric acid, and excess uric acid will lead to gout. A superactive glutathione reductase will not lead to an alteration in the activities of transketolase or transaldolase.

16 **The answer is E: 5.** Given the enzymes present, only the nonoxidative reactions of the HMP shunt would take place. In order for the nonoxidative reactions to occur, the glucose-6-phosphate (G6P, labeled in the 6th position with ^{14}C) must pass through glycolysis to produce fructose-6-phosphate (F6P, labeled in the 6th position) and glyceraldehyde-3-phosphate (labeled in the 3rd position). Transketolase will allow these two compounds to exchange carbons, which would generate erythrose-4-phosphate (E4P, labeled in the 4th position) and xylulose-5-phosphate (X5P, labeled in the 5th position). The X5P can then go to ribulose-5-phosphate (Ru5P) and ribose-5-phosphate (R5P), labeled in the fifth positions. The E4P (labeled in the 4th position) can react with another molecule of F6P (labeled in the 6th position) using transaldolase to generate sedoheptulose 7-phosphate (Se7P, labeled in the 7th position) and glyceraldehyde-3-phosphate (G3P), labeled in the 3rd position. Transketolase will then convert the Se7P and G3P to R5P and X5P, both labeled in the 5th positions. The nonoxidative reactions can be seen, schematically, in the figure below.

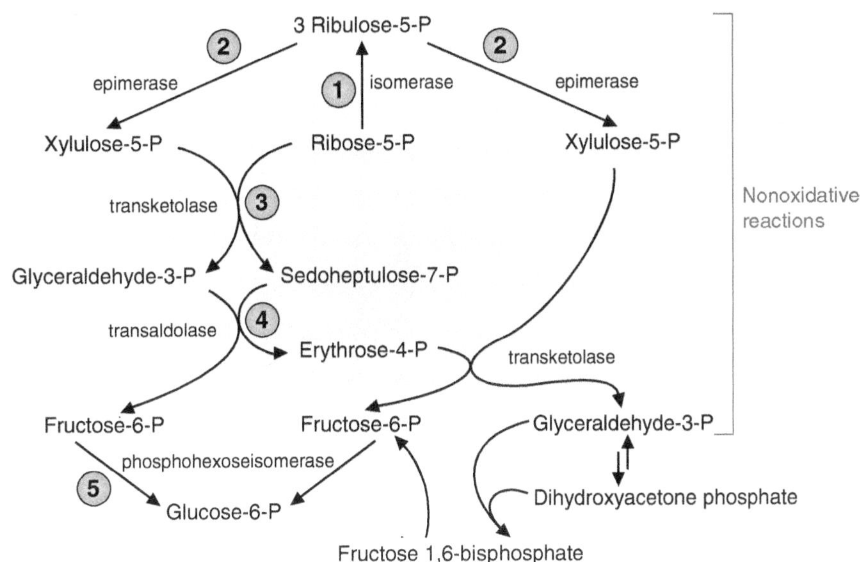

17 **The answer is B: Glucose-6-phosphatase deficiency.** The HMP shunt can have increased activity under two conditions, one being an increase in the cofactor $NADP^+$ levels and the other being an increase in the substrate levels (glucose-6-phosphate). The only enzyme listed, which when defective would lead to an increase in either glucose-6-phosphate or NADPH, is glucose-6-phosphatase. A deficiency in glycogen phosphorylase would not produce glucose-1-phosphate; thus, there would not be an increase in the HMP shunt under these conditions. A deficiency in fructose-1,6-bisphosphatase deficiency would impair gluconeogenesis and would not lead to the synthesis of glucose-6-phosphate. Deficiencies in either pyruvate carboxylase or pyruvate dehydrogenase would lead to pyruvate accumulation and NAD^+ accumulation, but not $NADP^+$ or glucose-6-phosphate accumulation.

18 **The answer is B: Inhibition of a detoxifying cytochrome P450 system.** The patient is suffering from the potential side effects of statins, namely, muscle damage and pain. This may occur due to an inhibition of coenzyme Q synthesis (which requires a product derived from mevalonic acid) and a lack of energy generation in the muscle. The reason this comes about is that statins are detoxified through a cytochrome P450 system, and the particular system that works on statins is inhibited by grapefruit juice. Thus, in the presence of grapefruit juice, the effective intracellular levels of statins are higher than in the absence of the juice, due to the decreased rate of destruction. The artificially induced higher levels of statins then lead to muscle damage. Statins inhibit the conversion of HMG-CoA to mevalonic acid (catalyzed by HMG-CoA reductase). Thus, answers indicating that mevalonic acid levels are increasing cannot be correct; they are reduced in the presence of a statin. Statins do not bring about calcium efflux from the sarcoplasmic reticulum.

19 **The answer is E: Glutathione.** Glutathione is the major antioxidant in the fluid lining the bronchial epithelium. It is essential for recovery of these tissues. Depletion of glutathione in the airway is thought to greatly increase a person's susceptibility to upper respiratory infections such as influenza. Glutathione is formed in the γ-glutamyl pathway, and oxidized glutathione is regenerated to reduced glutathione using NADPH produced by the HMP shunt pathway. None of the other answers (glycogen, sorbitol, pyruvate, and glucuronate) offer protection against oxidative damage. Glycogen is utilized for the storage of glucose. Pyruvate is the end product of glycolysis. Sorbitol is a product of the polyol pathway. Glucuronic acid is used for xenobiotic metabolism, in general, to increase the solubility of the xenobiotic and to prepare it for excretion.

20 **The answer is C: γ-Glutamyl cycle.** Glutathione is produced via the γ-glutamyl cycle; the HMP shunt pathway provides the NADPH that allows oxidized glutathione to be converted to reduced glutathione. The other pathways listed (TCA cycle, glycolysis, HMP shunt, and the polyol pathway) do not provide for glutathione synthesis. The TCA cycle is designed to oxidize acetyl-CoA to carbon dioxide and water. Glycolysis is the entry point of sugars into metabolism. The HMP shunt pathway generates five-carbon sugars and NADPH, and the polyol pathway generates sugar alcohols. The γ-glutamyl cycle is shown in the figure below.

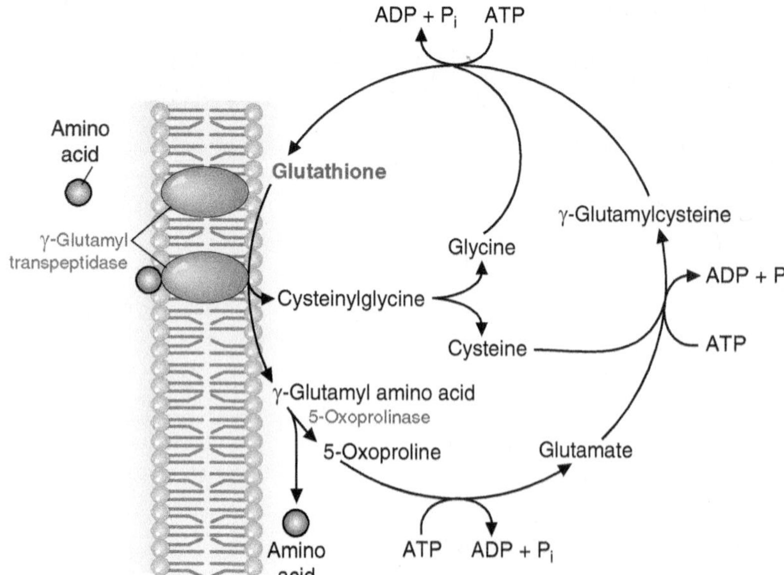

Answer 20: In cells of the intestine and kidney, amino acids can be transported across the cell membrane by reacting with glutathione to form a γ-glutamyl amino acid. The amino acid is released into the cell and glutathione is resynthesized. However, the major role of this cycle is glutathione synthesis because many tissues lack the transpeptidase and 5-oxoprolinase activities. Thus, the reactions performed by most cells include the condensation of cysteine and glutamate to form γ-glutamylcysteine and then the condensation of γ-glutamylcysteine with glycine to form glutathione.

Chapter 15

Amino Acid Metabolism and the Urea Cycle

This chapter quizzes the student on amino acid metabolism and products derived from amino acids.

QUESTIONS

Select the single best answer.

1 Routine newborn screening identified a child with elevated levels of phenylpyruvate and phenyllactate in the blood. Despite treating the child with a restricted diet, evidence of developmental delay became apparent. Supplementation with which of the following would be beneficial to the child?

(A) Tyrosine
(B) 5-hydroxytryptophan
(C) Melanin
(D) Phenylalanine
(E) Alanine

2 A newborn has milky white skin, white hair, and red-appearing eye color (see the figure below). This disorder

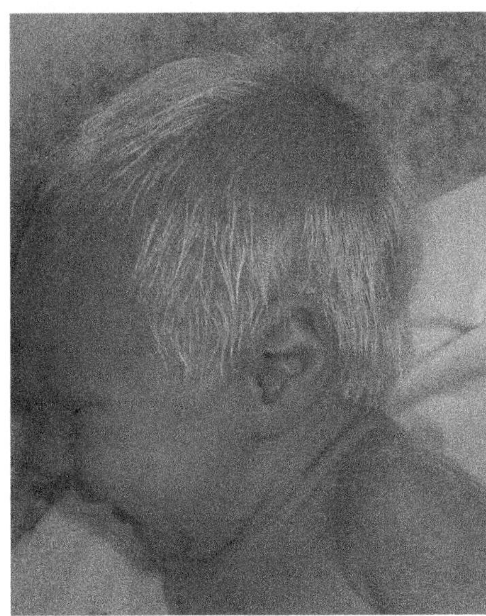

most often results from a defect in which of the following enzymes?

(A) Phenylalanine hydroxylase
(B) NADPH oxidase
(C) Dihydrofolate reductase
(D) Tyrosinase
(E) Homogentisic acid oxidase

3 A newborn becomes lethargic and drowsy 24 h after birth. Blood analysis shows hyperammonemia, coupled with orotic aciduria. This individual has an enzyme deficiency that leads to an inability to directly produce which of the following?

(A) Carbamoyl phosphate
(B) Ornithine
(C) Citrulline
(D) Argininosuccinate
(E) Arginine

4 Considering the patient in question 3, orotic acid levels are high in this patient due to which of the following?

(A) Elevated ammonia
(B) Elevated glutamine
(C) Bypassing carbamoyl phosphate synthetase II (CPS-II)
(D) Bypassing aspartate transcarbamoylase
(E) Inhibition of carbamoyl phosphate synthetase I (CPS-I)

5 Considering the patient discussed in the last two questions, a potential treatment for the patient is supplementation with which of the following?

(A) Arginine and glutamine
(B) Lysine and glutamine
(C) Arginine and benzoate
(D) Lysine and benzoate
(E) Glutamine and phenylbutyrate

6 Parents bring their 6-year-old son to the pediatrician due to the parents being concerned about "mental retardation." Blood work demonstrated a microcytic anemia and basophilic stippling. During the patient history, it became apparent that the boy often stayed with his grandparents, who owned a 150-year-old apartment. The boy admitted to eating paint chips from the radiators in the apartment. The boy's anemia is most likely the result of which one of the following?
(A) Inhibition of iron transport
(B) Reduction of heme synthesis
(C) Inhibition of the phosphatidyl inositol cycle
(D) Blockage of reticulocyte DNA synthesis
(E) Inhibition of β-globin gene expression

7 Routine newborn screening identified a child with elevated levels of α-ketoacids of the branched-chain amino acids. A certain subset of such children will respond well to which of the following vitamin supplementation?
(A) Niacin
(B) Riboflavin
(C) B_{12}
(D) B_6
(E) Thiamine

8 Another routine newborn screening identified a child with elevated levels of the branched-chain amino acids and their α-ketoacid derivatives. In addition, the child also exhibited lactic acidosis. Which enzyme listed below would you expect to be negatively affected (reduced activity) by this disorder?
(A) α-ketoglutarate dehydrogenase
(B) Isocitrate dehydrogenase
(C) Malate dehydrogenase
(D) Succinate dehydrogenase
(E) Acetyl-CoA carboxylase

9 A Russian child, 5 years old, was brought to the pediatrician for developmental delay. Blood analysis showed elevated levels of phenylalanine, phenyllactate, and phenylpyruvate. The developmental delay, in this condition, has been hypothesized to occur due to which of the following?
(A) Acidosis due to elevated phenyllactate
(B) Lack of tyrosine, now an essential amino acid
(C) Inhibition of hydroxylating enzymes due to accumulation of phenylalanine
(D) Lack of large, neutral amino acids in the brain
(E) Inhibition of neuronal glycolysis by phenylpyruvate

10 A 12-year-old boy is brought to the pediatrician because of behavioral problems noted by the parents. Upon examination, the physician notices brittle and coarse hair, red patches on the skin, long, thin arms and legs (reminiscent of Marfan syndrome patients), scoliosis, pectus excavatum, displaced lens, and muscular hypotonia. Blood work is likely to show an elevation of which of the following metabolites?
(A) Methionine
(B) Phenylpyruvate
(C) Cysteine
(D) Fibrillin fragments
(E) Homocystine

11 Considering the patient described in the previous questions, treatment with which of the following vitamins may be successful in controlling this disorder?
(A) B_1
(B) B_2
(C) B_3
(D) B_6
(E) B_{12}

12 A 13-year-old boy is admitted to the hospital due to flank and urinary pain. Analysis demonstrates the presence of kidney stones. The stones were composed of calcium oxalate. Family history revealed that the boy's father and mother had had similar problems. Oxalate accumulation arises in this patient due to difficulty in metabolizing which of the following?
(A) Alanine
(B) Leucine
(C) Lysine
(D) Glyoxylate
(E) Glycine

13 An 18-year-old boy was brought to the hospital by his mother due to a sudden onset of flank pain in his left side, radiating toward his pubic area. His urine was reddish-brown in color, and a urinalysis showed the presence of many red blood cells. When his urine was acidified with acetic acid, clusters of flat, hexagonal transparent crystals were noted. A radiograph of the abdomen showed radio-opaque stones in both kidneys. The boy eventually passed a stone whose major component was identified as cystine. A suggestion for treatment is which of the following?
(A) Increased ethanol consumption
(B) Restriction of dietary methionine
(C) Utilize drugs that acidify the urine
(D) Restrict dietary glycine
(E) Prescribe diuretics

14 You have an elderly patient with a history of heart attacks (MIs) and strokes (CVAs). Blood work indicates an elevated homocysteine level, which is reduced by the patient taking pharmacological doses of pyridoxamine. An enzyme that would benefit from such

treatment in lowering homocysteine levels is which of the following?
(A) Methionine synthase
(B) N5, N10 methylene tetrahydrofolate reductase
(C) Cystathionine β-synthase
(D) Cystathionase
(E) S-adenosyl homocysteine hydrolase

15 A 3-month-old boy of French–Canadian ancestry is seen by the pediatrician for failure to thrive and poor appetite. Physical exam denotes hepatomegaly and a yellowing of the eyes. The boy had been vomiting and had diarrhea, and a distinct cabbagelike odor was apparent. This disorder is due to a defect in the metabolism of which of the following amino acids?
(A) Alanine
(B) Tryptophan
(C) Tyrosine
(D) Histidine
(E) Lysine

16 Mr Smith had been prescribed a drug to treat his depression. One of the effects of the drug is to maintain elevated levels of a particular neurotransmitter that has been derived from which of the following amino acids?
(A) Tryptophan
(B) Tyrosine
(C) Glutamate
(D) Histidine
(E) Glycine

17 A patient has a "pill rolling" tremor, "cogwheel" rigidity, bradykinesis, speech difficulties, and a shuffling gait. The chemical that is lacking in this syndrome is a derivative of which of the following amino acids?
(A) Alanine
(B) Serine
(C) Tyrosine
(D) Tryptophan
(E) Phenylalanine

18 A patient presents with episodes of flushing, diarrhea, abdominal cramping, and wheezing. His blood pressure and pulse rate are normal during these episodes. Physical exam is normal except for scattered telangiectasias. In order to diagnose this problem, a 24-h urine collection for which of the following would be most appropriate?
(A) Vanillylmandelic acid (VMAs)
(B) Catechols
(C) Dopamine
(D) 5-hydroxyindoleacetic acid (5-HIAA)
(E) Cortisol

19 A patient taking a drug for depression experienced a greatly increased heart rate and sweating after eating red wine and gourmet, aged cheese. These symptoms appeared due to an inability to degrade which of the following?
(A) Tyrosine
(B) Tyramine
(C) Serotonin
(D) Glycine
(E) Glutamate

20 A 6-year-old boy is slightly anemic and is very sensitive to the sun, to the point where his skin blisters instead of healing normally from sunburn. His condition worsened when he was taking rifampin for a Methicillin Resistant Staph Aureus. The boy most likely has a defect in which of the following biochemical pathways?
(A) Glycogen synthesis
(B) Fatty acid oxidation
(C) DNA repair
(D) Transcription-coupled DNA repair
(E) Heme synthesis

ANSWERS

1 **The answer is B: 5-hydroxytryptophan.** The child has nonclassical phenylketonuria (PKU). Classical PKU is due to a defect in phenylalanine hydroxylase, leading to accumulation of phenylalanine derivatives. These interfere with amino acid transport into the brain and can lead to cognitive disorders if not treated, usually, by a low-phenylalanine diet. However, in nonclassical PKU, the required cofactor for the phenylalanine hydroxylase reaction, tetrahydrobiopterin, is deficient. This will lead to similar biochemical symptoms (elevation of phenylalanine derivatives), but, in addition, the catecholamines (dopamine, epinephrine, and norepinephrine) and serotonin cannot be synthesized as those pathways require tetrahydrobiopterin. Giving 5-hydroxytryptophan bypasses the block in serotonin biosynthesis, and would have to be a supplement for these children along with dihydroxyphenylalanine (DOPA), which is the hydroxylated precursor for catecholamine biosynthesis. Providing tyrosine will not overcome the block in neurotransmitter biosynthesis. Providing phenylalanine just makes the problem worse. Neither melanin nor alanine will bypass the metabolic block of this disease. The role of tetrahydrobiopterin, indicating its oxidation and subsequent reduction, in the phenylalanine hydroxylase reaction is shown below.

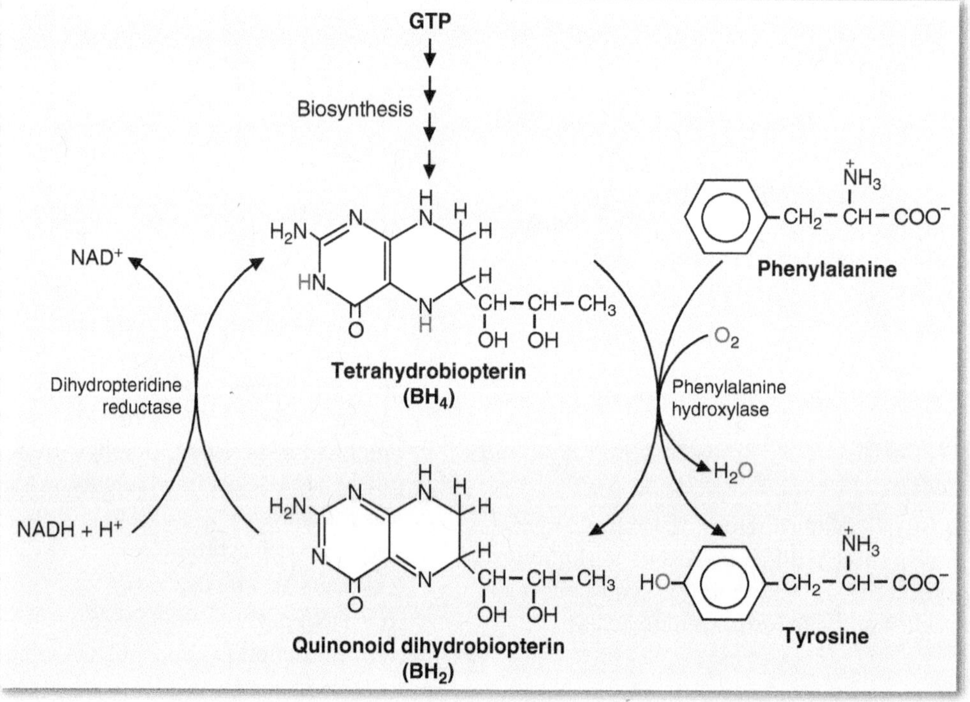

2 **The answer is D: Tyrosinase.** The child has albinism, a lack of pigment in the skin cells, which is produced by melanocytes. Melanocyte tyrosinase (a different isozyme than the neuronal tyrosinase that produces DOPA for catecholamine biosynthesis) is defective in albinism. The DOPA produced is then used for pigment production. A lack of phenylalanine hydroxylase leads to PKU. A lack of dihydrofolate reductase is most likely a lethal event as there are no reported cases of a lack of this enzyme. Tetrahydrofolate is not required for the conversion of tyrosine to DOPA in melanocytes. NADPH oxidase generates superoxide, which is not part of this pathway. Homogentisic acid is part of the phenylalanine and tyrosine degradation pathways, and is not involved in albinism.

3 **The answer is C: Citrulline.** The child has ornithine transcarbamoylase (OTC) deficiency, and cannot condense carbamoyl phosphate with ornithine to produce citrulline (see the figure on page 131). The excess carbamoyl phosphate produced leaks into the cytoplasm where it bypasses the regulated enzyme of de novo pyrimidine production, leading to excess orotic acid. Thus, in an OTC defect, carbamoyl phosphate can be produced, but citrulline cannot. Since citrulline cannot be produced, the later products of the urea cycle (argininosuccinate and arginine) are also produced at lower levels than normal, which is an indirect effect due to the inability to produce citrulline.

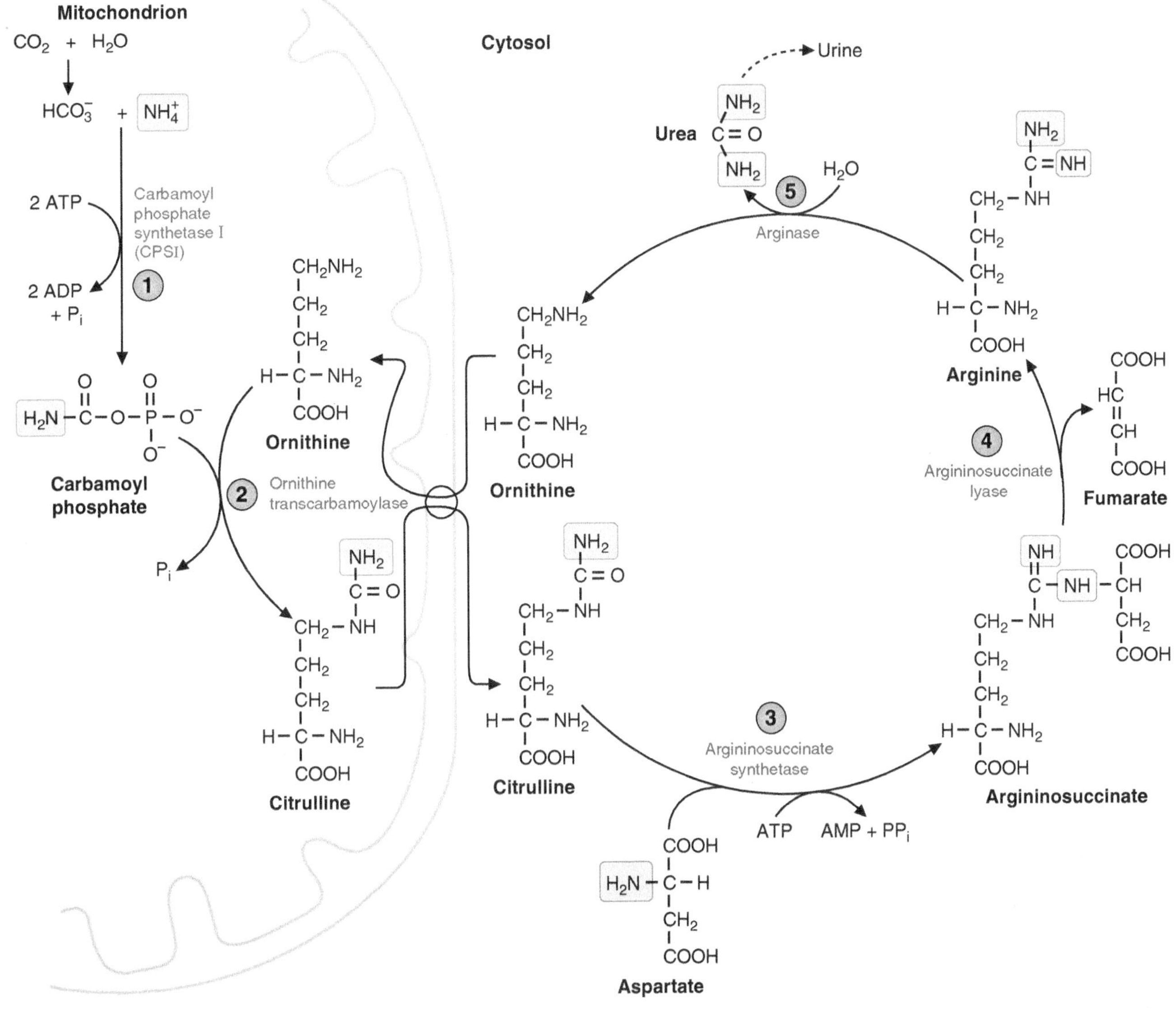

Answer 3: The urea cycle. Reaction 2 is defective in the disease described in this case.

4 **The answer is C: Bypassing carbamoyl phosphate synthetase II (CPS-II).** The rate-limiting step for de novo pyrimidine synthesis is carbamoyl phosphate synthetase II (CPS-II), which produces carbamoyl phosphate in the cytoplasm (see the figure on page 132). In an OTC deficiency, the carbamoyl phosphate produced in the mitochondria leaks into the cytoplasm, leading to orotic acid synthesis as the regulated step of the pathway is being bypassed. The elevated ammonia is not a substrate of CPS-II, and while glutamine is also elevated, and is a substrate of CPS-II, higher glutamine concentrations will not overcome enzyme inhibition by its allosteric inhibitor, UTP. Aspartate transcarbamoylase is the regulated step of pyrimidine biosynthesis in many prokaryotic cells, but not in humans. This step is necessary for pyrimidines to be synthesized starting with carbamoyl phosphate. CPS-I is a mitochondrial enzyme not involved in pyrimidine production.

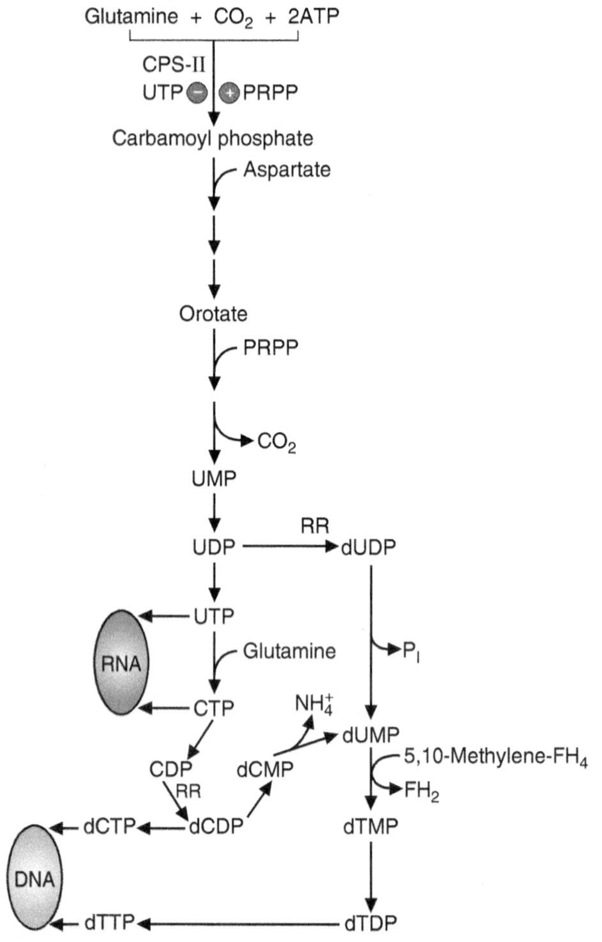

An overview of pyrimidine synthesis, indicating the regulation that occurs at the carbamoyl phosphate synthetase II step. If carbamoyl phosphate can be generated outside of this pathway (as in an ornithine transcarbamoylase deficiency), then pyrimidine synthesis will bypass its regulated step, and an overproduction of pyrimidines would result.

5 **The answer is C: Arginine and benzoate.** Whenever there is a urea cycle defect, arginine becomes an essential amino acid (as its route of synthesis is the urea cycle). Benzoate, along with phenylbutyrate, is given to patients with urea cycle defects to conjugate with a nitrogen carrying molecule (benzoate conjugates with glycine while phenylbutyrate, after activation to phenylacetate, conjugates with glutamine), which is then excreted. The reactions of benzoate and phenylbutyrate with nitrogen containing amino acids are shown above. The excretion of glycyl-benzoate reduces the glycine levels of the body, forcing more glycine to be produced and providing an alternative pathway for nitrogen disposal in the absence of a functional urea cycle. Giving lysine or glutamine will not help to reduce ammonia levels in the patient.

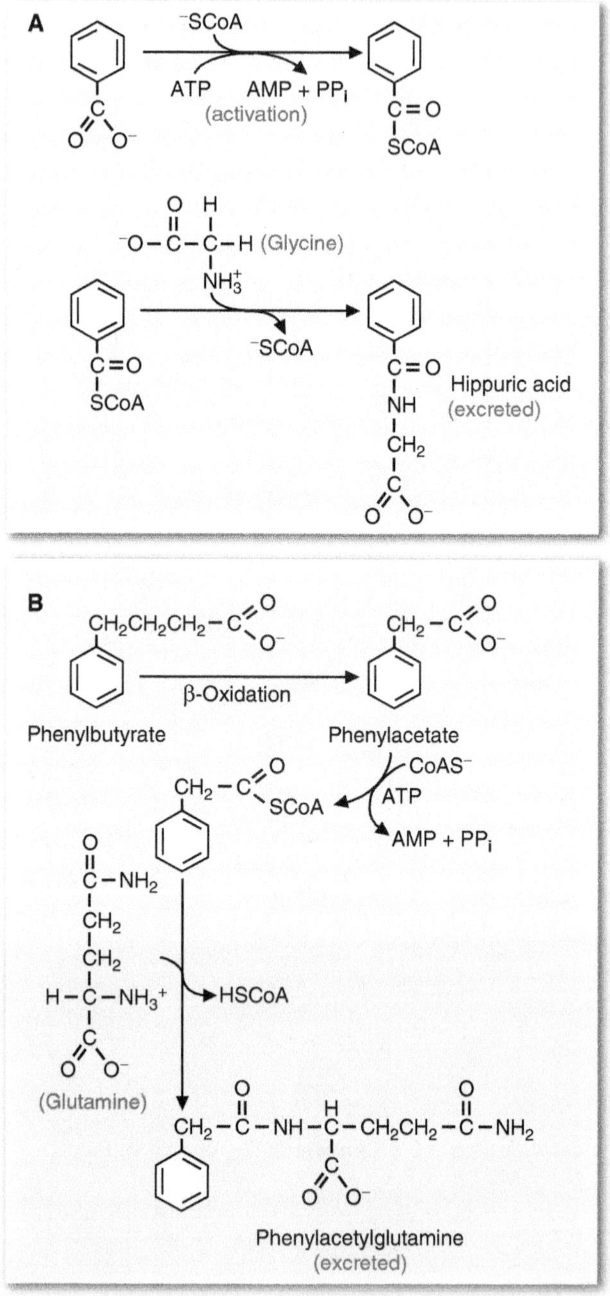

Removal of nitrogen using benzoic acid (**panel A**) and phenylbutyrate (**panel B**).

6 **The answer is B: Reduction of heme synthesis.** The boy is suffering from lead poisoning, which he obtained from eating the flaking paint chips. Lead inhibits the δ-aminolevulinic acid dehydratase step of heme synthesis, leading to reduced heme levels (see the figure on page 133). In addition, the ferrochelatase step (in which iron is inserted into the newly synthesized heme ring) is also inhibited by lead. The reduced heme levels reduce the amount of functional hemoglobin synthesized, leading

to the microcytic anemia observed in the child. Lead does not interfere with iron transport or inhibit part of the phosphatidyl inositol cycle (lithium is the metal that does that). DNA synthesis is not impaired by lead, nor does lead inhibit gene expression of the globin chains. Cytochrome synthesis is also decreased and may contribute to the lethargy observed in the child.

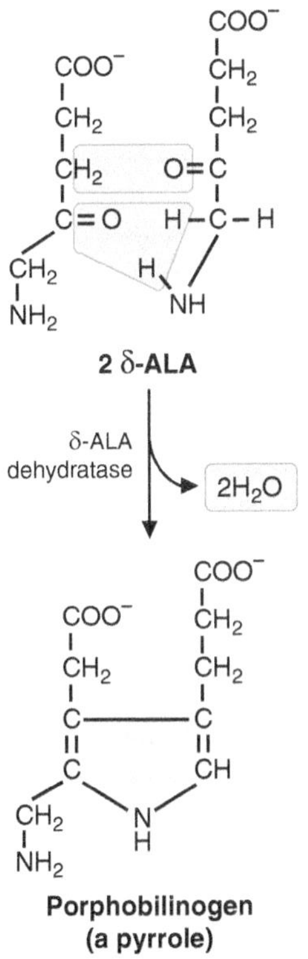

2 δ-ALA

δ-ALA dehydratase → $2H_2O$

Porphobilinogen (a pyrrole)

One of the two steps in heme biosynthesis that is sensitive to lead.

7 **The answer is E: Thiamine.** The child has maple syrup urine disease, a defect in the branched-chain α-keto acid dehydrogenase step that utilizes all three branched-chain α-keto acids as substrates. The reaction catalyzed by this enzyme is an oxidative decarboxylation reaction, which requires the same five cofactors as do pyruvate and α-ketoglutarate dehydrogenase; thiamine, NAD^+, FAD, lipoic acid, and coenzyme A. A subset of patients with this disorder has a mutation in the E1 subunit of the enzyme, which has reduced the affinity of the enzyme for vitamin B_1. Increasing the concentration of B1 can therefore overcome the effects of the mutation and allow the enzyme to exhibit sufficient activity to reduce the buildup of the toxic metabolites. While niacin and riboflavin are required for the enzyme, the mutation in the enzyme is such that the affinity of these cofactors for the enzyme has not been altered. B_{12} and B_6 are not required for this reaction.

8 **The answer is A: α-ketoglutarate dehydrogenase.** The child has a mutation in the shared E3 subunit of pyruvate dehydrogenase, α-ketoglutarate dehydrogenase, and the branched-chain α-ketoacid dehydrogenase. All three reactions are oxidative decarboxylation reactions and utilize a three-component enzyme complex, designated as E1, E2, and E3 (see the figure below). The E1 subunit binds thiamine pyrophosphate and catalyzes the decarboxylation reaction. The E2 subunit is a transacylase and is involved in the oxidation–reduction part of the reaction. The E3 component (dihydrolipoyl dehydrogenase) is shared among all three enzymes, and a mutation in this subunit will affect the activity of all three enzymes. This subunit reduces NAD^+, using electrons obtained from reduced lipoic acid. The key to solving the problem is the recognition that lactic acidosis occurs, which would happen when pyruvate dehydrogenase was defective. None of the other dehydrogenases listed (isocitrate dehydrogenase, malate dehydrogenase, and succinate dehydrogenase) require the E3 subunit for their activity, nor do they catalyze oxidative decarboxylation reactions. Acetyl-CoA carboxylase catalyzes a carboxylation reaction, and does not share subunits with the enzymes that catalyze oxidative decarboxylations.

Answer 8: Mechanism of α-keto acid dehydrogenase complexes. R represents the portion of the α-keto acid that begins with the β carbon. Three different subunits are required for the reaction: E1 (α-ketoacid decarboxylase), E2 (transacylase), and E3 (dihydrolipoyl dehydrogenase). TPP refers to the cofactor thiamine pyrophosphate. Lip refers to the cofactor lipoic acid.

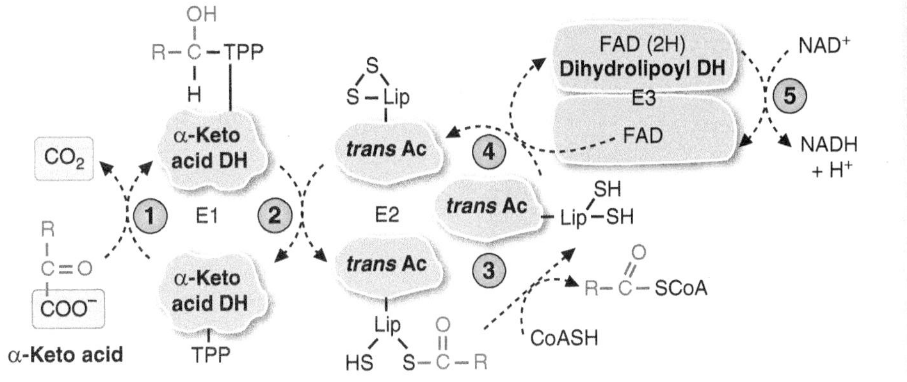

9 **The answer is D: Lack of large, neutral amino acids in the brain.** The child has PKU. The elevated phenylalanine levels in the blood are saturating the large, neutral amino acid transport protein in the nervous system (L-system), preventing other substrates from entering the brain (such as tryptophan, tyrosine, lysine, and leucine). This alters the ability of the brain to synthesize proteins, and leads to neurological problems. Providing large amounts of these large, neutral amino acids prevents saturation of the system by phenylalanine, and can be used as a treatment, along with restricted phenylalanine diet, for children with this disorder. (See J Inherit Metab Dis. 2006 Dec;29(6):732–738.) The developmental delay does not appear to be due to acidosis, lack of tyrosine, an inhibition of hydroxylating enzymes, or inhibition of neuronal glycolysis.

10 **The answer is E: Homocystine.** The boy is exhibiting the symptoms of homocystinuria, usually caused by a defect in cystathionine β-synthase. Cystathionine β-synthase will condense homocysteine with serine to form cystathionine. An inability to catalyze this reaction will lead to an accumulation of homocysteine, which will oxidize to form homocystine. The elevated serine can be metabolized back into the glycolytic pathway. Methionine will not increase in blood as the homocysteine produced is converted into homocystine. Phenylpyruvate is a diagnostic marker for PKU, but it is not relevant for homocysteine production or degradation. Fibrillin is mutated in Marfan syndrome, but this disorder is not Marfan syndrome.

11 **The answer is D: B_6.** Cystathionine β-synthase is a B_6 requiring enzyme (the reaction is a β-elimination of the serine hydroxyl group, followed by a β-addition of homocysteine to serine; both types of reactions require the participation of B_6). In some mutations, the affinity of the cofactor for the enzyme has been reduced, so significantly increasing the concentration of the cofactor will allow the reaction to proceed. The enzyme does not require the assistance of B_1, B_2, B_3 (niacin), or B_{12} to catalyze the reaction.

12 **The answer is D: Glyoxylate.** The boy has primary oxaluria type I, an autosomal recessive trait, which is a defect in a transaminase that converts glyoxylate to glycine. If this transaminase is defective, glyoxylate will accumulate. The glyoxylate will then be oxidized to oxalate, which, in the presence of calcium, will precipitate and form stones in the kidney. The metabolic pathway for glycine being converted to glyoxylate is shown below, and the enzyme that catalyzes this reaction is the D-amino acid oxidase. Alanine, leucine, and lysine metabolism do not give rise to oxalate.

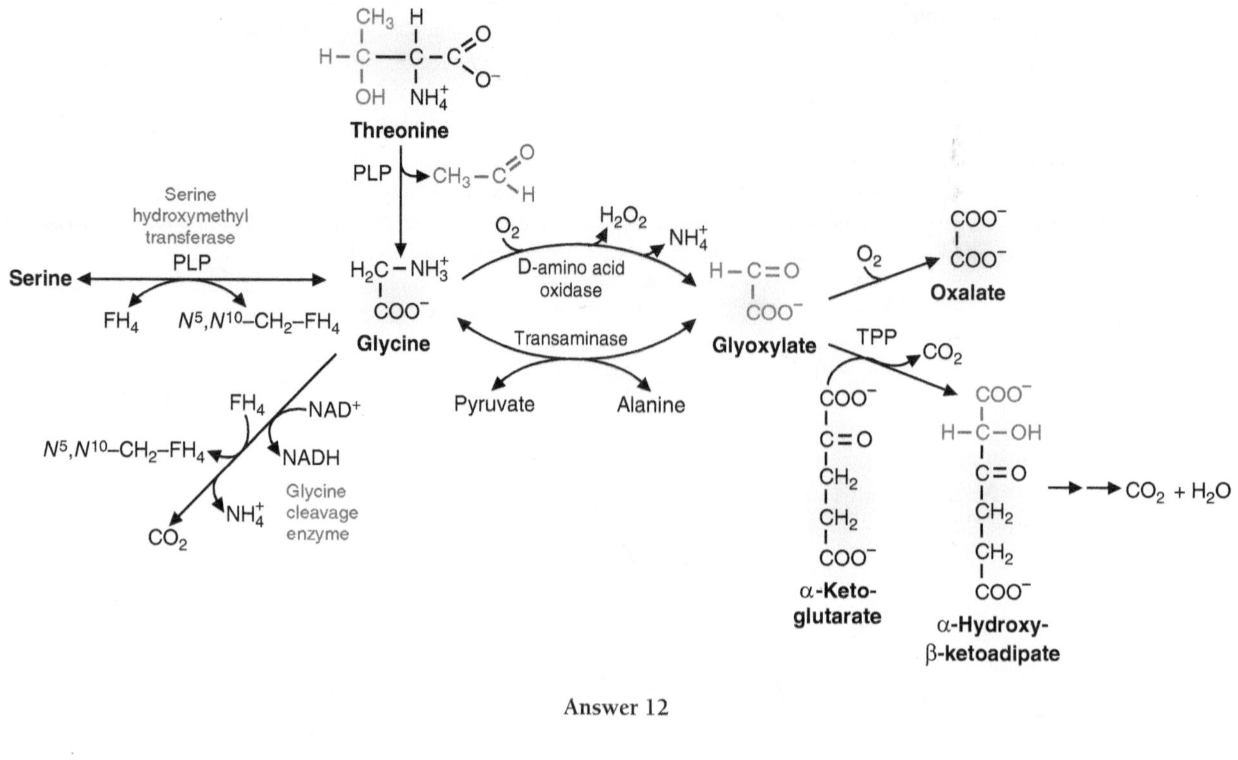

Answer 12

13 **The answer is B: Restriction of dietary methionine.** The boy has cystinuria, elevated levels of cystine in the urine, due to a defect in a kidney transporter that removes cystine from the urine and sends it back into the blood. Due to this, the concentration of cystine in the urine is higher than normal and reaches levels close to its solubility limit. Cysteine is derived from methionine, so a reduction in methionine levels will reduce cysteine levels, which then leads to a reduction in cystine levels. Increasing ethanol content will lead to dehydration, which will increase the concentration of cystine in the urine, leading to increased precipitation. This would also be the case if the urine were acidified (acidification also reduces the solubility of the cystine stones). Restricting glycine is not effective, as glycine is not a precursor of cysteine biosynthesis. Prescribing diuretics would force the boy to urinate more frequently, and would raise a risk for dehydration, which would lead to possible elevation of cystine concentrations.

14 **The answer is C: Cystathionine β-synthase.** Cystathionine β-synthase has a requirement of pyridoxal phosphate, and in about 50% of the cases of defective synthase enzymes, increasing the concentration of B_6 can overcome the effects of the mutation on the enzyme. While a defect in methionine synthase will lead to elevated homocysteine (see the figure below; cystathionine β-synthase is enzyme 3 and methionine synthase is enzyme 1), this enzyme requires B_{12}, not B_6. A defect in N5, N10 methylene tetrahydrofolate reductase will also lead to elevated homocysteine, but that enzyme has a requirement for NADH, not vitamin B_6. A defect in cystathionase (another B_6 requiring enzyme) will block the degradation of cystathionine, which will accumulate, but will not lead to significantly elevated homocysteine. S-adenosyl homocysteine hydrolase is the enzyme that converts S-adenosyl homocysteine to homocysteine and adenosine; lack of its activity will lead to a reduction, not an increase, in homocysteine levels.

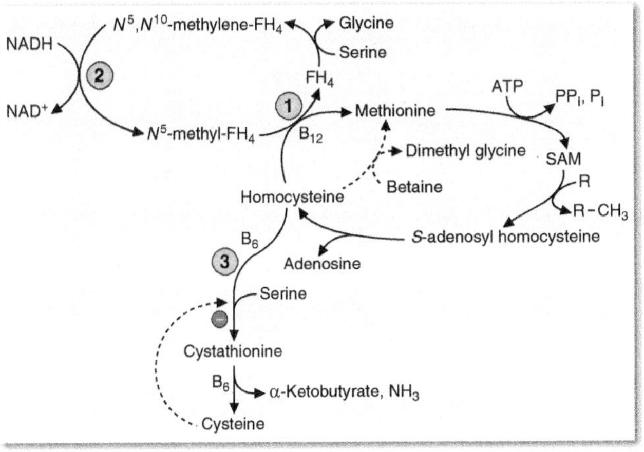

NADH
NAD⁺
(2)
N^5,N^{10}-methylene-FH_4
Glycine
Serine
FH_4
(1)
N^5-methyl-FH_4
B_{12}
Methionine
ATP
PP_i, P_i
Dimethyl glycine
SAM
Betaine
Homocysteine
R
R-CH_3
B_6
S-adenosyl homocysteine
(3)
Adenosine
Serine
Cystathionine
B_6
α-Ketobutyrate, NH_3
Cysteine

15 **The answer is C: Tyrosine.** The boy has the inherited disorder tyrosinemia type I, which is a defect in fumarylacetoacetate hydrolase, the last step in the degradation pathway for tyrosine (see the figure below). In its acute form, this disorder will lead to liver failure and death within 1 year of life. The accumulation of intermediates in the tyrosine degradation pathway triggers apoptosis

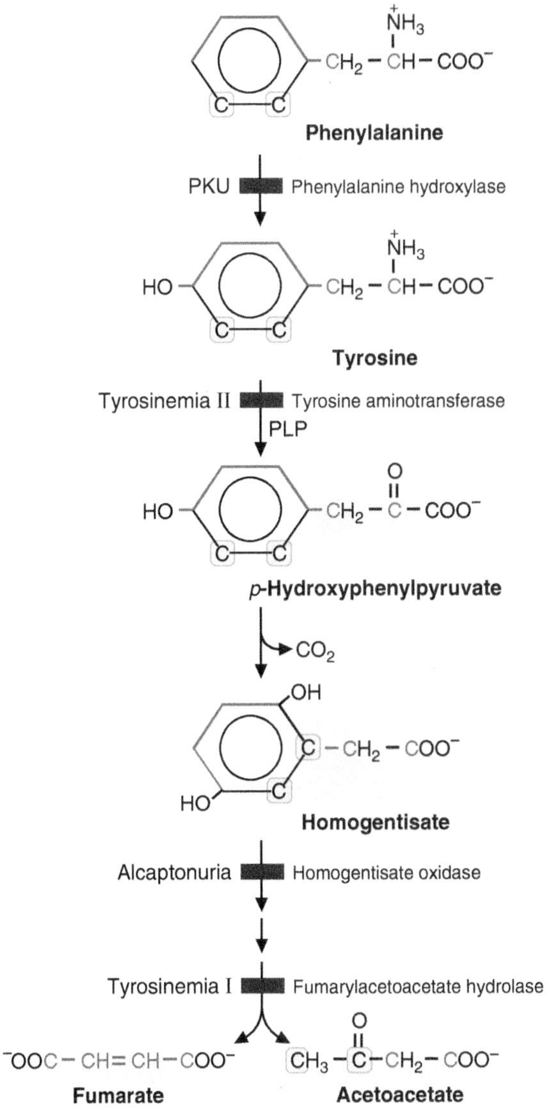

Phenylalanine
PKU
Phenylalanine hydroxylase
Tyrosine
Tyrosinemia II
Tyrosine aminotransferase
PLP
p-Hydroxyphenylpyruvate
CO_2
OH
HO
Homogentisate
Alcaptonuria
Homogentisate oxidase
Tyrosinemia I
Fumarylacetoacetate hydrolase
$^-OOC-CH=CH-COO^-$
Fumarate
$CH_3-C(=O)-CH_2-COO^-$
Acetoacetate

of the hepatocytes, leading to complete liver failure. The yellowing of the eyes (jaundice, due to accumulated bilirubin) is a result of liver failure. None of the other amino acids listed (alanine, tryptophan, histidine, and lysine) contribute to the formation of intermediates of the phenylalanine and tyrosine degradative pathways.

16 **The answer is A: Tryptophan.** Most drugs used to treat depression do so by elevating serotonin levels, and serotonin is derived from tryptophan (see the figure below). Tyrosine is the precursor for catecholamines, while glutamate is the precursor of GABA. Histidine is the precursor for histamine, while glycine itself acts as a neurotransmitter in the brain.

Nicotinamide moiety of NAD(P)

Tryptophan

O_2, BH_4, H_2O, BH_2 tryptophan hydroxylase

5-Hydroxytryptophan

PLP CO_2 DOPA decarboxylase

Serotonin

17 **The answer is C: Tyrosine.** This patient has Parkinson disease, which is a problem with dopamine synthesis in the substantia nigra. Dopamine is derived from tyrosine. Treatment with DOPA in the initial stages of the disease provides relief from the symptoms. DOPA cannot be synthesized from alanine, serine, tryptophan, or phenylalanine. The figure below indicates the biosynthetic pathway of DOPA and the catecholamines.

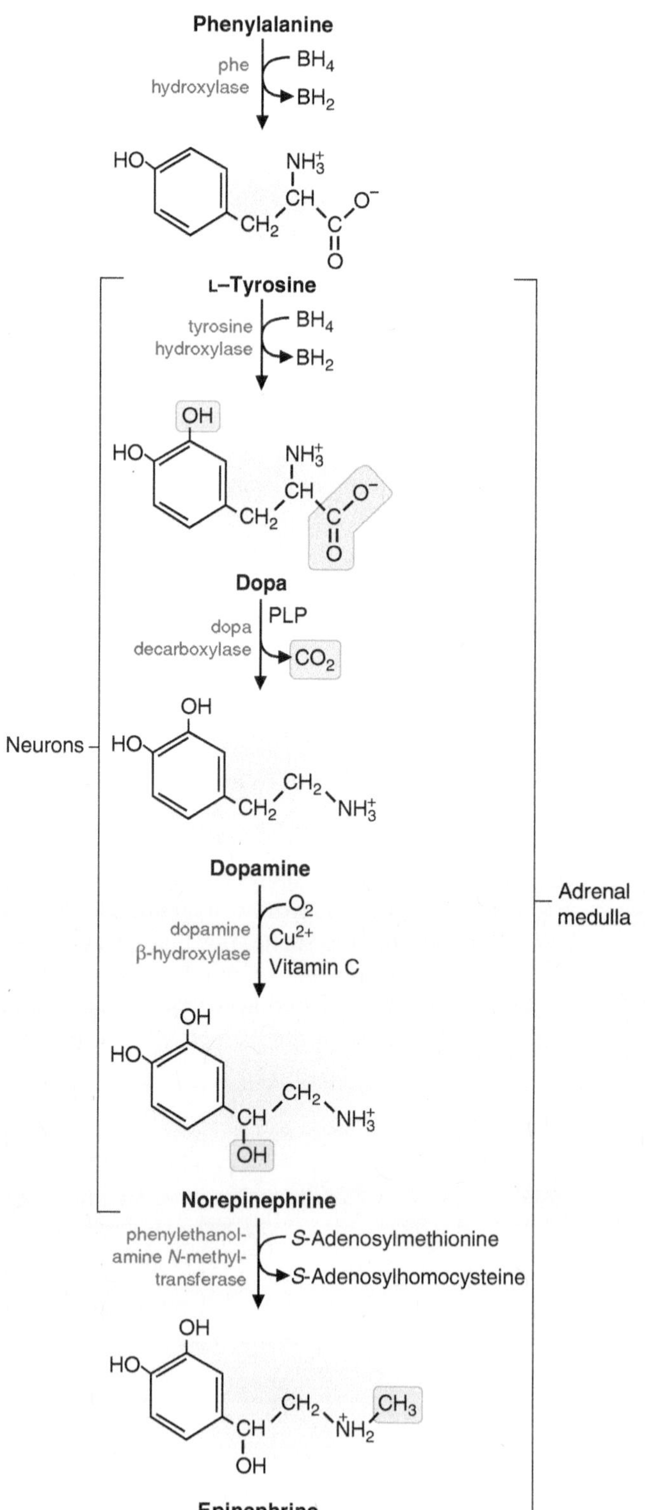

18 The answer is D: 5-hydroxyindoleacetic acid (5-HIAA). This patient has the classic presentation of a carcinoid tumor. This type of tumor secretes serotonin that causes these classic symptoms. The breakdown product of serotonin is 5-hydroxyindoleacetic acid (5-HIAA, see the figure below). Elevated levels of 5-HIAA in the urine confirms a high level of serotonin and the diagnosis of a carcinoid. VMA and/or catechols would be elevated if the patient had a pheochromocytoma producing epinephrine or norepinephrine (the VMAs are degradation products of these neurotransmitters, also seen in the figure below). The symptoms do not match a pheochromocytoma, particularly due to the lack of increase in heart rate or blood pressure. Dopamine is depleted in Parkinson disease, not in this condition. Cortisol levels would be high in Cushing syndrome, but not under these conditions.

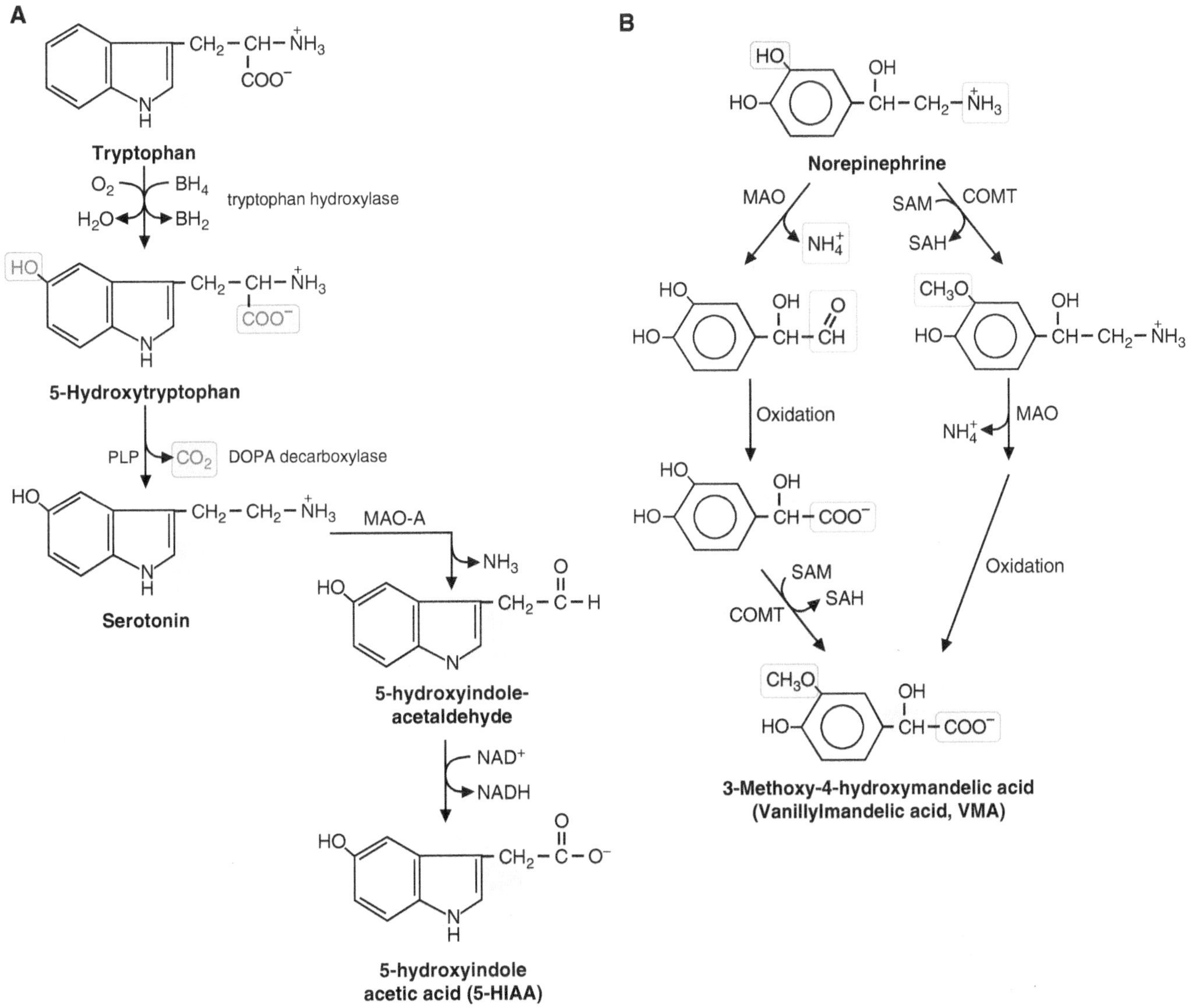

Panel A shows the generation of 5-HIAA from serotonin degradation, while **panel B** indicates the generation of VMA from catecholamine degradation.

19 The answer is B: Tyramine. Tyramine is a degradation product of tyrosine (decarboxylated tyrosine), which, when elevated, will lead to norepinephrine release. Tyramine is found in red wine and aged foods such as certain cheeses. When ingested, tyramine is degraded by monoamine oxidase to a harmless compound, and excessive norepinephrine release does not occur. However, if a patient is taking a monoamine oxidase inhibitor (MAOI), it is possible that tyramine does not get degraded appropriately. MAOIs which covalently modify (as opposed to being competitive inhibitors) the enzyme are very useful medications for atypical depression that is unresponsive to other modalities. Unfortunately, MAOIs have multiple interactions with many other medications and foods. A high tyramine level leads to a greatly elevated blood pressure due to the release of norepinephrine. Patients on MAOIs need to avoid foods high in tyramine, such as cheeses (aged and processed), red wine, caviar, brewer's yeast, miso soup, dried herring, and aged meats. MAOIs have no effect on glycoproteins or cholesterol.

20 **The answer is E: Heme synthesis.** The boy has porphyria, a reduced ability to synthesize heme. The supersensitivity to the sun is due to the presence of heme precursors in skin cells that are easily converted to radical form by the energy in sunlight, and which severely damage the cell. The drug the boy is taking is metabolized via a cytochrome P450 system, which is induced when the drug first enters the circulation. Induction of P450 systems induces the synthesis of heme, leading to increased concentrations of the heme intermediates and an increased sensitivity to the effects of these intermediates as induced by sunlight. The anemia is due to reduced heme levels in the red blood cells. This disorder is not due to defects in DNA repair, glycogen metabolism, or fatty acid metabolism.

Chapter 16

Phospholipid Metabolism

This chapter quizzes the reader on the biological roles of phospholipids, sphingolipids, and glycosaminoglycans. Diseases relating to these large molecules will be the focus of this chapter.

QUESTIONS

Select the single best answer.

1 A patient presents with rapidly progressive weakness of the lower extremities, loss of deep tendon reflexes, respiratory distress, and autonomic dysfunction following a flulike illness. This disease is an autoimmune inflammatory reaction to tissue made up chiefly of which of the following chemical structures?

(A) High-density lipoproteins
(B) Elastin
(C) Sphingolipids
(D) Glycoproteins
(E) Glycogen

2 The above patient is in the recovery phase of her illness. She wants to "naturally" help her body recover using dietary methods. Which of the following foods is best in providing the chemicals needed to regrow the affected tissues?

(A) Soybeans
(B) Calves' liver
(C) Pork kidney
(D) Green leafy vegetables
(E) Potatoes

3 A newborn infant had trouble breathing at birth. The infant was 3 months premature. The physicians treated the infant with a solution, which was directly injected into the lungs. Within seconds, the infant responded with much improved breathing. A major component of this solution is which one of the following?

(A) Dipalmitoyl phosphatidylcholine
(B) Palmitate containing ceramide
(C) Sphingosine
(D) Sphingomyelin
(E) Diacylglycerol

4 Considering the case in the previous question, the major function of the suspension utilized to improve breathing is which of the following?

(A) To allow oxygen exchange with red blood cells
(B) To facilitate carbon dioxide extraction from red blood cells
(C) To reduce surface tension at the air–water interface
(D) To stabilize the structure of lung cells
(E) To facilitate blood flow through the lung

5 A 9-month-old child is taken to the pediatrician for lethargy and poor feeding. The physician notes a cherry-red spot in the child's retina. The baby seemed fine for the first three to six months, then began to have problems swallowing, overreacted to loud sounds, seemed to have problems with her vision, and began losing muscle mass and strength. Measurements of which two metabolites is critical to correctly diagnose this disorder?

(A) GM2 and globoside
(B) GM2 and GM3
(C) GM1 and globoside
(D) GM1 and GM2
(E) Globoside and sphingomyelin

6 Considering the child described in the previous question, a diagnosis of Sandhoff disease was made. This results in a loss of which of the following enzymatic activities?

(A) Hexosaminidase A and Hexosaminidase C
(B) Hexosaminidase B and Hexosaminidase C
(C) Hexosaminidase A and Hexosaminidase B
(D) Hexosaminidase A and sphingomyelinase
(E) Hexosaminidase B and sphingomyelinase

7 Considering the child described in the last two questions, multiple enzymatic activities are lost. This is due to which of the following?
(A) A common operon for the two genes contains a mutation in the promoter region
(B) An inactivating mutation in an activator for the lost enzymatic activities
(C) A transcriptional activator is inactivated
(D) A common mutated subunit is present in the multiple activities
(E) A transcriptional repressor is activated

8 A 4-month-old infant is brought to the pediatrician for a variety of problems. The child is frequently irritable, small for age, vomits frequently, and displays hypotonia, as well as hyperesthesia (auditory, tactile, and visual). Liver and spleen size are normal. As the child ages, his condition worsens, with rapid psychomotor deterioration, seizures, and blindness. This disorder is caused by an accumulation of which of the following in neuronal lysosomes?
(A) Galactosylceramide
(B) Sulfatide
(C) Glucosylceramide
(D) Sphingomyelin
(E) Ceramide

9 A 6-month-old boy is brought to the pediatrician due to a large stomach. The doctor noticed splenomegaly, with no pain. The boy was always tired and had anemia. The boy also has thrombocytopenia and bruises easily. X-rays show a deformity of the distal femur, as shown below. This disorder is caused by an accumulation of which of the following in macrophage lysosomes?

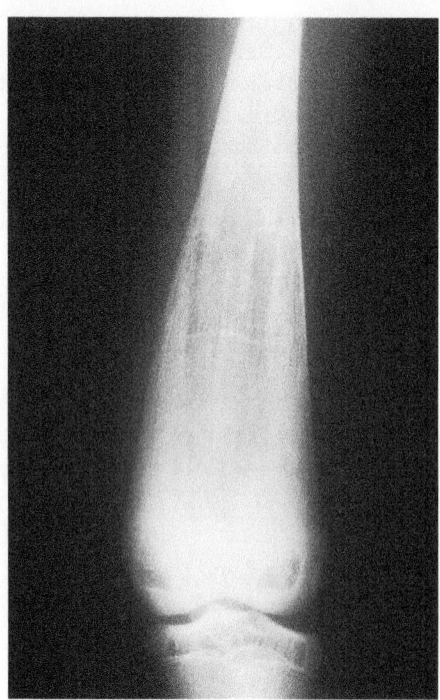

(A) Galactosylceramide
(B) Sulfatide
(C) Glucosylceramide
(D) Sphingomyelin
(E) Ceramide

10 The sphingolipidoses, as a class, are most similar to which one of the following disorders?
(A) Glucose-6-phosphate dehydrogenase deficiency
(B) von Gierke disease
(C) Zellweger syndrome
(D) MELAS
(E) I-cell disease

11 A child has been diagnosed with Tay–Sachs disease, in which a particular lipid accumulates within the lysosomes. The component of this lipid which cannot be removed in the lysosome is which of the following?
(A) Ceramide
(B) Sphingosine
(C) Fatty acid
(D) Glucose
(E) *N*-acetylgalactosamine

12 A depressed patient is prescribed lithium by his psychiatrist. The effect of lithium is to block the generation of which of the following?
(A) Diacylglycerol
(B) Inositol trisphosphate
(C) Inositol bisphosphate
(D) Inositol phosphate
(E) Inositol

13 An alcoholic patient with advanced cirrhosis presents with spur cell anemia. For virtually all cell types and organelles, the phospholipid composition of the inner and outer leaflets of the membrane is different. The spur cell anemia is the result of the loss of one potential benefit of such phospholipid asymmetry. Which of the following best explains this benefit?
(A) To vary the melting temperature of the membrane
(B) To represent all phospholipids species within the membrane
(C) To mark cells for recognition by outside systems
(D) To distinguish between intracellular organelles
(E) To prevent fusion of intracellular organelles

14 Phosphatidylinositol contributes to phospholipid bilayer asymmetry by being in the inner leaflet of membranes, facing the cytoplasm of the cell. This is most likely due to which of the following?

(A) The hydrophobic nature of inositol is unstable facing the cellular exterior
(B) Inositol is very similar in structure to glucose and could compete with glucose for binding of ligands to the extracellular surface
(C) Phosphatidylinositol acts as a substrate for intracellular processes
(D) Phosphatidylinositol binds to phosphatidylserine, another inner leaflet specific phospholipid
(E) Inositol interacts with intracellular actin, linking the inner leaflet to a cell's cytoskeleton

15 The use of proteoglycans in synovial fluid of joints is advantageous due to the ability of the proteoglycans to form which type of interactions with other components of the fluid?
(A) Disulfide and ionic bonds
(B) Hydrogen and ionic bonds
(C) Covalent and ionic bonds
(D) Covalent and hydrogen bonds
(E) Disulfide and hydrogen bonds

16 Your 52-year-old male patient, an avid soccer player in his youth, who had several knee injuries, has been complaining of knee pain for the past 6 months. The knees are tender, stiff, and feel warm when touched. He wants long-term relief, not just short-term relief. You suggest that the patient take which of the following to try and reduce the knee pain, for the long term?
(A) Aspirin
(B) Acetaminophen
(C) Sphingomyelin
(D) Glucosamine
(E) Inositol

17 Children with either I-cell disease or Hurler syndrome show very similar clinical features. One method to distinguish between the two is to find which of the following elevated in the blood?
(A) Heparan sulfate
(B) Short-chain dicarboxylic acids
(C) Lysosomal hydrolases
(D) Dermatan sulfate
(E) Cytochrome *c*

18 A 27-year-old woman sees her physician due to weakness and tiredness. She has tingling and numbness in her fingers and toes, loss of balance and falling, and blurry vision, sometimes double vision. Her ophthalmologist has diagnosed optic neuritis in her. An MRI of the brain shows "skip lesions." The component that is primarily defective in this patient is composed of which of the following?
(A) Phospholipids and proteins
(B) Triacylglycerol and protein
(C) Phospholipids and triacylglycerol
(D) Gangliosides and protein
(E) Triacylglycerol and gangliosides

19 A woman has a history of premature miscarriages (three), thrombocytopenia, and several episodes of deep vein thrombosis. She has a positive lupus anticoagulant but does not have systemic lupus erythematosus (SLE). Examination of the proteins in her blood should find antibodies directed against which of the following?
(A) Cytochrome *c*
(B) Phospholipids
(C) DNA
(D) RNA splicing proteins
(E) Ribosomes

20 An athlete presents to the ER with sudden pain in his calf after hearing a "popping noise," and inability to push off with his toes when he tries to run. He gives a history of having a "cortisol shot" in his heel area for Achilles tendonitis and he just finished a course of ciprofloxacin for chronic prostatitis. Physical exam reveals a mass in the superior posterior lower leg and an inability to plantar flex his foot. Biopsy of the Achilles tendon would be expected to reveal fibrotic areas, neovascularization, and an increase of which of the following in the extracellular matrix?
(A) Cholesterol
(B) Glycosaminoglycans
(C) Triglyceride
(D) Sphingosine
(E) High Density Lipoprotein (HDL)

ANSWERS

1 **The answer is C: Sphingolipids.** This patient has the classic symptoms of Guillain–Barré syndrome which is an inflammatory autoimmune neuritis wherein T-cells formed in response to a viral illness mistakenly attack the myelin sheath of peripheral nerves. The myelin sheaths are composed primarily of sphingolipids and phospholipids and do not contain high-density lipoproteins, elastin, glycogen, or a significant level of glycoprotein. A view of demyelination is shown below.

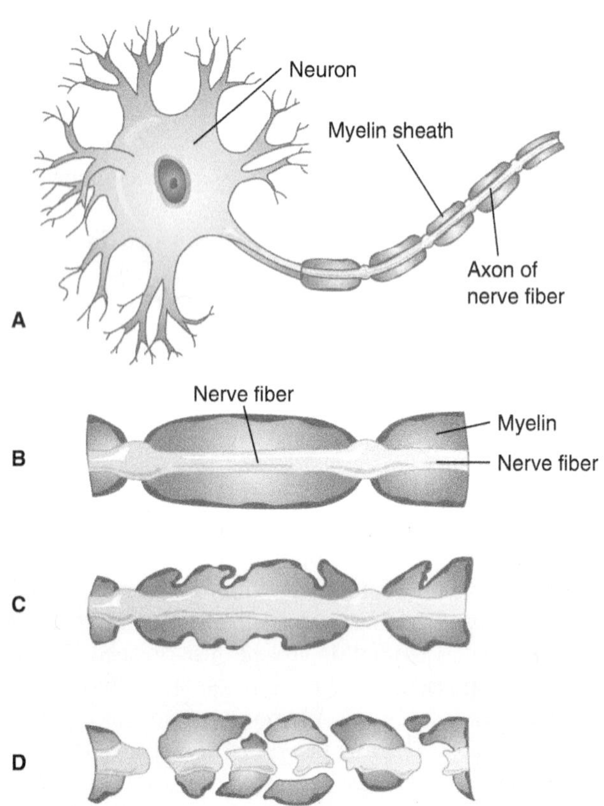

An overview of demyelination. **Panels A** and **B** depict normal conditions, whereas **panels C** and **D** show the slow disintegration of myelin, resulting in demyelination and a loss of axonal function.

2 **The answer is A: Soybeans.** Foods considered the highest sources of sphingolipids include dairy and soy products. Foods highest in phospholipids include those high in lecithin, such as eggs, soy, and wheat. Sphingolipids and phospholipids are found mostly in neural tissue. Other organs and muscle do not contain as high a quantity of these lipids as do neural tissues.

3 **The answer is A: Dipalmitoyl phosphatidylcholine.** The patient was treated with an artificial preparation of lung surfactant, which reduces surface tension within the lung at the air–water interface. In premature newborns, the type II cells within the lung have not yet begun synthesizing surfactant, so the application of surfactant to the baby will allow this compound to be present until the type II cells begin their synthesis of this complex. The major phospholipid in surfactant is dipalmitoyl phosphatidylcholine (DPPC), and it is complexed with a number of small proteins (surfactant proteins A, B, and C). While small amounts of sphingomyelin may be present in surfactant, DPPC is the major component. The structure of DPPC is shown below.

$CH_3-(CH_2)_{14}-C(=O)-O-CH(CH_2-O-C(=O)-(CH_2)_{14}-CH_3)-CH_2-O-P(=O)(O^-)-O-CH_2-CH_2-N^+(CH_3)_3$

Dipalmitoyl phosphatidylcholine, the major component of lung surfactant

4 **The answer is C: To reduce surface tension at the air–water interface.** The phospholipid–protein mixture of surfactant interacts at the surface of lung cells, allowing expansion and contraction due to reducing surface tension at the air–water interface (see the figure below). Surfactant does not affect oxygen exchange with the red blood cells, nor does it allow carbon dioxide removal from such cells. Surfactant does not stabilize lung cell structure (although it is essential for the function of the lung cell), nor does it facilitate blood flow through the lung.

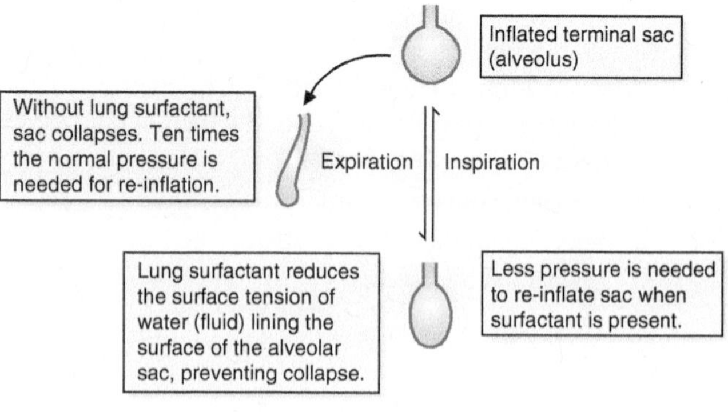

The effect of lung surfactant

5 **The answer is A: GM2 and globoside.** The cherry-red spot is indicative of either Tay–Sachs disease (an autosomal recessive disorder leading to a loss of hexosaminidase A [hex A] activity) or Sandhoff disease (an autosomal recessive disorder leading to a loss of both hexosaminidase A and B [hex B] activity). With just a

loss of hex A activity, GM2 would accumulate. With a loss of hex B activity, globoside and GM2 would accumulate. Thus, by measuring the levels of GM2 and globoside, one can distinguish between Tay–Sachs and Sandhoff disease. A loss of either hex A or hex B would not affect GM1 or GM3 degradation.

6 **The answer is C: Hexosaminidase A and Hexosaminidase B.** In Sandhoff disease, both hex A and hex B activities are lost. The mutation in Sandhoff disease does not affect sphingomyelinase activity, and there is no hexosaminidase C activity. Sandhoff disease is one of many which affect sphingolipid metabolism. An overview of the sphingolipidoses is shown in the figure below.

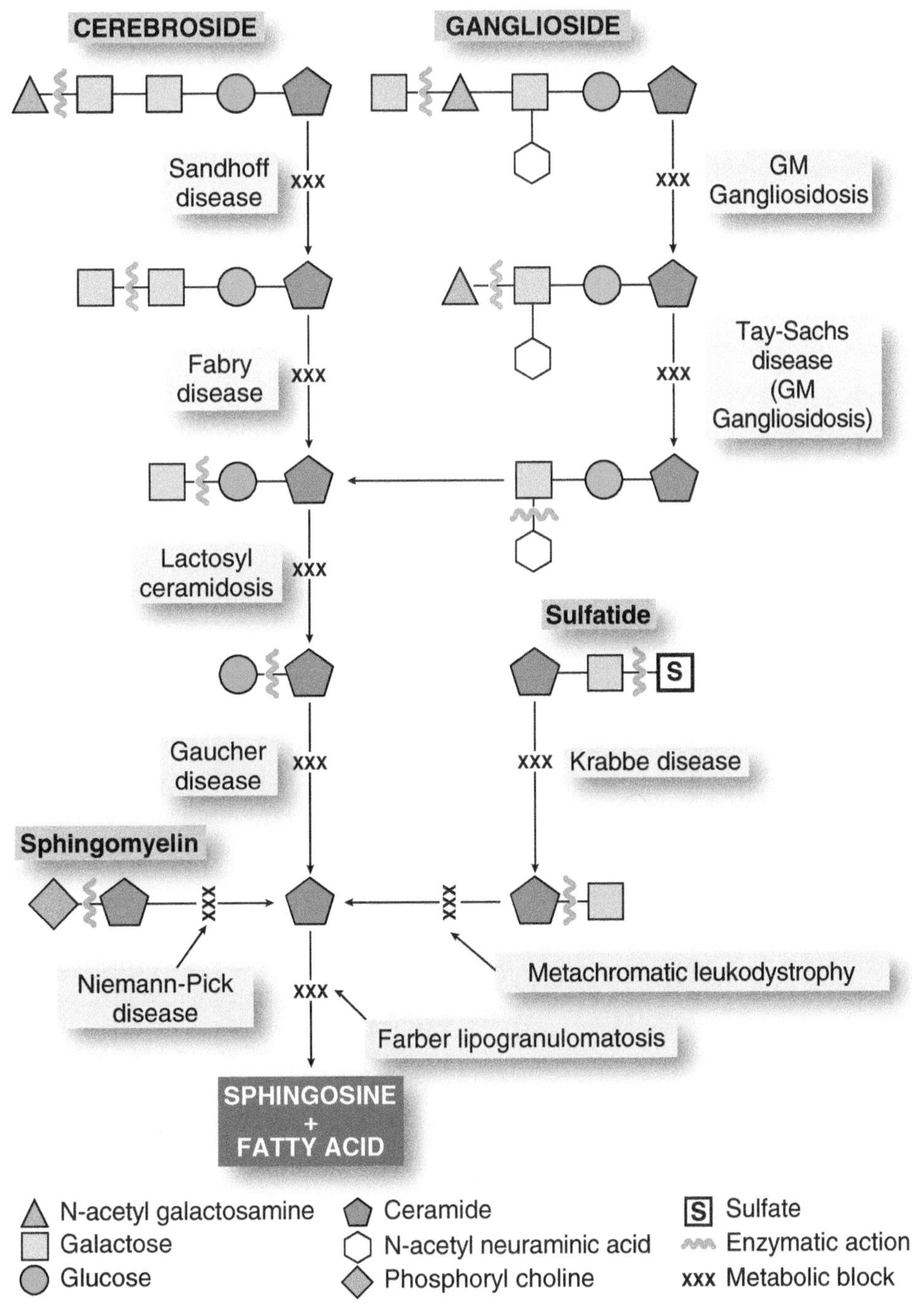

Answer 6: A summary of the sphingolipidoses in diagrammatic form.

7 **The answer is D: A common mutated subunit is present in the multiple activities.** The hexosaminidase A gene encodes the hex A protein, and the hexosaminidase B gene encodes the hex B protein. Hexosaminidase A activity requires a complex of hex A and hex B proteins; hexosaminidase B activity only requires a complex of hex B proteins. Tay–Sachs disease is a defect in the hex A protein, affecting only hex A activity. Sandhoff disease is a defect in the hex B protein, which affects both hex A and hex B activity, due to the sharing of a common subunit between the two proteins. hex A and hex B are not in an operon (which is only operative in bacteria); in fact, the genes are on different chromosomes. There is an activating protein for hex A activity, but not hex B activity (a loss of the activating protein is known as Sandhoff activator disease, with symptoms very similar to Tay–Sachs disease). There are no mutations in transcriptional control proteins (either an activator or inhibitor) in Tay–Sachs or Sandhoff disease. The interactions of the hex A and hex B proteins are shown in the figure below.

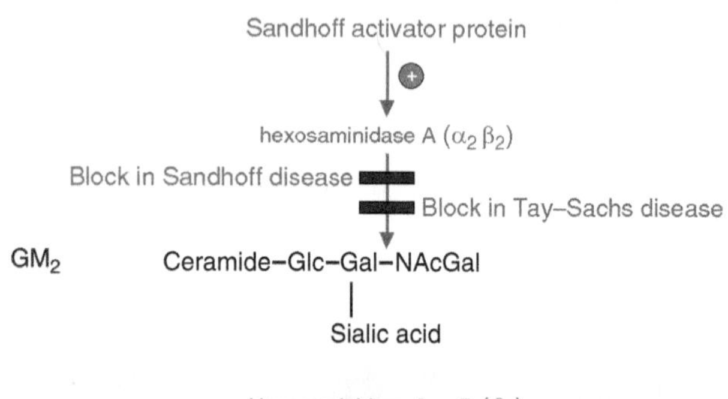

Substrate specificities of hexosaminidase A and B, and the function of the activator protein. Defects in the β-subunit inactivate both hex A and hex B activities, leading to GM2 and globoside accumulation. A defect in Sandhoff activator protein also leads to GM2 accumulation, as hex A activity is reduced. Defects in the α-subunit only inactivate hex A activity, such that hex B activity toward globoside is unaffected. Glc, glucose; Gal, galactose; NAcGal, *N*-acetylgalactosamine.

8 **The answer is A: Galactosylceramide.** The child has Krabbe disease, a mutation in a galactosidase, which cannot remove galactose from galactose cerebroside (an inability to break the bond between galactose and ceramide). The buildup of galactose–ceramide leads to the neuronal and muscle damage seen in the child. An inability to degrade a sulfatide would lead to metachromatic leukodystropy, which has very different symptoms than Krabbe disease. An inability to degrade glucosylceramide leads to Gaucher disease, again, with a very different disease progression than that seen with Krabbe disease. A defect in the degradation of sphingomyelin leads to Niemann–Pick disease, with a different set of symptoms than that seen with Krabbe disease. A defect in degrading ceramide leads to Farber disease, a defect in ceramidase. Farber disease is similar to Krabbe disease, but often presents with hepatomegaly and splenomegaly. See Table 16.1 in the next answer for a summary of all the sphingolipidoses and the material that accumulates within the lysosomes. Additionally, the figure associated with the answer to question 6 of this chapter depicts the metabolic blocks of the sphingolipidoses.

9 **The answer is C: Glucosylceramide.** The child has a form of Gaucher disease, which is a defect in a glucosidase which removes glucose from glucosylceramide. The accumulation of glucosylcerebroside in the lysosomes leads to the observed symptoms. Defects in degrading galactosylceramide lead to Krabbe disease, which does not result in hepatomegaly and splenomegaly. A defect in degrading sulfatide leads to metachromatic leukodystrophy, which has different symptoms than what the child is experiencing. A defect in the degradation of sphingomyelin leads to Niemann–Pick disease, with a different set of symptoms than that seen with Gaucher disease. A defect in degrading ceramide leads to Farber disease, a defect in ceramidase, with more severe symptoms than those observed in Gaucher disease. Table 16-1 summarizes the sphingolipidoses, the enzyme defect, and the material that accumulates. Utilize this table with the figure associated with the answer to question 6 of this chapter for a thorough understanding of the consequences of the sphingolipidoses.

10 **The answer is E: I-cell disease.** The sphingolipidoses and I-cell disease are both lysosomal storage diseases, whereas the other disorders listed do not involve lysosomal dysfunction. Mitochondrial myopathy, encephalopathy, lactic acidosis, and stroke (MELAS) is a mitochondrial disorder, and Zellweger's is a disorder of peroxisomal biogenesis. G6PDH (glucose-6-phosphate dehydrogenase) deficiency and von Gierke disease are single gene mutations which do not alter lysosomal function (although type II glycogen storage disease, Pompe disease, is a lysosomal storage disease).

11 **The answer is E: *N*-acetylgalactosamine.** Tay–Sachs is a defect in hexosaminidase A, which removes the terminal *N*-acetylgalactosamine residue from ganglioside GM2, producing the free sugar and GM3. Hexosaminidase A does not cleave glucose, ceramide, sphingosine, or the fatty acyl component of ceramide from GM2; it is specific for N-acetylgalactosamine.

12 **The answer is E: Inositol.** Lithium primarily inhibits the phosphatase which converts inositol phosphate to free inositol, thereby disrupting the phosphatidylinositol cycle, leading to increased levels of the intermediates of the cycle, which are often signaling molecules. Lithium does not affect the generation of diacylglycerol, inositol trisphosphate (IP_3), inositol bisphosphate (IP_2), or

Table 16-1. Defective enzymes in the gangliosidoses

Disease	Enzyme Deficiency	Accumulated Lipid
Fucosidosis	α-Fucosidase	Cer–Glc–Gal–GalNAc–Gal:Fuc H-isoantigen
Generalized gangliosidosis	G_{M1}-β-galactosidase	Cer–Glc–Gal(NeuAc)–GalNAc:Gal GM1 ganglioside
Tay–Sachs disease	Hexosaminidase A	Cer–Glc–Gal(NeuAc):GalNAc GM2 ganglioside
Tay–Sachs variant or Sandhoff disease	Hexosaminidase A and B	Cer–Glc–Gal–Gal:GalNAc Globoside plus GM2 ganglioside
Fabry disease	α-Galactosidase	Cer–Glc–Gal:Gal Globotriaosylceramide
Ceramide lactoside lipidosis	Ceramide lactosidase (β-galactosidase)	Cer–Glc:Gal Ceramide lactoside
Metachromatic leukodystrophy	Arylsulfatase A	Cer–Gal:OSO_3 3-Sulfogalactosylceramide
Krabbe disease	β-Galactosidase	Cer:Gal Galactosylceramide
Gaucher disease	β-Glucosidase	Cer:Glc Glucosylceramide
Niemann–Pick disease	Sphingomyelinase	Cer:P–choline Sphingomyelin
Farber disease	Ceramidase	Acyl: sphingosine Ceramide

NeuAc, *N*-acetylneuraminic acid; *Cer*, ceramide; *Glc*, glucose; *Gal*, galactose; *Fuc*, fucose: site of deficient enzyme reaction.

inositol phosphate (IP); it affects just the conversion of IP to free inositol and a phosphate.

13 **The answer is C: To mark cells for recognition by outside systems.** By having different phospholipid compositions of the inner and outer leaflets of membranes, one can utilize phospholipid head groups (which face the aqueous phase of their leaflet) as markers for "inside" and "outside" the membrane structure. For example, the exposure of phosphatidyl serine on the "outside" of red blood cells as is seen in spur cell anemia is a signal for the removal of the cells from circulation by the spleen, as the serine residue should be facing the "inside" of the red blood cell. Spur cells are large red blood cells covered with spikelike projections from preferential overexpansion of outer membrane components, leading to a spurlike shape. Movement of the phospholipid is a signal of cell aging. The melting temperature of the membrane is better determined by the fatty acid composition of the phospholipids, not the head group composition. Not all phospholipids are represented in all membranes (for example, cardiolipin is found almost exclusively in the mitochondria). Assymetric phospholipid compositions do not distinguish one organelle from another (that is primarily due to protein content), and assymetry in phospholipid composition may promote fusion (vesicles need to bud from and fuse with other membranes, particularly in the Golgi apparatus).

14 **The answer is C: Phosphatidylinositol acts as a substrate for intracellular processes.** Phosphatidylinositol is used as the substrate to provide signaling molecules in response to the appropriate stimuli (the phosphatidylinositol cycle). As such, it must face the cytoplasm of the cell such that when the inositol phosphate derivatives are produced, such as IP_3, they can move to their target receptors to elicit a cellular response. Inositol contains six hydroxyl groups and is a very hydrophilic molecule. Inositol's structure is quite different from glucose (there is no carbonyl group in inositol), so it is unlikely that glucose and inositol would compete for binding to the same receptors. Phosphatidylinositol does not bind to phosphatidylserine in the inner leaflet of membranes. Inositol also does not interact with the actin cytoskeleton.

15 **The answer is B: Hydrogen and ionic bonds.** The high concentration of negative charges provided by the proteoglycans attracts cations that create a high osmotic pressure within cartilage, drawing water into this specialized connective tissue and placing the collagen network under tension. The water remains due to hydrogen bond formation with the proteoglycans. At equilibrium, the resulting tension balances the swelling pressure caused by the proteoglycans. Cartilage can thus withstand the compressive load of weight bearing and then re-expand to it previous dimensions when that load is relieved. Disulfide bonds and covalent bonds do not play a role in proteoglycan stabilization of joints.

16 **The answer is D: Glucosamine.** While aspirin and acetaminophen may provide short-term relief, the use of glucosamine may help to rebuild the proteoglycan layer in the knees, reducing the osteoarthritis (although medical studies are controversial concerning the use of glucosamine and glucosamine sulfate, in terms of providing relief from joint pain). Sphingomyelin and inositol are not important components of the cartilage in joints. Proteoglycans contain long carbohydrate chains, which consist of repeating disaccharide units (see the figure below). Note the inclusion of glucosamine derivatives in three of the five repeating disaccharide units.

Hyaluronate

Glucuronic acid β(1→3) N-acetyl-glucosamine

Chondroitin-6-sulfate

Glucuronic acid β(1→3) N-acetyl-galactosamine

Heparin

Iduronic acid α(1→4) Glucosamine

Keratan sulfate

Galactose β(1→4) N-acetyl-glucosamine

Dermatan sulfate

Glucuronic acid β(1→3) N-acetyl-galactosamine

Repeating disaccharide units found in glycosaminoglycans.

17 **The answer is C: Lysosomal hydrolases.** In I-cell disease, the lysosomal hydrolases are mistargeted and are excreted from cells into the circulation. As the pH of the blood is above 7 and the pH optimum of these enzymes is around 5, there is no activity of the hydrolases in blood. In Hurler syndrome, a defect in the degradation of mucopolysaccharides, there is an accumulation of dermatan and heparan sulfate in the urine, but not in the blood. Short-chain dicarboxylic acids are produced with a defect in medium chain acyl-CoA dehydrogenase, and cytochrome *c* release into the cytoplasm of cells from mitochondria is the signal to initiate apoptosis.

18 **The answer is A: Phospholipids and proteins.** The woman is experiencing the symptoms of multiple sclerosis, a demyelinating disease. In this disorder, the myelin sheath around nerves degenerates, eventually interfering with nerve conduction due to a lack of insulation (see the figure below for a schematic representation of the myelin sheath in the central nervous system). The myelin sheath is composed primarily of phospholipids and proteins. Triacylglycerol and gangliosides are not found in the sheath.

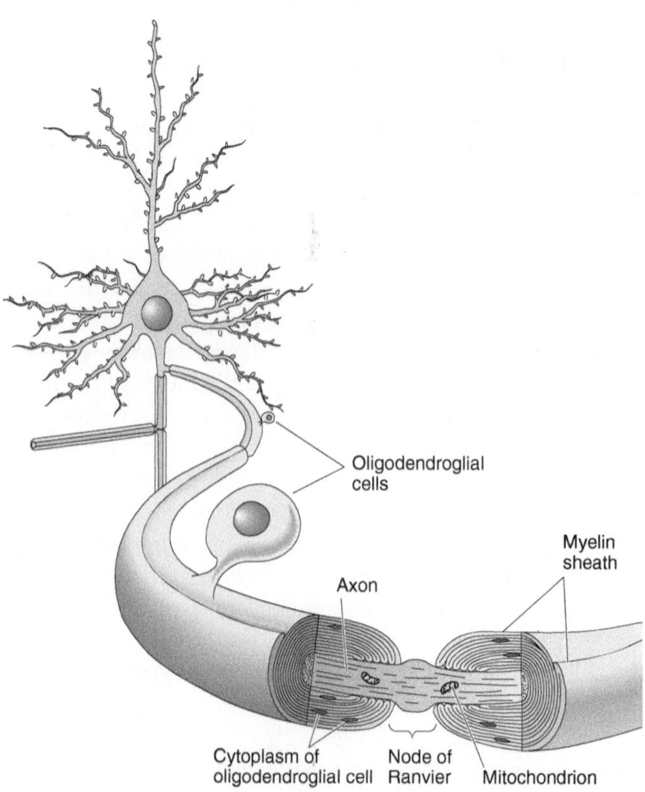

The oligodendroglial cells synthesize the myelin sheath found surrounding the neurons in the central nervous system.

19 **The answer is B: Phospholipids.** The woman has primary antiphospholipid syndrome (Hughes syndrome), in which the body produces antibodies against its own phospholipids and protein/phospholipid complexes (the major one being an anticardiolipin antibody). These antibodies will bind to proteins involved in coagulation and increase the risk of blood clots. Antibodies directed against cytochrome *c*, DNA, RNA splicing proteins (which occurs in SLE), or ribosomes are not observed in this disorder.

20 **The answer is B: Glycosaminoglycans.** Fluoroquinolones have been associated with spontaneous tendon rupture yielding the classic histopathologic findings as described in the case. Other risk factors for Achilles tendon rupture include steroid injections into the tendon, gout, rheumatoid arthritis, and renal transplantation. During tendon degeneration, glycosaminoglycan synthesis is increased in the extracellular matrix material of the tendon. Cholesterol, HDL, and triglyceride have no function in the tendon rupture. In addition, sphingosine is also not found in the extracellular matrix of the tendon.

Chapter 17

Whole-body Lipid Metabolism

This chapter quizzes the student on the flow and storage of lipids (primarily cholesterol and triglyceride) throughout the body.

QUESTIONS

Select the single best answer.

1 You have a patient whose blood work indicates high total cholesterol and elevated liver enzymes. You place him on cholestyramine to lower his cholesterol. Cholestyramine acts to lower cholesterol by inhibiting which of the following enzymes/pathways?

(A) HMG-CoA reductase
(B) Hepatic cholesterol synthesis
(C) Release of bile salts from the gall bladder
(D) Enterohepatic circulation reabsorption of bile salts
(E) The production of chylomicrons

2 You have placed a patient on Pravachol pravastatin to reduce her cholesterol. This class of drugs is effective due to a direct inhibition of which of the following?

(A) Medium chain acyl-CoA dehydrogenase (MCAD)
(B) HMG-CoA synthase
(C) HMG-CoA reductase
(D) Carnitine acyltransferase 1 (CAT-1)
(E) Citrate lyase

3 A knockout mouse was created in which the ability to create conjugated bile salts was greatly impaired. The net result of this mutation in a mouse fed a normal diet is which of the following?

(A) Steatorrhea
(B) Elevated levels of chylomicrons
(C) Deficiency of B vitamins
(D) Reduced pH in the intestinal lumen
(E) Reduced secretion of pancreatic zymogens

4 A patient has enlarged orange tonsils, hepatosplenomegaly, loss of sensation in hands and feet, and clouding of the corneas. His HDL levels are 18 mg/dL. The molecular defect in this patient is present in which of the following proteins?

(A) HMG-CoA reductase
(B) AMP-activated protein kinase
(C) Lecithin cholesterol acyltransferase
(D) ABC1
(E) Cholesterol ester transfer protein

5 Current American Heart Association Guidelines indicate that an adult male should have HDL levels equal to or greater than 40 mg/dL. A necessary enzyme contributing to HDL's protective effect is which of the following?

(A) CETP
(B) LCAT
(C) ACAT
(D) AMP-activated protein kinase
(E) Protein kinase A

6 Many clinical labs report lipid values using a calculated value for LDL. This calculation estimates the cholesterol content in which of the following particles under fasting conditions?

(A) HDL
(B) LDL
(C) IDL
(D) VLDL
(E) Chylomicron

7 Statins are ineffective in lowering cholesterol levels in individuals with homozygous familial hypercholesterolemia due to which of the following?

(A) HMG-CoA reductase is resistant to statins
(B) Statins cannot enter the liver cells
(C) LDL receptors are nonfunctional
(D) Reverse cholesterol transport is inoperative in these patients
(E) LCAT is resistant to statin action

8 You see a patient who has steatorrhea, with very low levels of chylomicrons and VLDL in the circulation. Circulating triglyceride levels are extremely low. Examination of intestinal epithelial cells shows lipid-laden cells. A possible enzymatic defect leading to these findings is which of the following?

(A) LPL
(B) Apolipoprotein CII
(C) MTTP
(D) LCAT
(E) CETP

9 A type 1 diabetic who has neglected to take his insulin for a few days displays both hyperglycemia and hypertriglyceridemia. The hypertriglyceridemia is due, in part, to which of the following?

(A) Reduced synthesis of VLDL
(B) Reduced production of apolipoprotein CII
(C) Increased fatty acid oxidation
(D) Reduced secretion of LPL
(E) Increased synthesis of B100

10 A 12-year-old female presented with severe abdominal pain and was found to have a markedly elevated plasma triglyceride concentration (750 mg/dL). A lipoprotein analysis revealed elevated levels of chylomicrons and VLDL and reduced levels of HDL. Which protein might be defective in this patient?

(A) Apo B100
(B) Apo B48
(C) Apo CII
(D) Pancreatic lipase
(E) LCAT

11 A 43-year-old woman presents with steatorrhea. Fecal analysis reveals the presence of elevated triglycerides, phospholipids, and cholesterol esters. Levels of carbohydrate and protein were normal. Physical exam is unremarkable. A possible defect in the release of which of the following would lead to these results?

(A) Cholecystokinin
(B) Insulin
(C) Glucagon
(D) Secretin
(E) Cortisol

12 A 46-year-old man has been progressively having trouble breathing while walking. Walking from his car to his office has become difficult, and he has to stop to rest along the way. He visits his physician, who orders an angiogram, which shows blockage of major arteries leading to the heart. An initiating factor for the development of the blockage is which of the following?

(A) LDL
(B) Oxidized LDL
(C) Triglycerides
(D) HDL
(E) Oxidized HDL

13 Your 27-year-old male patient, with a BMI of 34, has a total cholesterol of 450 mg/dL and triglycerides of 610 mg/dL. He exhibits planar xanthomas and has already had one angioplasty last year. This patient may be exhibiting a rare autosomal recessive disorder which generates a mutation in which of the following proteins?

(A) LPL
(B) Apolipoprotein CII
(C) Apolipoprotein E
(D) Apolipoprotein B100
(E) Apolipoprotein B48

14 A 44-year-old man displayed elevated cholesterol levels and was prescribed a statin to reduce such levels. Statin treatment has the potential to interfere with the synthesis of which of the following?

(A) Heme
(B) Coenzyme Q
(C) Ketone bodies
(D) Glycogen
(E) Dihydrobiopterin

15 A 57-year-old man has been taking low-dose aspirin to reduce his risk of heart disease. He adds phytosterols to his daily regime for which of the following?

(A) To reduce circulating triglyceride levels
(B) To reduce circulating cholesterol levels
(C) To reduce endogenous cholesterol synthesis
(D) To decrease insulin secretion
(E) To reduce fatty acid biosynthesis

16 Concerning the patient in the previous question, phytosterols have the same general mechanism of action as which of the following drugs?

(A) Atorvastatin
(B) Ezetimibe
(C) Pravastatin
(D) Simvastatin
(E) Metformin

17 Macrophages found in arterial fatty streaks are often lipid filled and become foam cells. Such large amounts of cholesterol uptake into these cells is possible due to which of the following?

(A) Increased activity of ACAT within the foam cell
(B) Increased activity of LCAT within the foam cell
(C) Constant SR-A1 expression on the cell surface
(D) Upregulation of HMG-CoA reductase
(E) Increased activity of the LDL receptor

18 A patient, 45-year-old male, BMI of 25, has had a history of elevated cholesterol (~300 mg/dL), with normal triglyceride levels (~125 mg/dL), and HDL levels (48 mg/dL). Treatment with statins has reduced his serum cholesterol to 180 mg/dL. The patient's father had a similar history and died of a heart attack at age 48. A potential mutation in this patient would be in which of the following proteins?
(A) LCAT
(B) CETP
(C) ABC1
(D) Apo B100
(E) LDL receptor

19 A patient sees his or her physician for continuing treatment of hypercholesterolemia. Recent blood work has indicated a substantial increase in the level of lipoprotein (a). Such a result would suggest which of the following?
(A) Substantially reduced risk for cardiovascular complications
(B) No change in risk for cardiovascular complications
(C) Increased risk for cardiovascular complications
(D) Increased platelet count
(E) Decreased platelet count

20 A 16-year-old male presents to you with xanthomas on the extensor tendons of the hand and Achilles tendon and arthritis of the knees. He has had one previous heart attack, despite normal cholesterol levels. Further analysis of his serum showed greatly elevated levels of plant sterols. The molecular defect in this patient is most likely in which of the following proteins?
(A) Apo B100
(B) Apo B48
(C) ABC1
(D) ABCG5
(E) MTTP

ANSWERS

1 **The answer is D: Enterohepatic circulation reabsorption of bile salts.** Because of the elevated liver enzymes (suggestive of liver damage), a statin would be relatively contraindicated in this patient, as a potential side effect of statins is liver damage. Cholestyramine would be a reasonable alternative to statins. Cholestyramine is one of the "bile acid binders" and prevents the reabsorption of bile salts. Since cholesterol is the precursor of bile salts, and 95% of bile salts are usually reabsorbed back into the enterohepatic circulation, losing bile salts in the feces would require increased synthesis of bile salts, thereby reducing the levels of free cholesterol in the body. Statins work by inhibiting HMG-CoA reductase. Cholestyramine does not reduce hepatic cholesterol synthesis, inhibit the release of bile salts, or interfere with the production of chylomicrons. Its sole action is in the lumen of the intestine, where it binds the bile salts so that they cannot be resorbed and sent back to the liver. The enterohepatic circulation is diagrammed below.

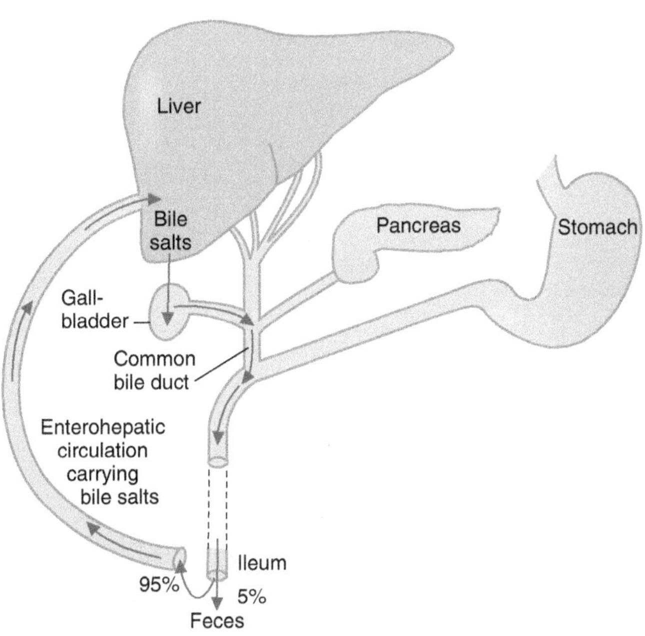

2 **The answer is C: HMG-CoA reductase.** The first stage of cholesterol synthesis leads to the production of the intermediate mevalonate. Two molecules of acetyl-CoA condense to form acetoacetyl-CoA which condenses with another acetyl-CoA to form β-hydroxymethylglutaryl-CoA (HMG-CoA). HMG-CoA synthase catalyses this step. Next, HMG-CoA reductase catalyzes the reduction of HMG-CoA to mevalonate. Statins (the class of drugs to which pravastatin belongs) directly inhibit HMG-CoA reductase, so mevalonate cannot be formed and cholesterol synthesis cannot continue. Statins do not inhibit the enzymes MCAD (required for fatty acid oxidation), CAT-1 (required for acyl-CoA transport into the mitochondria), or citrate lyase (needed to provide acetyl-CoA in the cytoplasm). The reactions required to produce HMG-CoA are shown below.

$CH_3-C(=O)-SCoA$
Acetyl CoA

+ $CH_3-C(=O)-SCoA$ → CoA-SH

$CH_3-C(=O)-CH_2-C(=O)-SCoA$
Acetoacetyl CoA

HMG-CoA synthase: + $CH_3-C(=O)-SCoA$ → CoA-SH

$^{-}O-C(=O)-CH_2-C(CH_3)(OH)-CH_2-C(=O)-SCoA$
β-hydroxy-β-methyl-glutaryl CoA (HMG-CoA)

HMG-CoA reductase: 2NADPH + 2H⁺ → 2NADP⁺; → CoA-SH

STEP INHIBITED BY STATINS

$^{-}O-C(=O)-CH_2-C(CH_3)(OH)-CH_2-CH_2OH$
Mevalonate

3 **The answer is A: Steatorrhea.** The primary reason for synthesizing conjugated bile acids is to lower the pK_a of the acid, so that a higher percentage of the acid will be ionized in the intestine. The greater a bile acid is ionized, the more efficient the emulsification is for the digestion of the triglyceride. Without conjugation with glycine or taurine, the pK_a of the bile salts is about 6.0; at a pH of 6.0, only 50% of the bile salts will be ionized in the intestinal lumen, which would produce inefficient triglyceride digestion, and the triglyceride content of the stool would increase. By reducing the pK_a to 4.0 (conjugated with glycine) or 2.0 (conjugated with taurine), greater than 99% of the bile acids will be ionized, and triglyceride digestion will be maximal. If an inability to conjugate the bile acids leads to inefficient triglyceride digestion, then intestinal chylomicron formation will be reduced, not

elevated (due to reduction of lipid uptake into the enterocyte). Transport of the water soluble B vitamins into the intestinal cells is not dependent on lipid digestion, as is fat-soluble vitamin absorption. The conjugation of bile acids will not affect the pH of the intestinal lumen, nor will it affect the secretion of zymogens from the pancreas to the intestine. The reactions involved in the conjugation of the bile acids are shown below.

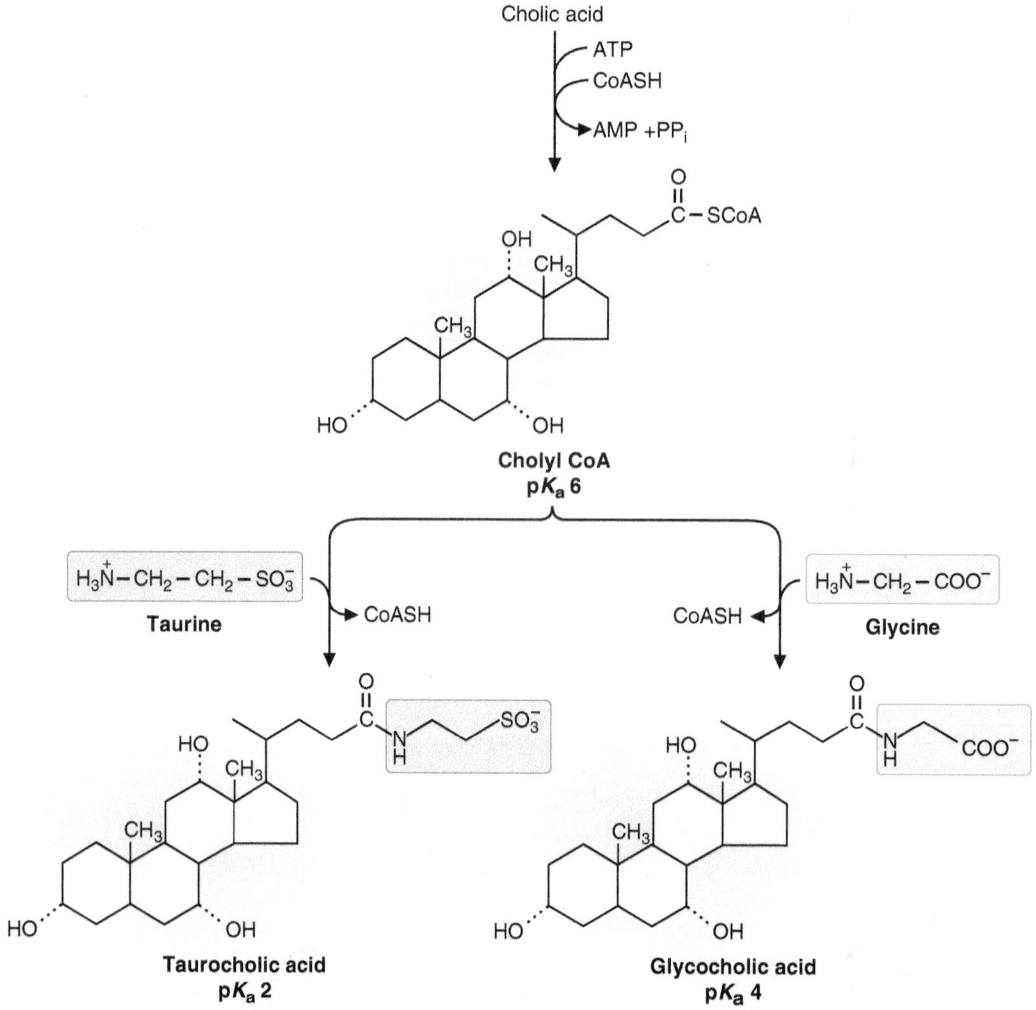

Cholic acid

ATP

CoASH

AMP + PP_i

Cholyl CoA

pK_a 6

$H_3\overset{+}{N}-CH_2-CH_2-SO_3^-$

Taurine

CoASH

$H_3\overset{+}{N}-CH_2-COO^-$

Glycine

CoASH

Taurocholic acid

pK_a 2

Glycocholic acid

pK_a 4

4 **The answer is D: ABC1.** The patient has Tangier disease, which is a defect in the ATP-binding cassette protein 1 (ABC1), a transporter in cell membranes which allows cholesterol efflux from the membrane into the HDL particle. Once inside the HDL particle, the cholesterol is trapped through esterification into a cholesterol ester. The HDL particle can then return the cholesterol to the liver for further recycling. The defect in the patient is not in HMG-CoA reductase (required for the biosynthesis of cholesterol), the AMP-activated kinase (a regulator of HMG-CoA reductase), LCAT (lecithin-cholesterol acyltransferase, the enzyme which esterifies cholesterol in the HDL particle), or CETP (cholesterol ester transfer protein, a protein which exchanges HDL cholesterol esters for VLDL triglyceride).

5 **The answer is B: LCAT.** HDL is protective, in part, due to its ability to remove excess cholesterol from cell membranes and return it to the liver. In order to accomplish this, the cholesterol, after transport to the HDL particle via the participation of ABC1, needs to be trapped within the core of the HDL particle, and this is accomplished by esterification and converting the cholesterol to a cholesterol ester. LCAT (lecithin cholesterol acyl transferase) is the enzyme that creates a cholesterol ester. The reaction, on page 153, is the transfer of a fatty acid from phosphatidyl choline (lecithin) to cholesterol, creating the cholesterol ester and lysophosphatidyl choline. ACAT (acyl-CoA cholesterol acyl transferase) creates cholesterol esters in cells, but not in the HDL particles. CETP exchanges HDL cholesterol esters for VLDL triglyceride.

Protein kinase A is not involved in cholesterol transfer throughout the body. The AMP-activated protein kinase is not utilized in HDL action. The LCAT reaction is shown below.

Lecithin (PC)

LCAT

Cholesterol

Cholesterol ester

Lysolecithin

6 **The answer is D: VLDL.** Under fasting conditions, the total cholesterol measured will be the sum of the cholesterol in the HDL particles, the LDL particles, and VLDL. Chylomicrons should be nil under fasting conditions. The total cholesterol is measured, as are HDL and triglycerides. Since the VLDL is the primary triglyceride carrier under these conditions, the cholesterol content of the VLDL is estimated to be 20% that of the triglyceride content. Thus, the formula for calculating LDL values is LDL = total cholesterol – HDL – [(TG)/5].

7 **The answer is C: LDL receptors are nonfunctional.** Statins are effective in lowering circulating cholesterol levels due to a series of events. First, the statins inhibit HMG-CoA reductase, reducing intracellular synthesis of cholesterol. The reduced cholesterol levels in the cell then upregulate the synthesis of LDL receptors, which remove LDL from circulation, thereby reducing circulating cholesterol levels. Familial hypercholesterolemia (FH) is a mutation in the LDL receptor, making the receptor unable to bind LDL. In homozygous familial hypercholesterolemia, both LDL receptor genes are mutated, and the LDL receptors are nonfunctional. Upregulating nonfunctional LDL receptors will not lead to a reduction of LDL in the circulation, so such individuals are resistant to statin action. FH is not due to a resistant HMG-CoA reductase, nor an inability of statins to reach their target. FH is not related to reverse cholesterol transport, nor to LCAT. A diagram of receptor-mediated endocytosis, indicating the role of the receptor, is shown below.

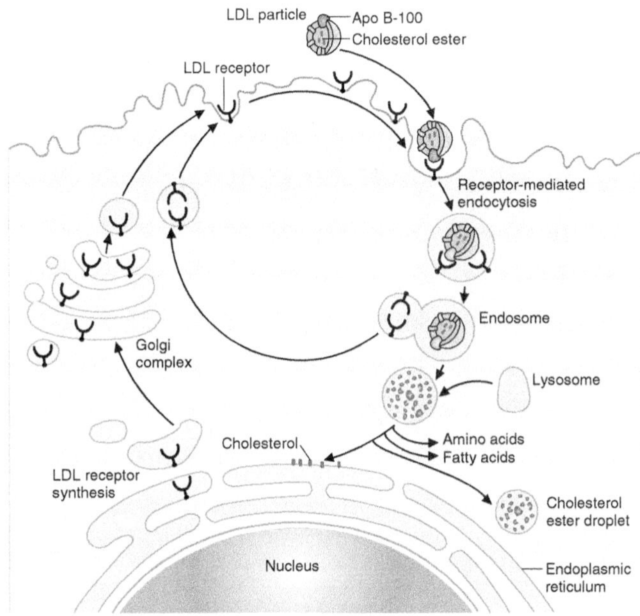

8 **The answer is C: MTTP.** The patient has abetalipoproteinemia, an absence of apo B-containing proteins in the circulation. This leads to low chylomicron and VLDL levels. The problem is the synthesis of the chylomicrons and VLDL, both of which require the activity of the microsomal triglyceride transfer protein (MTTP). In the absence of MTTP activity, triglycerides cannot be transferred to the core particle as it is being synthesized, leading to little, if any, synthesis of these particles. The intestinal cells become laden with lipids obtained from the diet and those which cannot be exported due to the inability to produce chylomicrons. Mutations in LPL or apolipoprotein CII will not interfere with chylomicron or VLDL synthesis; mutations in those proteins would lead to an inability to remove triglyceride from those circulating particles. Deficiencies in LCAT or ABC1, which are related to HDL metabolism, would not affect the synthesis of

chylomicrons or VLDL. A schematic of MTTP action is shown below.

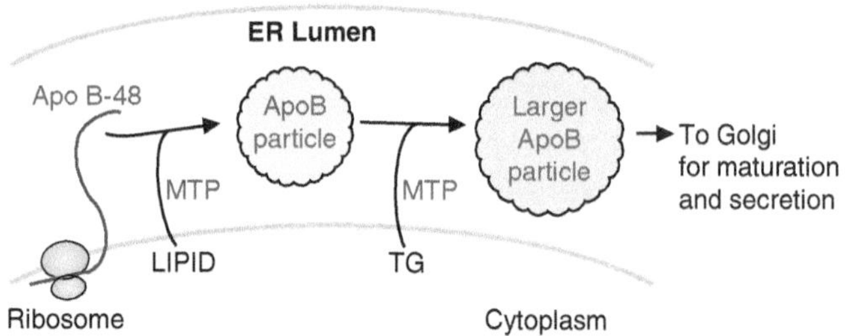

A model of microsomal triglyceride transfer protein (MTTP) action. MTTP is required to transfer lipid to apo B48 as it is synthesized, and to transfer lipid from the cytoplasm to the lumen of the endoplasmic reticulum as the particle (chylomicrons in the intestine, and VLDL in the liver) is being synthesized.

9 **The answer is D: Reduced secretion of LPL.** Insulin release stimulates the secretion of lipoprotein lipase (LPL) from fat and muscle cells such that the capillaries infiltrating these tissues have the lipase bound to extracellular matrix material. Then, as the triglyceride-rich particles move through the tissues, they bind to LPL via apolipoprotein CII, and the triglyceride is digested and the fatty acids used by the tissues. In the absence of insulin, LPL levels are low, and the particles have a longer half-life in circulation due to the reduced rate of digestion, which contributes to hypertriglyceridemia. If there were reduced synthesis of VLDL, triglycerides in the circulation would be reduced, not increased. Insulin does not alter the rate of apolipoprotein CII production. The release of insulin decreases fatty acid oxidation (promoting fatty acid synthesis), but if increased fatty acid oxidation did occur, then triglycerides would not accumulate in the circulation. Insulin also does not alter the synthesis of apolipoprotein B100 in the liver, which is required for VLDL synthesis.

10 **The answer is C: Apo CII.** A lack of apolipoprotein CII would mean that lipoprotein lipase could not be activated, and the triglyceride in both chylomicrons and VLDL would be unable to be digested. This would lead to elevated levels of these particles, and a very high serum triglyceride level. Since VLDL is not being converted to IDL or LDL cholesterol levels are not elevated. Defects in either apo B100 or apo B48 would lead to a loss of either VLDL or chylomicrons, which is not observed. A defect in pancreatic lipase would lead to steatorrhea, as the dietary triglycerides would not be able to be digested. A defect in LCAT would affect HDL metabolism, but not triglyceride metabolism. An overview of the functions of the lipoproteins is presented in Table 17-1.

Table 17-1. Characteristics of the major apoproteins

Apoprotein	Primary Tissue Source	Molecular Mass (Daltons)	Lipoprotein Distribution	Metabolic Function
Apo A-1	Intestine, liver	28,016	HDL (chylomicrons)	Activates LCAT; structural component of HDL
Apo A-II	Liver	17,414	HDL (chylomicrons)	Unknown
Apo A-IV	Intestine	46,465	HDL (chylomicrons)	Unknown
Apo B-48	Intestine	264,000	Chylomicrons	Assembly and secretion of chylomicrons from small bowel
Apo B-100	Liver	540,000	VLDL, IDL, LDL	VLDL assembly and secretion; structural protein of VLDL, IDL, and LDL; ligand for LDL receptor
Apo C-1	Liver	6,630	Chylomicrons, VLDL, IDL, HDL	Unknown; may inhibit hepatic uptake of chylomicron and VLDL remnants
Apo C-II	Liver	8,900	Chylomicrons, VLDL, IDL, HDL	Cofactor activator of lipoprotein lipase (LPL)
Apo C-III	Liver	8,800	Chylomicrons, VLDL, IDL, HDL	Inhibitor of LPL; may inhibit hepatic uptake of chylomicrons and VLDL remnants
Apo E	Liver	34,145	Chylomicron remnants, VLDL, IDL, HDL	Ligand for binding of several lipoproteins to the LDL receptor, to the LDL receptor-related protein (LRP) and possibly to a separate apo-E receptor
Apo(a)	Liver		Lipoprotein "little" a (Lp(a))	Unknown

11 **The answer is D: Secretin.** Secretin is released from the intestine when food enters, and it signals the pancreas to release a watery mixture of bicarbonate into the intestine, in order to help neutralize the acid present from the digestion that occurred in the stomach. If the pH of the intestinal lumen is too low, the bile salts will not be ionized, and emulsification of the dietary fats will be inefficient, as will be the formation of mixed micelles to allow intestinal absorption of fat components. Digestion of carbohydrates and protein is not dependant on bile salt ionization. A loss of cholecystokinin would result in no pancreatic zymogens being secreted, and there would be no digestion of carbohydrates, proteins, or lipids within the intestine. A lack of insulin secretion, or glucagon secretion, does not affect digestion in the intestinal lumen. Cortisol secretion also does not alter intestinal digestion of nutrients.

12 **The answer is B: Oxidized LDL.** Oxidized LDL is taken up by macrophages, which eventually turn into foam cells in the development of an atherosclerotic plaque. The higher one's LDL levels are, the more likely that oxidized LDL will form, leading to plaque formation. The receptor which recognizes and takes up oxidized LDL, SR-A1, is not downregulated, so the macrophage has an unlimited capacity to take up and store the oxidized LDL. Plaque formation does not occur due to elevated levels of nonoxidized LDL, HDL of any form, or triglycerides. A cartoon depiction of a normal and an atherosclerotic artery is shown below.

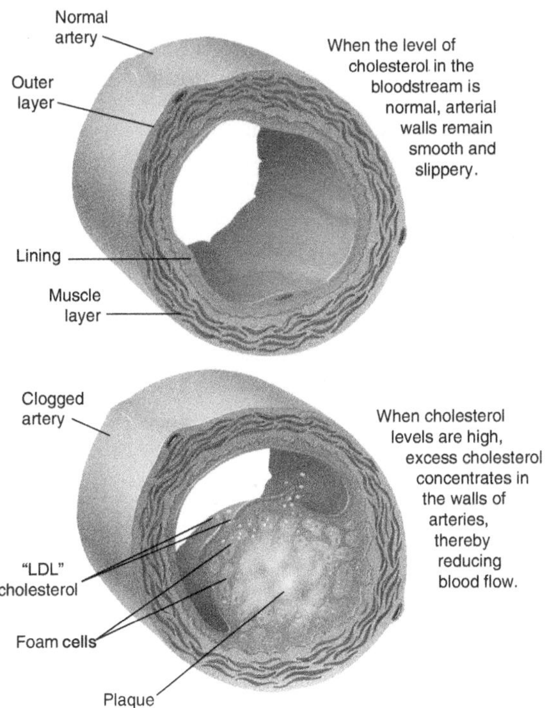

13 **The answer is C: Apolipoprotein E.** The patient has dysbetalipoproteinemia, a mutation in apolipoprotein E, such that the patient exhibits the rare E2 form instead of the normal E3 form. Apolipoprotein E has affinity for the LDL receptor and the LDL receptor-related protein and, as such, is important for chylomicron remnant and IDL uptake from the circulation by the liver. With the homozygous E2 form, binding of the particles to their receptors is weak, and the particles circulate longer than normal, contributing to the high cholesterol and triglyceride levels seen in the circulation. Only about 10% of the individuals who are homozygous for E2 will develop this condition, and in those, obesity (BMI of 34) is a key factor which links the condition to the mutation. This disorder is not a problem with lipoprotein lipase (LPL) digesting triglycerides from particles, so neither LPL nor apo CII is defective. As both chylomicrons and VLDL are produced, it is not a defect in either apo B48 or B100 production or function.

14 **The answer is B: Coenzyme Q.** Coenzyme Q is derived from isoprene units, which are produced in the pathway of cholesterol biosynthesis, after the HMG-CoA reductase step. If HMG-CoA reductase is inhibited (as it is by statins), then the production of the isoprenes is also reduced, and both Coenzyme Q and dolichol levels could become limiting. The biosynthesis of heme, ketone bodies, glycogen, or dihydrobiopterin is not dependent on isoprene units.

15 **The answer is B: To reduce circulating cholesterol levels.** Phytosterols interfere with cholesterol absorption in the intestine (through blockage of cholesterol incorporation into the mixed micelles, which are necessary for intestinal epithelial cells to absorb dietary cholesterol), thereby leading to a reduction in circulating cholesterol levels. The phytosterols do not interfere with the biosynthesis of cholesterol, nor do they alter the secretion of insulin. Phytosterols are also not capable of altering the rate of fatty acid biosynthesis, nor do they affect circulating triglyceride levels. The effect of phytosterols is specific for the inhibition of cholesterol absorption from the intestine.

16 **The answer is B: Ezetimibe.** Ezetimibe reduces circulating cholesterol levels by blocking cholesterol absorption in the intestine, which is similar to the mechanism of action of phytosterols. Atorvastatin is a statin, and its mechanism of action is inhibition of HMG-CoA reductase. Pravastatin is also a statin and works as does atorvastatin. Simvastatin is yet another statin. Metformin is a lipid- and glucose-lowering drug which works via activation of the AMP-activated protein kinase and does not alter cholesterol absorption

Table 17-2. Mechanism(s) of action and efficacy of lipid-lowering agents

		Percentage Change in Serum Lipid Level (monotherapy)			
Agent	**Mechanism of Action**	**Total Cholesterol**	**LDL Cholesterol**	**HDL Cholesterol**	**Triacylglycerols**
Statins	Inhibit HMG-CoA reductase activity	↓15%–60%	↓20%–60%	↑5%–15%	↓10%–40%
Bile acid resins	Increase fecal excretion of bile salts	↓15%–20%	↓10%–25%	↑3%–5%	Variable, depending on pretreatment level of triacylglycerols (may increase)
Niacin	Activates LPL; reduces hepatic production of VLDL; reduces catabolism of HDL	↓22%–25%	↓10%–25%	↑15%–35%	↓20%–50%
Fibrates	Antagonizes PPAR-α, causing an increase in LPL activity, a decrease in apoprotein C-III production, and an increase in apoprotein A-I production.	↓12%–15%	Variable, depending on pretreatment levels of other lipids	↑5%–15%	↓20%–50%
Ezetimibe	Reduces intestinal absorption of free cholesterol from the gut lumen	↓10%–15%	↓15%–20%	↑1%–3%	↓5%–8% if triacylglycerols are high pretreatment

LPL, lipoprotein lipase; *LDL*, low-density lipoprotein; *HDL*, high-density lipoprotein; triacylglycerols, triglycerides; *PPAR*, peroxisome proliferator-activated receptor.

Adapted from Circulation. Grundy SM, Becker D, Clark LT etal. 2002;106:3145–3457.

in the intestine. Table 17-2 summarizes the action of cholesterol lowering drugs.

17 The answer is C: Constant SR-A1 expression on the cell surface. The macrophages take up oxidized LDL using a scavenger receptor, SR-A1, which is not downregulated. This allows the receptor to remain on the cell surface and to constantly import oxidized LDL into the cell. The high levels of cholesterol in the foam cells is not due to a change in activity of ACAT or LCAT (which is found in HDL particles), nor is there upregulation of HMG-CoA reductase (which would produce more endogenous cholesterol, which is unlikely since the cell is filled with cholesterol and cholesterol esters). Macrophages do not use the LDL receptor for importing oxidized LDL.

18 The answer is E: LDL receptor. The patient is heterozygous for a mutation in the LDL receptor (familial hypercholesterolemia). This condition leads to elevated LDL levels since there are insufficient receptors available to remove LDL from the circulation. If left untreated, heart attacks are common in such patients before the age of 50. This condition is treated with statins, which reduce endogenous cholesterol synthesis, thereby leading to an upregulation of LDL receptors, which allows for normal LDL uptake from the circulation. Mutations in LCAT (familial LCAT deficiency) are rare and do not often lead to premature atherosclerotic disease (although some exceptions are noted), but do lead to kidney and corneal damage due to large amounts of unesterified cholesterol present in those tissues. HDL level in these individuals is usually less than 10 mg/dL, which is not observed in our patient. Mutations in CETP (cholesterol ester transfer protein) lead to elevations in HDL levels and would not be responsive to statin action. Mutations in ABC1 lead to Tangier disease, which would lead to a reduction in HDL levels, which is not seen in this patient. A deficiency in apo B100 would impair VLDL synthesis and would actually reduce circulating LDL levels since there is less VLDL present to be converted to LDL. The diagram on page 157 depicts potential problems which result from defects in the LDL receptor.

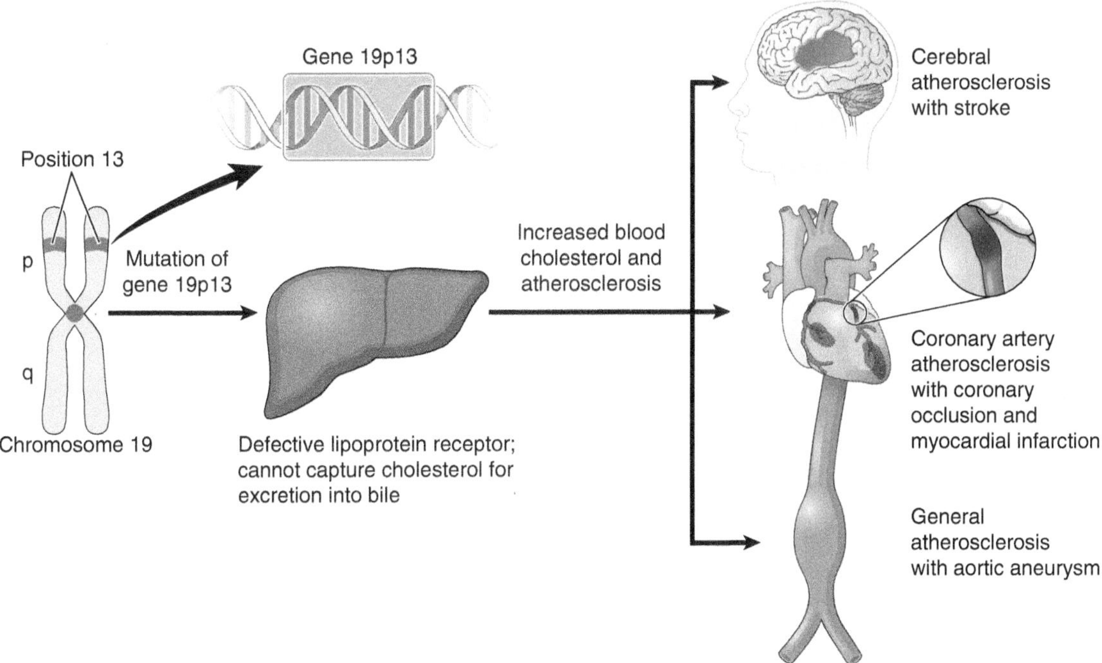

Answer 18: Potential results of mutations within the LDL receptor.

19 **The answer is C: Increased risk for cardiovascular complications.** Lipoprotein (a) is an LDL particle with a covalently linked apoprotein A (linked to apoprotein B100) attached to the particle. The presence of this unusual lipoprotein particle has been positively correlated with the presence of heart disease. The role of this particle is unknown, but may be related to coagulation, since apoprotein A resembles plasminogen in structure. Lp (a) levels do not regulate the levels of platelets in the circulation.

20 **The answer is D: ABCG5.** The patient has sitosterolemia, an accumulation of plant sterols (phytosterols) in cells and tissues. Under normal conditions, phytosterols can diffuse into the epithelial cells, but they are actively transported back into the intestinal lumen by an ABC-cassette (ATP-binding) containing protein, ABCG5 (the other protein responsible for phytosterol efflux is ABCG8).Those sterols which make it to the liver are exported by the same proteins in the liver to the bile duct, where they will be released along with the bile during fat digestion. In the absence of activity of either ABCG5 or ABCG8, the phytosterols are packaged into chylomicrons and are eventually delivered to the liver, where they are packaged into VLDL. While human cells cannot utilize phytosterols, their increased presence interferes with the synthesis of cholesterol and the normal cholesterol recycling within the affected patient. Patients with this disorder develop premature coronary artery disease. It has been hypothesized that the high levels of plant sterols in the circulating lipoprotein particles accelerate the deposition of these sterols in the walls of the arteries, promoting atherosclerosis. This disorder is not due to mutations in either apo B100 or apo B48, as both VLDL and chylomicrons are synthesized normally in the patient. The defect is not in ABC1, as the patient does not display the symptoms of Tangier disease. The defect is also not in MTTP, as a defect in that protein leads to abetalipoproteinemia.

Chapter 18

Purine and Pyrimidine Metabolism

The questions in this chapter will test ones knowledge concerning de novo and salvage pathways related to nucleotide metabolism, as well as the relevance of these pathways to human disease, and the treatment of human disease.

QUESTIONS

Select the single best answer.

1 Your 56-year-old male patient presents with intense redness, heat, and pain over his right great toe at the metatarsophalangeal joint. Fluid from this joint shows bifringent crystals. An X-ray of the foot is shown below. This disease is caused by the degradation of an excessive amount of which of the following?

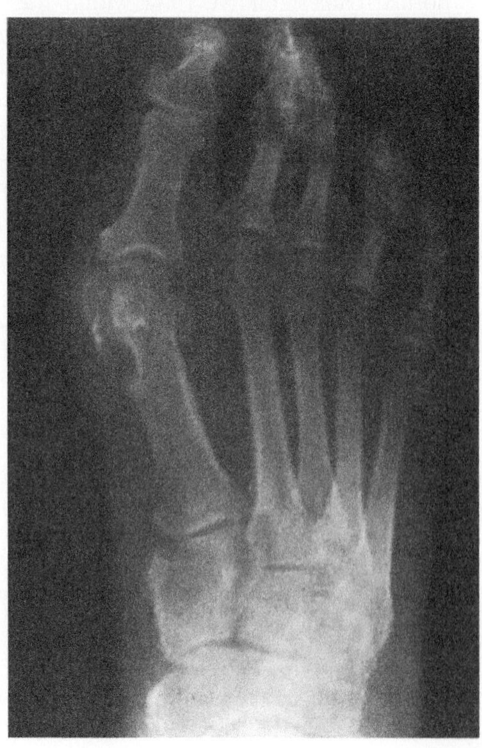

(A) Adenine
(B) Thymine
(C) Uracil
(D) Cytosine
(E) Ribose-5-phosphate

2 Your 60-year-old female patient has psoriasis and has been treated with methotrexate for several years. She has no other medical problems and her preventive screenings, including fecal occult blood tests and colonoscopy, have all been normal. She has developed an anemia. Which of the following would you expect to find when working up her anemia?

(A) A macrocytic anemia
(B) A microcytic anemia
(C) Thalassemia
(D) Spherocytes
(E) A low vitamin B_{12} level

3 A researcher wants to develop a method of labeling purines with ^{15}N for use in future spectroscopic studies. Purine synthesis will be done in a test tube using only the enzymes necessary to synthesize purines via the de novo pathway. Which starting materials should be labeled with the heavy nitrogen in order to maximize ^{15}N incorporation into purines?

(A) Aspartate, glycine, and glutamate
(B) Aspartate, glycine, and N5-formimino tetrahydrofolate
(C) Asparagine, glycine, and glutamine
(D) Asparagine, glutamate, and glutamine
(E) Aspartate, glycine, and glutamine

4 A patient has been recently diagnosed with colorectal cancer. The physician treats the patient with a combination of chemotherapeutic drugs, one of which is 5-fluorouracil (5-FU). 5-FU is effective as an anticancer drug because it inhibits which one of the following enzymes?

(A) Dihydrofolate reductase
(B) Thymidylate synthase
(C) Amidophosphoribosyl transferase
(D) 5′-phosphoribosyl 1′-pyrophosphate (PRPP) synthetase
(E) UMP synthase

5 A patient exhibits fasting hypoglycemia and lactic acidosis under fasting conditions. Hepatomegaly is also evident. A glucagon challenge only releases about 10% of the expected level of glucose from the liver. The patient has also developed gout due to an increase in the levels of which of the following metabolites?
(A) PRPP
(B) Glutamine
(C) ATP
(D) NADH
(E) dTTP

6 A 6-month-old infant is seen by the pediatrician for developmental delay. Blood work shows megaloblastic anemia, although measurements of B_{12} and folate are in the high normal range. Urinalysis demonstrates, upon standing, the formation of a crystalline substance. Supplementation of the child's diet with uridine reversed virtually all of the clinical problems. The crystalline substance was most likely composed of which of the following?
(A) Uracil
(B) Thymine
(C) Orotate
(D) Aspartate
(E) Cytosine

7 Considering the patient in the previous question, after uridine treatment the crystals were no longer found in the urine. This is due to which of the following?
(A) Inhibition of the enzyme producing the crystalline molecule
(B) Bypassing the mutated step of the pathway
(C) Inhibition of aspartate transcarbamoylase
(D) Inhibition of nitrogen fixation by carbamoyl phosphate synthetase I
(E) Inhibition of carbamoyl phosphate synthetase II

8 Considering the patient in the last two problems, the observed megaloblastic anemia results from which of the following?
(A) Interference with folate metabolism
(B) Interference with B_{12} absorption
(C) Inhibition of ribonucleotide reductase
(D) Lack of thymidine for DNA synthesis
(E) Lack of adenine for DNA synthesis

9 Your patient has sickle cell disease and is being treated with hydroxyurea. After 2 weeks on the drug, you find greatly reduced levels of most blood cell types, and the patient is removed from the drug to allow his blood cell counts to stabilize. One potential reason for this side effect of hydroxyurea treatment is its ability to alter the synthesis of which of the following metabolites?
(A) N5-methyltetrahydrofolate
(B) 5′ phosphoribosyl 1′ amine
(C) PRPP
(D) Adenosylcobalamin
(E) dUMP

10 An 18-month-old infant has had a history of recurrent bacterial and viral infections. The child has failure to thrive, developmental delay, and tremors. Physical exam shows a lack of peripheral lymphoid tissue. Blood work shows lymphopenia, but normal levels of B-cells and circulating immunoglobulins. This child most likely has a defect in which of the following enzymes?
(A) Hypoxanthine guanine phosphoribosyltransferase (HGPRT)
(B) Adenine phosphoribosyltransferase (APRT)
(C) Adenosine deaminase (ADA)
(D) Adenosine kinase
(E) Purine nucleoside phosphorylase

11 Considering the child in the previous question, which one of the following metabolites would you expect to accumulate in the thymocytes?
(A) dCTP
(B) dTTP
(C) dIMP
(D) dGTP
(E) dUTP

12 Individuals with gout are given allopurinol for long-term management of the disease. In such individuals, which of the following bases would accumulate in the urine?
(A) Urate and xanthine
(B) Guanine and adenine
(C) Hypoxanthine and guanine
(D) Xanthine and guanine
(E) Hypoxanthine and xanthine

13 A 1-year-old boy was brought to the pediatrician due to a developmental delay, biting of his lips and fingers, and the presence of orange crystals in his diapers. Enzymatic analysis shows loss of 99% of the activity of a particular enzyme. The defective enzyme in this disorder would normally utilize which of the following as a substrate?

(A) Adenine
(B) Guanine
(C) Adenosine
(D) Guanosine
(E) GMP

14 Considering the patient in the previous question, the orange sand in the diapers was composed of which of the following?
(A) Xanthine
(B) Hypoxanthine
(C) Guanine
(D) Adenine
(E) Urate

15 A 6-month-old boy was brought to the pediatrician due to frequent bacterial and viral infections. Blood work shows the complete absence of B and T cells. Radiographic analysis shows a greatly reduced thymic shadow. Treatment of the child with a stabilized protein reverses the deficiencies. This protein has which of the following activities?
(A) Converts IMP to XMP
(B) Converts adenine to AMP
(C) Converts guanine to GMP
(D) Converts adenosine to inosine
(E) Converts guanosine to inosine

16 Concerning the patient in the previous questions, which metabolite will accumulate in the blood cells?
(A) dUTP
(B) dCTP
(C) dATP
(D) dGTP
(E) dTTP

17 Concerning the patient discussed in the last two questions, one possible reason for the lack of immune cells is inhibition of which of the following enzymes?
(A) ADA
(B) Purine nucleoside phosphorylase
(C) Hypoxanthine guanine phosphoribosyltransferase
(D) Adenine phosphoribosyltransferase
(E) Ribonucleotide reductase

18 A penicillin-allergic child was given a sulfonamide for otitis media. Human cells are resistant to sulfonamides due to which of the following?
(A) Sulfonamides are specific for prokaryotic DNA polymerases
(B) Sulfonamides are specific for prokaryotic RNA polymerases
(C) Sulfonamides inhibit a metabolic pathway not present in eukaryotic cells
(D) Sulfonamides inhibit bacterial ribonucleotide reductase, but not eukaryotic ribonucleotide reductase
(E) Sulfonamides inhibit prokaryotic mismatch repair, but not eukaryotic mismatch repair

19 The primary route of carbon entry into the tetrahydrofolate (THF) pool is via the serine hydroxymethyl transferase reaction. Which of the following is required to convert that initial form of the THF into the form that can donate carbons to de novo purine synthesis?
(A) Glycine
(B) FAD
(C) Water
(D) B_{12}
(E) B_6

20 Many anticancer drugs are given to patients in their nucleoside form, rather than the nucleotide form. Which enzyme below will be required in the conversion of deoxyguanosine to dGTP?
(A) Pyrimidine nucleoside phosphorylase
(B) Deoxyguanosine kinase
(C) Ribonucleotide reductase
(D) Adenine phosphoribosyltransferase
(E) 5′-nucleotidase

ANSWERS

1 **The answer is A: Adenine.** This person has gout. Gout is caused by uric acid crystallization into a joint and an intense inflammatory reaction to those crystals. The X-ray demonstrated soft-tissue swelling over the first metatarsophalangeal joint and typical gouty erosion. Uric acid is an insoluble breakdown product of purines (adenine, hypoxanthine, or guanine). Pyrimidines (thymine, uracil, and cytosine) breakdown to different water-soluble products that do not crystallize. Ribose-5-phosphate is also degraded to very water-soluble products. The pathway of uric acid formation is shown below.

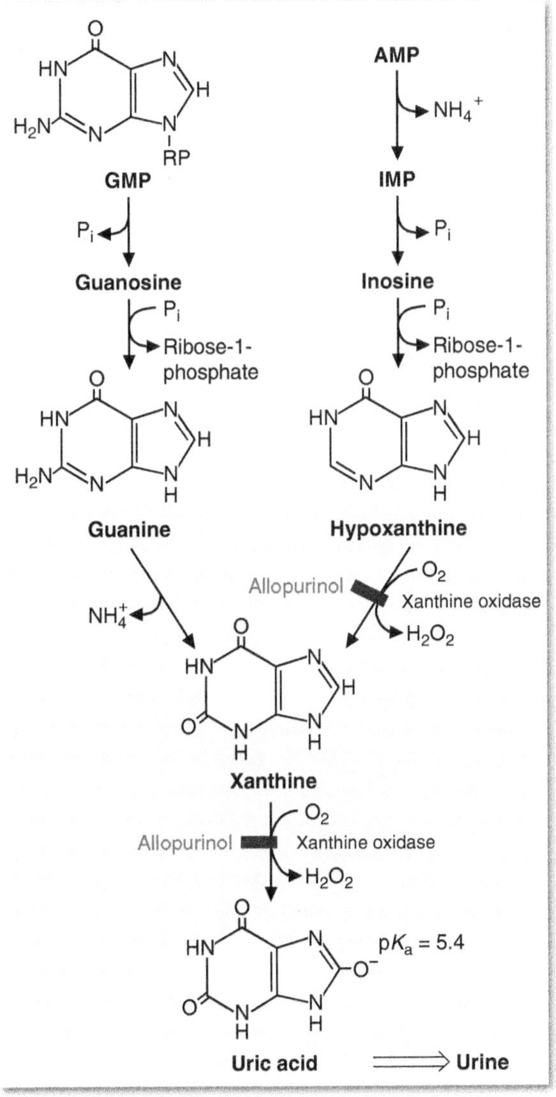

The degradative pathway for purines. Note how allopurinol, a drug used to treat gout, inhibits the enzyme xanthine oxidase, which reduces uric acid production.

2 **The answer is A: A macrocytic anemia.** Methotrexate acts by inhibiting dihydrofolate reductase such that THF cannot be formed (either from folate or dihydrofolate), and a functional folate deficiency results (see the figure below). The folate deficiency then results in a macrocytic anemia due to the lack of DNA synthesis. Red cell precursors increase in mass but cannot divide due to the lack of precursors for DNA replication. As a result, larger than normal cells are released into the circulation, although the overall red cell number decreases, resulting in an anemia. Both thalassemia and spherocytosis lead to microcytic anemia. Vitamin B_{12} levels would not be affected, and the normal occult blood tests and colonoscopy indicate that there is no bleeding leading to the anemia.

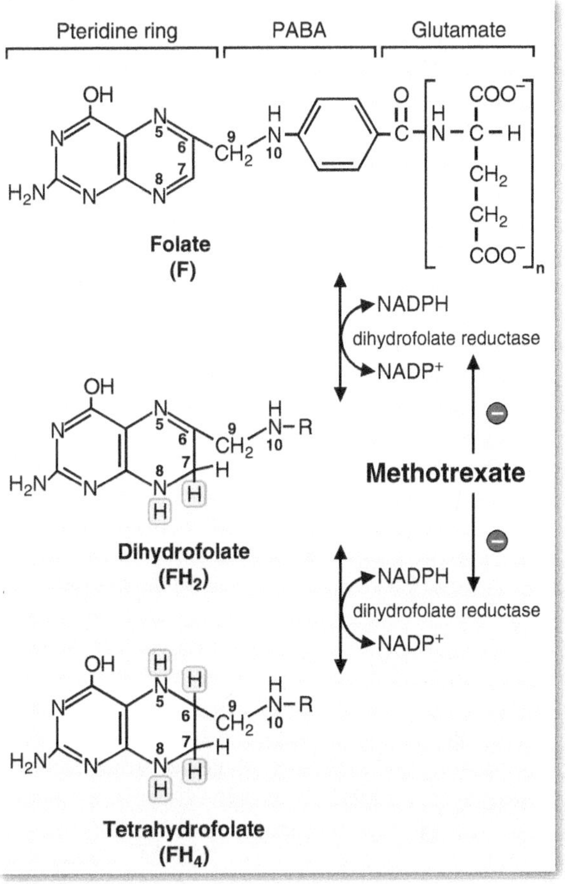

3 **The answer is E: Aspartate, glycine, and glutamine.** As shown in the figure below, the nitrogen in a purine ring is directly derived from glycine, glutamine, and aspartic acid. Glutamate, N5-formimino tetrahydrofolate, and asparagine do not directly donate nitrogen to the ring.

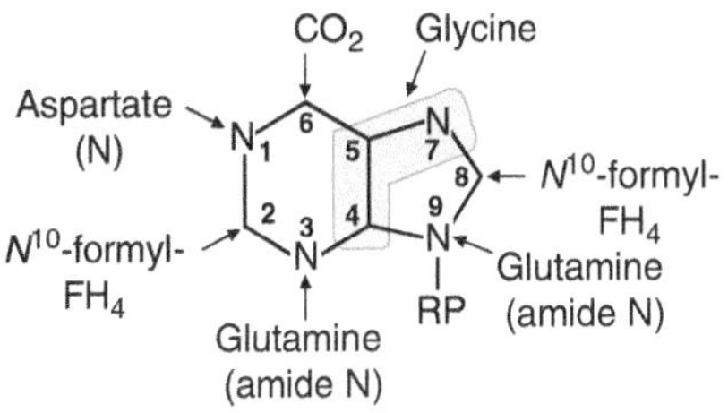

4 **The answer is B: Thymidylate synthase.** 5-fluorouracil is a thymine analog (thymine is 5-methyl uracil), which, after activation in the cells to F-dUMP, binds tightly to thymidylate synthase and blocks the enzyme from converting dUMP to dTMP (see the figure below). By blocking thymidine synthesis, cells can no longer synthesize DNA and will not replicate. 5-FU has no direct effect on dihydrofolate reductase, amidophosphoribosyl transferase, PRPP synthase, or UMP synthase. The figure also indicates the effect of methotrexate on dihydrofolate reductase.

5-Fluorouracil

5-Fluorouracil

thymidylate synthase

Deoxyribose-P dUMP

N^5,N^{10}-Methylene FH_4

Deoxyribose-P dTMP

FH_2 Dihydrofolate

Methotrexate

NADPH

dihydrofolate reductase

Glycine

Serine

FH_4

$NADP^+$

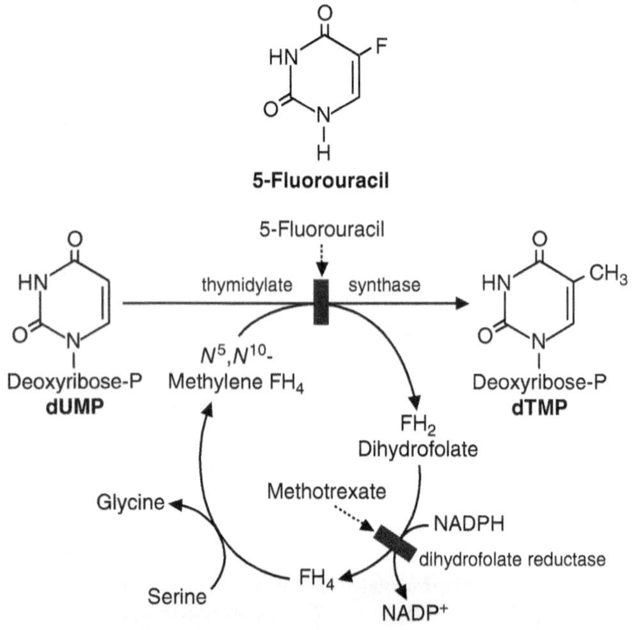

5 **The answer is A: PRPP.** The patient has von Gierke disease, a lack of glucose-6-phosphatase activity. When this individual tries to produce glucose for export in the liver, glucose-6-phosphate accumulates, which then goes through either glycolysis (generating lactate) or the HMP shunt pathway, producing excess ribose-5-phosphate. The excess ribose-5-phosphate is converted to PRPP, which then stimulates the amidophosphoribosyl transferase reaction (the rate-limiting step of purine production) to produce 5′-phosphoribosyl 1′-amine. This last reaction occurs because under normal cellular conditions, the concentrations of PRPP and glutamine are significantly below the *Km* values for amidophosphoribosyl transferase. Any cellular perturbation that increases PRPP levels, then, will increase the rate of the reaction, producing purines that are not required by the cell. This leads to degradation of the excess purines, producing urate and leading to gout. The lactic acidosis associated with von Gierke disease also blocks the transport of urate from the blood into the urine, which contributes to the elevated uric acid levels seen in these patients. Von Gierke disease does not lead to elevated glutamine, ATP, NADH, or dTTP levels.

6 **The answer is C: Orotate.** The child has hereditary orotic aciduria, a mutation in the UMP synthase that leads to orotic acid accumulation in the urine (see the figure below). Treatment with uridine bypasses the block and allows UTP, CTP, and dTTP synthesis. Uridine treatment also has the beneficial effect of blocking

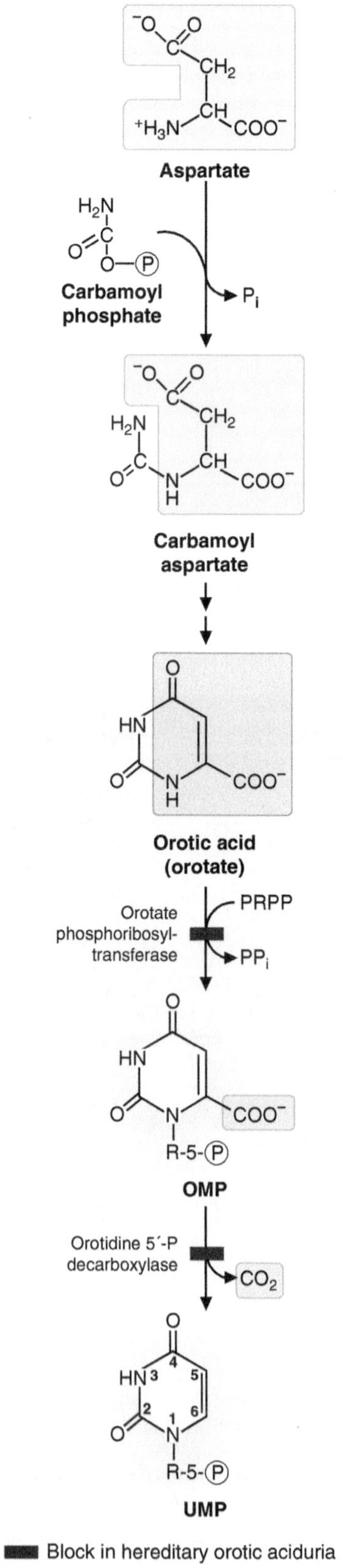

Aspartate

Carbamoyl phosphate

P_i

Carbamoyl aspartate

Orotic acid (orotate)

Orotate phosphoribosyl-transferase

PRPP

PP_i

R-5-(P)

OMP

Orotidine 5′-P decarboxylase

CO_2

R-5-(P)

UMP

Block in hereditary orotic aciduria

further orotate production, as UTP inhibits carbamoyl phosphate synthetase II, the rate-determining step of pyrimidine production. As CPS-II is inhibited, less orotate is produced. The megaloblastic anemia is the result of inadequate DNA synthesis in the red cell precursors due to the lack of dTTP and dCTP. The crystals are made of orotate, as that is the compound that is accumulating. Uracil, thymine, and cytosine would not be synthesized in a patient with this disorder. Aspartate is very soluble and would not form crystals if it were to accumulate.

7 **The answer is E: Inhibition of carbamoyl phosphate synthetase II.** Uridine bypasses the mutated step of the pathway, allowing UTP to be produced. UTP inhibits the rate-determining step of the pathway, carbamoyl phosphate synthetase II, which halts the production of orotic acid, thereby lowering the concentration of orotate in the urine. This is the mechanism whereby the crystals no longer form. Uridine is not inhibiting the enzyme that directly forms orotate, nor does it inhibit aspartate transcarbamoylase or CPS-I. While adding uridine does bypass the regulated step, it is the synthesis of UTP from the uridine that leads to the drop in orotate production. The pathway of orotate synthesis is shown in the answer to the previous question.

8 **The answer is D: lack of thymidine for DNA synthesis.** When UMP synthesis is inhibited, there are insufficient precursors for dTMP synthesis (which is derived from dUMP via the thymidylate synthase reaction). The lack of dTTP (which is derived from dTMP) leads to an inhibition of DNA synthesis in red blood cell precursors, leading to the megaloblastic anemia. The mutation in hereditary orotic aciduria does not affect folate or B_{12} metabolism. Since this is a mutation in a pyrimidine biosynthetic pathway, there is no effect on adenine synthesis. This mutation also does not affect the activity of ribonucleotide reductase.

9 **The answer is E: dUMP.** Hydroxyurea, in addition to inducing γ-chain synthesis of hemoglobin, is also an inhibitor of ribonucleotide reductase. If ribonucleotide reductase is inhibited, the cells' ability to generate deoxyribonucleotides will be impaired, and DNA synthesis will be hindered. Since blood cells are regenerated at a rapid rate, they are one of the first cells affected by an inhibition of DNA synthesis, and the result is a decrease of blood cells in the patient. Of the answers listed, the synthesis of only dUMP requires the activity of ribonucleotide reductase. Hydroxyurea does not interfere with the synthesis of N5-methyltetrahydrofolate, 5′-phosphoribosyl 1′-amine, PRPP, or adenosylcobalamin.

10 **The answer is E: Purine nucleoside phosphorylase.** The child has purine nucleoside phosphorylase deficiency, which, for reasons not yet fully elucidated, specifically reduces T-cell counts but not B-cells. Purine nucleoside phosphorylase is one of the salvage enzymes that converts guanosine or inosine to the free base plus ribose-1-phosphate (adenosine is not a substrate for this enzyme). HGPRT deficiency leads to Lesch–Nyhan syndrome, whose symptoms are quite different (there is no immune deficiency with an HGPRT defect). APRT deficiency leads to a buildup of an insoluble metabolite (2, 8-dihydroxyadenine) that precipitates in the kidney and will lead to renal failure. ADA deficiency will lead to an immune disorder, but in ADA deficiency, both B and T cells are deficient. An adenosine kinase deficiency has not been reported in humans. An overview of the purine salvage pathway is shown below.

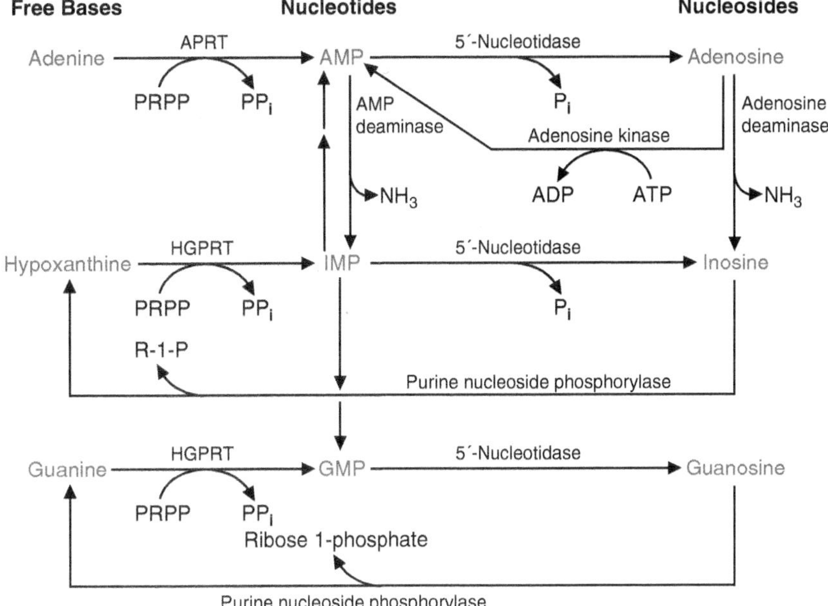

Answer 10: Salvage of bases. The purine bases hypoxanthine and guanine react with PRPP to form the nucleotides inosine and guanosine monophosphate, respectively. HGPRT catalyzes this reaction. Adenine forms AMP in a similar type of reaction catalyzed by APRT. Nucleotides are converted to nucleosides by 5′-nucleotidase. Free bases are generated from nucleosides by purine nucleoside phosphorylase (although note that adenosine is not a substrate of this enzyme). Deamination of the base adenine occurs with AMP and ADA. Of the purines, only adenosine can be phosphorylated by adenosine kinase directly back to a nucleotide.

11 **The answer is D: dGTP.** With a purine nucleoside phosphorylase deficiency, guanosine will accumulate (see the figure in the answer to the previous question), which will inhibit the conversion of GMP to guanosine via the actions of 5′-nucleotidase (this is also true for dGMP). As dGMP accumulates, it will be phosphorylated to form dGTP. Concurrently, inosine will accumulate, blocking the conversion of adenosine to inosine and also leading to an increase in dATP levels. The combination of dATP and dGTP leads to inhibition of ribonucleotide reductase in the thymocytes, leading to T-cell depletion. It has also been reported that the accumulation of deoxyguanosine triggers apoptosis in T cells, providing another mechanism for T-cell depletion. This does not affect the B cells in this disorder. None of the other nucleotides listed (dCTP, dTTP, dIMP, and dUTP) will accumulate in this disorder.

12 **The answer is E: Hypoxanthine and xanthine.** As shown below, the target of allopurinol, the enzyme xanthine oxidase, catalyzes two reactions. The first is the conversion of hypoxanthine (which is produced during the degradation of adenine) to xanthine and the second is the conversion of xanthine (which is produced during the degradation of guanine) to uric acid. Thus, in the presence of allopurinol, hypoxanthine accumulates from the degradation of adenine and xanthine accumulates via the guanine degradative pathway. Both of these compounds are more soluble than urate, thus alleviating the major problem in gout.

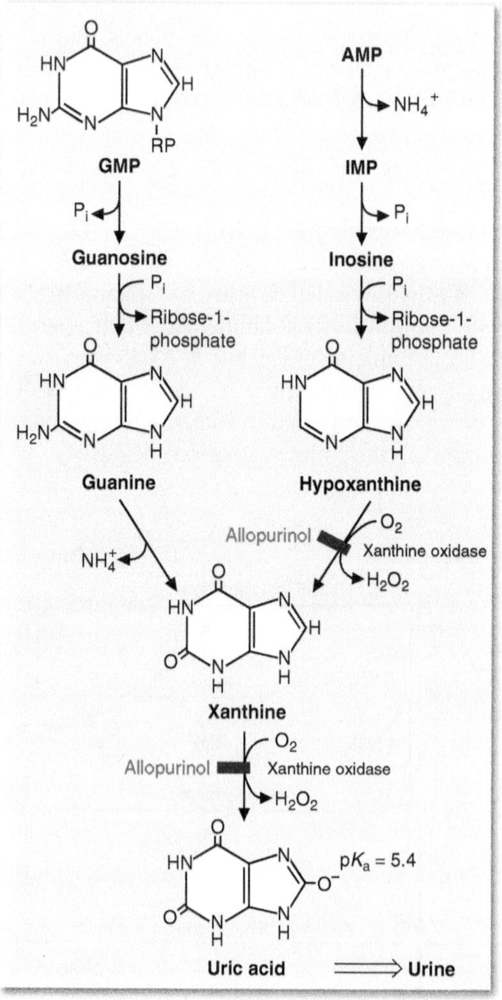

The degradative pathway for purines. Note how allopurinol, a drug used to treat gout, inhibits the enzyme xanthine oxidase, which reduces uric acid production.

13 **The answer is B: Guanine.** The patient has Lesch–Nyhan syndrome, a deficiency in HGPRT activity. HGPRT utilizes as substrates hypoxanthine, guanine, and PRPP, converting the free base to a nucleoside monophosphate (IMP and GMP). The enzyme does not utilize adenine, adenosine, guanosine, or GMP as a substrate. The reason for the aberrant behavior and developmental delay observed in this disorder has not yet been elucidated.

14 **The answer is E: Urate.** Patients with Lesch–Nyhan syndrome develop severe gout as the free bases, guanine and hypoxanthine, can no longer be salvaged. As these bases accumulate, urate is produced in excess, leading to gout. This is frequently seen in infants with this disorder as an orange sand-like compound. Xanthine, hypoxanthine, guanine, and adenine are not accumulating in the urine, as these molecules are metabolized to produce urate.

15 **The answer is D: Converts adenosine to inosine.** The patient has the symptoms of ADA deficiency, which leads to severe combined immunodeficiency syndrome. ADA catalyzes the conversion of adenosine to inosine. IMP dehydrogenase converts IMP to XMP. APRT converts adenine to AMP. HGPRT converts guanine to GMP, and there is no enzyme that can convert guanosine to inosine in one step (guanase can convert guanine to xanthine in one step, but does not work on nucleoside substrates).

16 **The answer is C: dATP.** Due to the lack of ADA activity, adenosine accumulates and is converted to AMP by adenosine kinase (and deoxyadenosine is converted to dAMP). The dAMP will eventually be converted to dATP, which accumulates within the cell. There is no accumulation of dUTP, dCTP, dGTP, and dTTP under these conditions. Adenosine and deoxyadenosine levels are also high in the blood, as all tissues of the body release these compounds when they can be no longer metabolized, due to ADA deficiency. This leads to accumulation of these toxic intermediates in the lymphocytes, which are the tissues that manifest the clinical aspects of the disease.

Table 18-1. Effectors of ribonucleotide reductase activity

Preferred Substrate	Effector Bound to Overall Activity Site	Effector Bound to Substrate Specificity Site
None	dATP	Any nucleotide
CDP	ATP	ATP or dATP
UDP	ATP	ATP or dATP
GDP	ATP	dTTP
ADP	ATP	dGTP

Notes: Ribonucleotide reductase contains two allosteric sites. One regulates the overall activity of the enzyme (with dATP blocking activity and ATP stimulating activity). The other site regulates which substrate will be reduced (thus, with ATP bound to the substrate specificity site, pyrimidine diphosphates will be reduced by the enzyme).

17 **The answer is E: Ribonucleotide reductase.** The increase in dATP, which occurs when ADA is defective, leads to the binding of dATP to the allosteric activity site of ribonucleotide reductase, which leads to the inhibition of overall enzyme activity. Thus, deoxyribonucleotides cannot be produced for the synthesis of DNA, and cells are not capable of replication. Elevated levels of dATP do not have an inhibitory effect on purine nucleoside phosphorylase, hypoxanthine guanine phosphoribosyltransferase, APRT, or ADA. The regulation of ribonucleotide reductase is summarized in Table 18-1.

18 **The answer is C: Sulfonamides inhibit a metabolic pathway not present in eukaryotic cells.** Sulfonamides inhibit the synthesis of THF, a compound that eukaryotic cells cannot synthesize (which is why folic acid is a required vitamin in the human diet). Via inhibition of THF synthesis, the target prokaryotic cells can no longer synthesize dTMP and purines and are unable to grow and replicate. Sulfonamides do not affect DNA polymerases directly, nor do they alter mismatch repair. Sulfonamides also have no effect on ribonucleotide reductase.

19 **The answer is C: Water.** Serine donates a carbon to THF to form N5, N10-methylene THF. This is oxidized to form N5, N10-methenyl THF, which is then hydrolyzed with water to form N10-formyl THF (see the figure below). As such, glycine, FAD, B_{12}, and B_6 are not required for these conversions to take place. The pathway for folate metabolism is shown below.

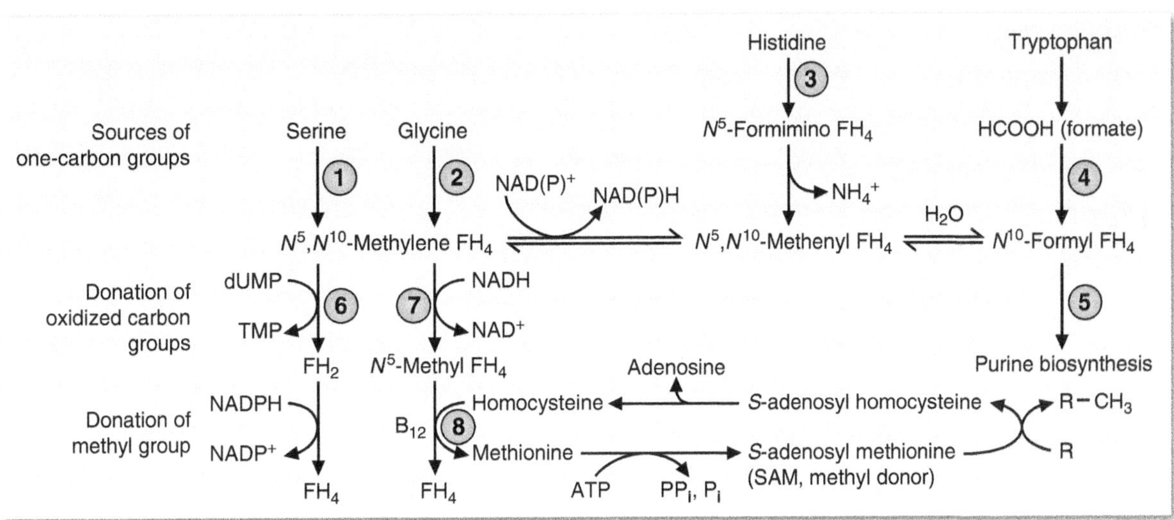

Answer 19

20 **The answer is C: Ribonucleotide reductase.** Deoxyguanosine would be first acted on by purine nucleoside phosphorylase, which would produce guanine and deoxyribose-1-phosphate. The guanine would be converted to GMP by HGPRT, and the GMP phosphorylated to GDP. The GDP would be reduced by ribonucleotide reductase to dGDP, which is then phosphorylated again to produce dGTP. Since guanine is a purine, pyrimidine nucleoside phosphorylase is not required in this pathway. There is no deoxyguanosine kinase (the only purine nucleosides that can be phosphorylated by adenosine kinase are adenosine and deoxyadenosine). APRT only works for the adenine base, not guanine. The 5′-nucleotidase is not required as there are no dephosphorylation events in the pathway outlined.

Chapter 19

Diabetes and Metabolic Syndrome

This chapter also presents questions involving overall whole-body metabolism, emphasizing the integration of biochemical pathways, which do not specifically address diabetes or metabolic syndrome.

QUESTIONS

Select the single best answer.

1 Your diabetic patient has recently been placed on pramlintide (Symlin) to help control his diabetes. Which of the following best describes the mechanism of action of this medication?

(A) It decreases glucose-6-phospate
(B) It increases hexokinase
(C) It stimulates glycogen phosphorylase
(D) It inhibits glucagon secretion
(E) It inhibits insulin secretion

2 Your 20-year-old male patient has had multiple episodes of lightheadedness, sweating, fatigue, tremor, and intense hunger. He had one seizure. During two of these episodes, his blood glucose was 40 mg/dL. This patient was desperately trying to get a discharge from the military, and you suspected he was inducing his symptoms by doing which of the following?

(A) Self injection of glucagon
(B) Self injection of insulin
(C) "Carb loading" before exercise
(D) Taking metformin before exercise
(E) Taking an amylin blocker

3 A patient had new glasses prescribed by his optometrist. Less than a week later, his prescription was inadequate and he could not see well with his new glasses. His optometrist checked his vision twice more over the next week and the patient's prescription was different both times. His optometrist refers the patient to an ophthalmologist. What is the reason the patient is having such rapid changes in his glasses prescription?

(A) Elevated levels of galactose in the lens
(B) Elevated levels of glucose in the lens
(C) Elevated levels of sorbitol in the lens
(D) Cataract formation
(E) Increased intraocular pressure from hyperglycemia

4 A type 2 diabetic has been taking metformin to help regulate blood glucose levels. What effect will metformin also exert within the muscle?

(A) Reduce glucose uptake from the circulation
(B) Enhance fatty acid oxidation
(C) Reduce fatty acid oxidation
(D) Stimulate glucose release
(E) Enhance gluconeogenesis

5 Your patient with type 2 diabetes mellitus is usually in good control with an HbA1C of 7.1 and fasting blood glucose values between 90 and 100 mg/dL. His problem is with his 1-h postprandial glucose levels at lunch and dinner. A recall of his usual diet reveals some type of meat, potato, broccoli, milk, and diet drink at these meals. Which of these foods is most likely responsible for his postprandial high blood glucose?

(A) Meat
(B) Potato
(C) Broccoli
(D) Milk
(E) Diet drink

6 You see a 56-year-old female patient in follow-up after discharge from the hospital. She was treated for ketoacidosis and hyperglycemia and now is on basal and rapid acting insulins. You wonder if she really has type 1 diabetes mellitus and was in ketoacidosis or has type 2 diabetes mellitus and had a hyperosmolar state with lactic acidosis. Which of the following lab tests would help you determine whether this patient has type 1 or type 2 diabetes mellitus?

(A) Insulin levels
(B) C-peptide levels
(C) Fasting blood glucose levels
(D) Random blood glucose levels
(E) Hemoglobin A1C levels

7 Your patient, with a BMI of 36 and a waist circumference of 44 in., has a fasting blood glucose level of 145 mg/dL. One reason for the elevated blood glucose is which of the following?
(A) Enhanced release of glucose from the intestinal epithelial cells
(B) Stimulation of GLUT4 transporters in muscle
(C) Activation of pyruvate carboxylase
(D) Inhibition of liver GLUT4 transporters
(E) Activation of protein kinase B

8 Considering the patient in the previous question, the primary energy source being used by the muscle is which of the following (in the untreated state)?
(A) Glucose
(B) Amino acids
(C) Lactate
(D) Glycerol
(E) Fatty acids

9 Considering the patient described in the last two questions, it is likely that your patient is now leptin resistant. This has occurred due to which of the following?
(A) Activation of SMAD4
(B) Downregulation of the leptin receptor
(C) Activation of the insulin receptor
(D) Activation of SOCS3
(E) Downregulation of anorexigenic factors

10 Sequelae of insulin resistance in type 2 diabetes mellitus and metabolic syndrome is reduced secretion of insulin in response to increases in blood glucose. Insulin release from the pancreas appears to be dependent upon increase in concentration of which pair of metabolites?
(A) ATP and CO_2
(B) ATP and NADH
(C) ATP and NADPH
(D) Glucose-6-phosphate and CO_2
(E) Glucose-6-phosphate and NADH

11 An increase in serum free fatty acid levels, as evident in individuals exhibiting metabolic syndrome, occurs due to which of the following?
(A) Increased activity of lipoprotein lipase
(B) Increased activity of pancreatic lipase
(C) Substrate-induced activation of hormone-sensitive lipase
(D) Increased transcription of colipase
(E) Activation of microsomal triglyceride transfer protein

12 Your patient with metabolic syndrome is in for a checkup. His HbA1C is 9.0 and his fasting triglycerides are 325 mg/dL. You prescribe pioglitazone (Actos) to better treat his diabetes, but nothing else specific for the high lipids. A month later, the fasting triglyceride levels have dropped to 155 mg/dL due to a direct activation of which of the following?
(A) AMP-activated protein kinase
(B) PPAR-γ
(C) Leptin
(D) Adiponectin
(E) LKB1

13 Your type 2 diabetic patient has been taking metformin for the past 6 months and has reduced fasting blood glucose levels from 185 to 112 mg/dL. This occurs due to which of the following effects of metformin?
(A) Activation of adenylate cyclase
(B) Inhibition of the electron transfer chain
(C) Activation of LKB1
(D) Stimulation of amidophosphoribosyl transferase
(E) Stimulation of adenylate kinase

14 The major, defining difference between a type 1 diabetic and a type 2 diabetic is which of the following?
(A) Weight
(B) Ability to produce insulin
(C) LDL levels
(D) Blood glucose levels
(E) Serum triglyceride levels

15 Your type 1 diabetic patient was managing their disease using a combination of Humulin R and Humalog. The Humalog is more rapid acting than the Humulin R due to which of the following?
(A) Humalog is taken orally, rather than subcutaneously
(B) Humulin R is complexed with zinc, which slows its absorption
(C) Humalog is complexed with manganese, which accelerates its absorption
(D) Humulin R is taken orally, which slows its absorption
(E) Humalog is taken through an insulin pump mechanism

16 The biochemical difference between Humulin R and Humalog is which of the following?

(A) The C-peptide remains in Humalog and is removed from Humulin R
(B) Disulfide bond formation is prevented in Humalog and is present in Humulin R
(C) The amino acid sequence is completely reversed in Humalog as compared to Humulin R
(D) The position of two amino acids is reversed in Humalog as compared to Humulin R
(E) Humulin R contains genetically engineered histidine residues so it can complex with nickel, which is not present in Humalog

17 Type 1 diabetics, prior to diagnosis, display polydipsia, polyuria, and polyphagia. The polyuria is due to which of the following?

(A) Insulin stimulation of urea production
(B) Osmotic imbalance due to elevated ketones in the blood
(C) Osmotic imbalance due to reduced glucose levels in the urine
(D) Osmotic imbalance due to increased glucose levels in the urine
(E) Insulin stimulation of glucose resorption in the kidney

18 The polyphagia observed in the untreated type 1 diabetic, who has lost 6 lb in the last 2 weeks, is due to which of the following?

(A) Glucagon stimulation of triacylglycerol production
(B) Cortisol stimulation of amino acid release from the muscle
(C) Insulin-induced inhibition of fatty acid oxidation
(D) AMP kinase-induced activation of GLUT4 transporters
(E) Activation of muscle acetyl-CoA carboxylase-2

19 A pregnant patient has developed gestational diabetes. One of the consequences of gestational diabetes is fetal macrosomia. Which of the following is the mechanism that causes these large for gestational age babies?

(A) The anabolic effects of glucose
(B) The anabolic effects of insulin
(C) The anabolic effects of glucagon
(D) The anabolic effects of growth hormone
(E) The anabolic effects of thyroid hormone

20 A patient who had gestational diabetes has just delivered a 10 lb baby. The baby appears "jittery" and a heel stick glucose is 30 mg/dL. Which of the following mechanisms is the explanation for the newborn's blood glucose reading?

(A) The mother's relative hyperinsulinemia
(B) The baby's relative hyperinsulinemia
(C) The mother's hyperglycemia
(D) The baby's hyperglycemia
(E) Placental insulin production

ANSWERS

1 **The answer is D: It inhibits glucagon secretion.** Pramlintide is an amylin agonist used to lower postprandial blood glucose. Amylin is a peptide hormone secreted by the beta cells of the pancreas (with insulin), and inhibits glucagon secretion when blood glucose levels are elevated after a meal (thus aiding insulin action). Glucagon stimulates release of glucose from glycogen and further raises blood glucose. Insulin stimulates glycogenesis and storage of glucose which lowers blood glucose. Inhibiting insulin secretion would worsen the problem of high blood glucose levels. Decreasing glucose-6-phosphate or stimulating hexokinase or glycogen phosphorylase would increase glycogenolysis and raise blood glucose, which is opposite what one wants to accomplish in a diabetic patient.

2 **The answer is B: Self injection of insulin.** This patient could inject exogenous insulin to simulate an insulinoma. The symptoms and lab findings would be identical unless a C-peptide analysis was done. Injecting insulin between meals leads to hypoglycemia as the insulin stimulates glucose transport from the blood into the peripheral tissues, in the absence of dietary glucose. The figure below compares the effects of hypoglycemia (what is occurring in this case) versus hyperglycemia (as in an untreated diabetic) on a patient. Injecting glucagon would cause release of glucose from glycogenolysis (and gluconeogenesis), resulting in a higher blood glucose level. Amylin is a compound which blocks the action of glucagon, so an amylin blocker would be the same as injecting glucagon (blocking amylin activity would increase glucagon activity, since amylin is no longer active). Carbohydrate loading is an attempt to raise glycogen stores for more glucose availability during prolonged exercise and would not lead to hypoglycemic episodes. Metformin blocks liver gluconeogenesis during the fasting state, so more fatty acids are utilized. It also reduces insulin resistance. It does not stimulate insulin release and does not produce hypoglycemia.

	Hypoglycemia	Hyperglycemia
Signs and symptoms	Nervous Shaky Sweaty Confused	Dry mouth Thirsty Frequent urination Fatigue Blurred vision
Possible causes	Eating less or later than usual Being more active than usual Taking too much diabetes medicine Alcohol	Eating too much Being less active than usual Taking too little diabetes medicine
Treatment	10–15 g carbohydrates : • 2–3 sugar packets • 0.5 cup (4 oz) fruit juice • 0.5 cup (4 oz) soda (not diet) • 3–5 pieces hard candy	Following prescribed regimen • diet and exercise • oral hypoglycemics • insulin • special care when sick

3 **The answer is C: Elevated levels of sorbitol in the lens.** Sorbitol synthesis from glucose in the polyol pathway occurs in the lens of the eye. Aldose reductase converts glucose to sorbitol which then accumulates in the lens. Sorbitol dehydrogenase can convert the sorbitol to fructose, which can also accumulate within the lens. In diabetes mellitus, fluctuating levels of glucose lead to fluctuating levels of sorbitol, which change the consistency of the lens and therefore the glasses prescription. Glucose and galactose by themselves do not directly affect the lens. Chronically, high glucose and sorbitol

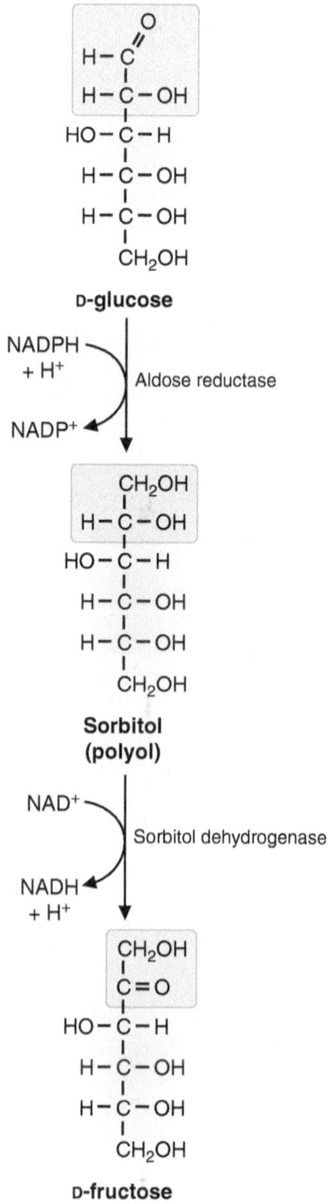

H–C=O
H–C–OH
HO–C–H
H–C–OH
H–C–OH
CH_2OH
D-glucose

$NADPH + H^+$ → $NADP^+$ Aldose reductase

CH_2OH
H–C–OH
HO–C–H
H–C–OH
H–C–OH
CH_2OH
Sorbitol (polyol)

NAD^+ → $NADH + H^+$ Sorbitol dehydrogenase

CH_2OH
C=O
HO–C–H
H–C–OH
H–C–OH
CH_2OH
D-fructose

levels can increase cataract formation, but this patient is experiencing an acute problem. Hyperglycemia does not increase intraocular pressure; however, the conversion of glucose to sorbitol will. The polyol pathway of sugar metabolism is shown on page 170.

4 **The answer is B: Enhance fatty acid oxidation.** Metformin, through its activation of the AMP-activated protein kinase, will stimulate glucose entry into the muscle (thus, answer choice A is incorrect) and also increase fatty acid oxidation. The AMP-activated protein kinase will phosphorylate and inhibit acetyl-CoA carboxylase and will phosphorylate and activate malonyl-CoA decarboxylase. Thus, malonyl-CoA levels drop, leading to enhanced entry of fatty acids into the mitochondria, and an increase in fatty acid oxidation. This occurs as the malonyl-CoA inhibition of carnitine palmityl transferase 1 is now lifted due to the reduction of malonyl-CoA levels (see the figure below). Metformin does not stimulate glucose release from the muscle, as the muscle lacks glucose-6-phosphatase activity. Metformin also reduces gluconeogenesis in the liver at a transcriptional level.

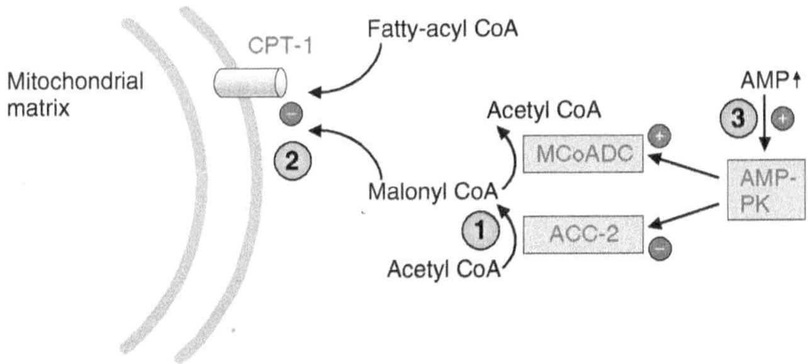

Regulation of fatty acyl-CoA entry into muscle mitochondria. (1) Acetyl-CoA carboxylase-2 (ACC-2) converts acetyl-CoA to malonyl-CoA, which inhibits carnitine palmitoyl transferase I (CPT-I), thereby blocking fatty acyl-CoA entry into the mitochondria. (2) However, as energy levels drop, AMP levels rise because of the activity of the adenylate kinase reaction. (3) The increase in AMP levels activates the AMP-activated protein kinase (AMPK), which phosphorylates and inactivates ACC-2, and also phosphorylates and activates malonyl-CoA decarboxylase (MCoADC). The decarboxylase converts malonyl-CoA to acetyl-CoA, thereby relieving the inhibition of CPT-1 and allowing fatty acyl-CoA entry into the mitochondria. This allows the muscle to generate ATP via the oxidation of fatty acids.

5 **The answer is B: Potato.** Amounts of simple carbohydrates in a meal are the most reliable indicators of postprandial rise in blood glucose. As the HbA1C nears normal or target values, fasting blood glucose values are usually normal and postprandial glucose values have a much more important effect on the HbA1C. Proteins, fats, and complex carbohydrates are absorbed more slowly than simple carbohydrates. This can be viewed as the glycemic index (the ability of a food to rapidly raise blood glucose). A higher number for the glycemic index means a more rapid and higher rise of blood glucose. Potatoes have the highest glycemic index of the mentioned foods and are composed of simple carbohydrates. Broccoli has more complex carbohydrates and a much lower glycemic index. Meat is mostly proteins and fats. Milk contains proteins and so has a lower glycemic index than potatoes (whole milk also has fats and an even lower glycemic index). Diet drinks contain no carbohydrates or calories. A table of the glycemic index of common foods is listed in Table 19-1, with the values adjusted to a white bread level of 100.

Table 19-1.

Breads		**Cookies**	
Whole wheat	100	Oatmeal	78
Pumpernickel (whole grain rye)	88	Plain water crackers	100
Cereal Grains		**Fruit**	
Barley (pearled)	36	Apple	52
Rice (instant, boiled 1 min)	65	Apple juice	45
Rice, polished, (boiled 10–25 min)	81	Orange	59
Sweet corn	80	Raisins	93
Root Vegetables		**Dairy Products**	
Potatoes (instant)	120	Ice cream	69
Potato (new, white, boiled)	80	Whole milk	44
Potato chips	77	Skim milk	46
Yam	74	Yogurt	52
Legumes		**Sugars**	
Baked beans (canned)	70	Fructose	26
Butter beans	46	Glucose	138
Garden peas (frozen)	85	Lactose	57
Kidney beans (dried)	43	Sucrose	83
Kidney beans (canned)	74		
Peanuts	15		
Pasta		**Breakfast Cereals**	
Spaghetti, white, boiled	67	All bran	74
		Cornflakes	121
		Muesli	96

6 **The answer is B: C-peptide levels.** It is difficult, at times, to differentiate type 1 diabetes mellitus and ketoacidosis from type 2 diabetes mellitus hyperosmolar state and lactic acidosis unless testing for acetate and/or β-hydroxybutyrate (ketone bodies) are specifically ordered when acidosis is noticed. At this point in the

patient's disease process, ketone bodies should be normal. The patient is already on insulin, so insulin levels would not be helpful. Measurement of blood glucose levels, whether fasting or not, and determination of Hb1AC levels cannot differentiate type 1 from type 2 diabetes (since the patient is on insulin). Since insulin is secreted as a macromolecule and does not become active until C-peptide is cleaved from the macromolecule, a C-peptide level would be helpful in this differentiation (see the figure below for an overview of insulin biosynthesis). Type 1 diabetes mellitus (no endogenous insulin produced) should give a very low or nonexistent level of C-peptide, whereas type 2 diabetes mellitus (insulin resistance) should give a normal or high level of C-peptide. Exogenous (commercial) insulin lacks the C-peptide, so the injected insulin will not interfere with this measurement.

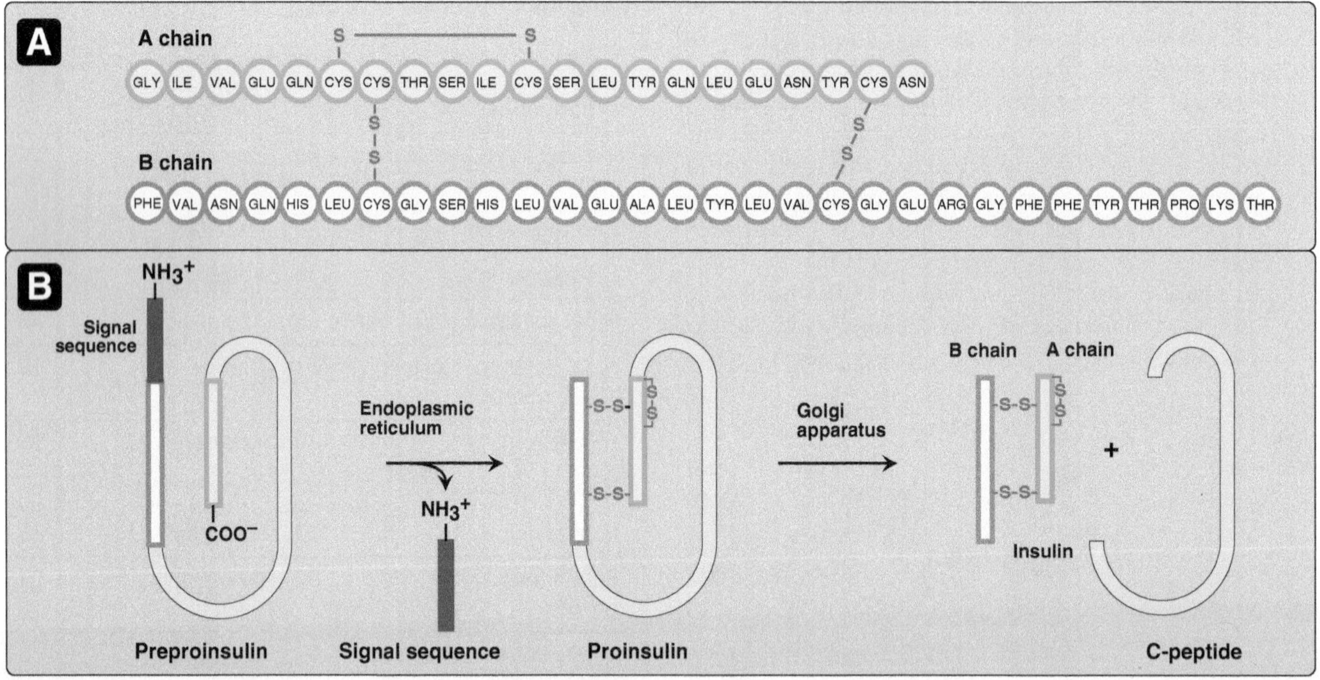

Panel A indicates the amino acid sequence of mature insulin, while **panel B** indicates the steps involved in converting preproinsulin to mature insulin. Note the release of the C-peptide as insulin is converted to its mature form.

7 **The answer is C: Activation of pyruvate carboxylase.** The patient most likely has metabolic syndrome, and the liver has become resistant to the action of insulin. Because of this, gluconeogenesis is enhanced in the liver. Due to the large size of the adipocytes, free fatty acid levels in the portal circulation are high (visceral adipocytes release compounds into the portal vein), and the liver is oxidizing fatty acids for energy, generating acetyl-CoA. The acetyl-CoA is an activator for pyruvate carboxylase, and an inhibitor of pyruvate dehydrogenase. The activation of pyruvate carboxylase contributes to the activation of gluconeogenesis, and high blood glucose levels. The intestinal epithelial cells release glucose, obtained from the diet, down its concentration gradient, so enhanced release would only occur when blood glucose levels were very low. If GLUT4 transporters were stimulated in muscle, blood glucose levels would drop, as the muscle would be capable of removing glucose from the circulation. The insulin-resistance that is occurring also affects the muscle, such that insulin can no longer stimulate glucose transport into that tissue. Liver utilizes both GLUT1 and GLUT4 transporters, but due to the insulin resistance, the liver is exporting glucose rather than using it. Activation of protein kinase B occurs when insulin binds to its receptor; since the liver is resistant to insulin action, the level of protein kinase B activation is reduced.

8 **The answer is E: Fatty acids.** Since the patient is exhibiting signs of metabolic syndrome, a key component of which is insulin resistance, the muscle has difficulty in transporting glucose from the circulation into the tissue. This means that the muscle will use fatty acids as its primary energy source. When abundant fatty acids are available, the muscle will utilize the fatty acids preferentially and will not use amino acids as an energy source. The muscle (other than the heart) does not utilize lactate for energy, and glycerol can only be metabolized in the liver, as that is the only tissue which contains glycerol kinase. The use of fatty acids by the muscles, instead of

glucose, also contributes to the hyperglycemia observed in these patients.

9 **The answer is D: Activation of SOCS3.** Large adipocytes release leptin as a satiety signal. The leptin travels to the hypothalamus and binds to receptors which signal the release of anorexigenic neuropeptides, which signal "stop eating." However, leptin also induces the expression of suppressor of cytokine signaling (SOCS3), which blocks the action of leptin. With constant leptin release, SOCS3 levels are raised, and leptin can no longer induce the release of anorexigenic signals, leading to overeating. The leptin pathway (a JAK/STAT receptor and signaling mechanism) does not involve SMAD4 (a component of the TGF-β signaling pathway). The leptin resistance is not due to downregulation of the leptin receptors, or the activation of the insulin receptor. The downregulation of the release of anorexigenic factors is a consequence of leptin resistance, not a cause.

10 **The answer is C: ATP and NADPH.** The β-cells of the pancreas monitor both ATP and NADPH levels in order for insulin release to occur. The NADPH levels are increased through enhanced pyruvate cycling (see the figure below), which occurs when pyruvate levels increase (which is correlated with an increase in glucose levels within the β-cell). Increased glucose also leads to an increase in ATP, which leads to changes in ion fluxes across the membrane, resulting in insulin release. Glucose-6-phosphate, carbon dioxide, and NADH are not necessary for insulin release in response to glucose.

11 **The answer is C: Substrate-induced activation of hormone-sensitive lipase.** Individuals with metabolic syndrome have a high concentration of triglyceride in their adipocytes. Hormone-sensitive lipase has a low basal activity in the absence of activation by phosphorylation via protein kinase A. If you combine the high substrate level (triglyceride) with the low level of activity of hormone-sensitive lipase, one sees a release of fatty acids from the adipocyte which is greater than normal (when triglyceride levels are low). The increase in free fatty acid levels then aids in promoting insulin resistance in both the adipocytes and muscle cells. This occurs because the muscle and fat cells will use fatty acids as an energy source instead of glucose, thereby contributing to high blood glucose levels. The increased serum free fatty acid levels do not affect the activity of lipoprotein lipase (which removes fatty acids from VLDL and chylomicrons), nor pancreatic lipase (which digests dietary triglycerides in the intestinal lumen). The fatty acids do not affect the transcription rate of colipase, and while the levels of fatty acids within the liver may alter the activity of microsomal triglyceride transfer protein (MTTP), an alteration in MTTP activity does not lead to the increase in free fatty acid levels in the blood.

12 **The answer is B: PPAR-γ.** Thiazolidinediones (TZDs), of which pioglitazone is a member bind to peroxisome proliferator activated receptor-γ (PPAR-γ) in the adipocyte and activate the synthesis and release of adiponectin, which acts on target cells to reduce blood glucose levels (by upregulating GLUT4 content of the membranes) and to reduce circulating triglyceride levels (through phosphorylation and inhibition of acetyl-CoA carboxylase 2, which relieves the inhibition of carnitine palmitoyl transferase I). While adiponectin levels rise, which leads to a stimulation of the AMP-activated

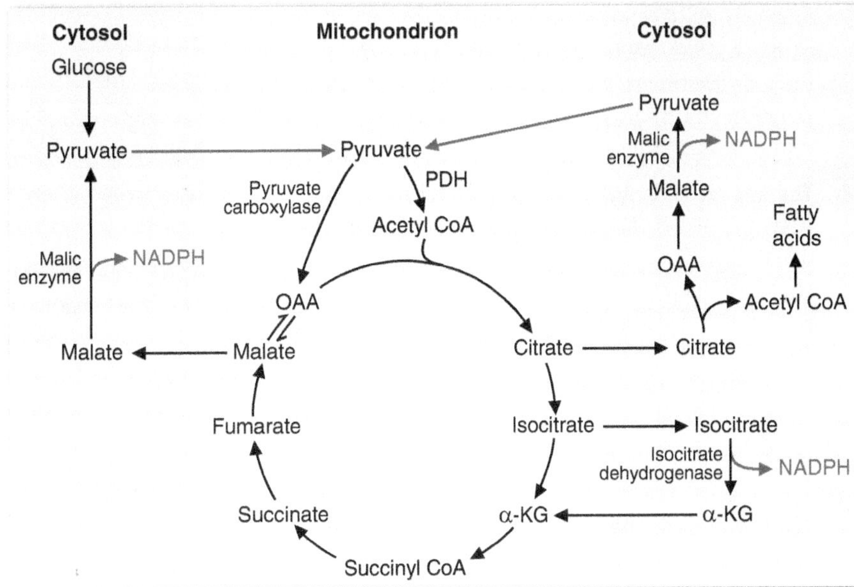

Answer 10: Pyruvate cycling: An increase in pancreatic glucose levels leads to an increase in pyruvate, which enters the mitochondria. The pyruvate can be converted to oxaloacetate, then malate, which re-enters the cytoplasm and is converted back to pyruvate via malic enzyme, generating NADPH in the process. Conversely, pyruvate can be converted to acetyl-CoA, generate citrate, which can then leave the mitochondria and regenerate pyruvate, also generating NADPH in the reaction sequence. The pancreas also contains a cytoplasmic, $NADP^+$ dependent, isocitrate dehydrogenase, which provides a third mechanism for raising NADPH levels when pyruvate levels are increased within the pancreatic β-cell.

protein kinase, neither of those effects is due to a direct interaction with the TZD. LKB1, an upstream kinase responsible for activating the AMP-activated protein kinase, and leptin are not involved in the response to TZDs. The structure of Actos (pioglitazone) is shown below.

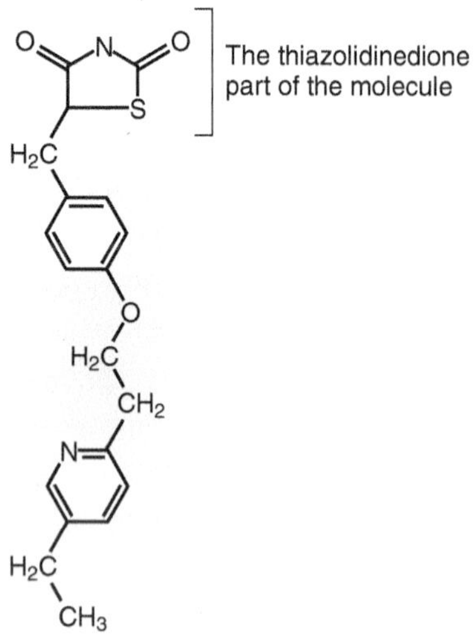

The thiazolidinedione part of the molecule

Pioglitazone

13 **The answer is B: Inhibition of the electron transfer chain.** Metformin partially inhibits complex I of the electron transport chain. This leads to reduced ATP production, which, as energy is required, rapidly increases AMP levels due to the adenylate kinase reaction. The increase in AMP levels leads to the activation of the AMP-activated protein kinase (AMPK), which is the primary messenger for metformin's effects. Metformin does not activate adenylate cyclase, nor does LKB1 (it has been postulated that LBK1 is constantly phosphorylating the AMP-activated protein kinase, but a phosphatase is always inactivating the AMPK. When AMP levels rise, however, AMP inhibits the phosphatase, leading to fully active AMPK). Metformin also has no direct effect on the rate-limiting step of purine production, amidophosphoribosyltransferase, or of adenylate kinase.

14 **The answer is B: Ability to produce insulin.** By definition, a type 1 diabetic cannot produce insulin. A type 2 diabetic produces insulin, but has become resistant to the effects of insulin. Weight does not differentiate between type 1 and 2 diabetics (although most type 2 diabetics are overweight). Blood glucose levels are elevated in both types of diabetes and cannot differentiate between them. Neither LDL levels nor triglyceride levels will differentiate between these two major forms of diabetes.

15 **The answer is B: Humulin R is complexed with zinc, which slows its absorption.** Humulin R (regular acting) is a hexamer complexed with zinc. After injection, the concentration of the insulin has to be reduced (through diffusion) for monomers and dimers of insulin to leave the zinc complex. This dramatically slows the time of insulin appearing in the circulation. Humalog, with a slightly different amino sequence, is not complexed with zinc and is absorbed much more rapidly from the injection site than Humulin R. Both types of insulin are taken subcutaneously, not orally, even when using an insulin pump. Pumps will not alter absorption, just delivery and time of delivery of the insulin. Humalog is not complexed with manganese.

16 **The answer is D: The position of two amino acids is reversed in Humalog as compared to Humulin R.** The sequence of Humulin R is the same as native insulin, but Humalog has switched the positions of amino acids 28 and 29 of the B chain (see the figure in the answer to question 6 of this chapter) and is designated as lys–pro insulin, for the two amino acids that have switched positions (regular insulin has the sequence pro–lys at these positions, whereas lys–pro insulin has lys–pro at these positions). The C-peptide is removed from both forms of insulin (insulin would have no biological activity if the C-peptide were not removed), and both contain the same disulfide bonds. There are no his-tags present on Humulin. This minor difference in insulin structure allows Humulin to be absorbed much faster than Humalog, yet still retain its normal affinity for the insulin receptor.

17 **The answer is D: Osmotic imbalance due to increased glucose levels in the urine.** In an untreated type 1 diabetic, glucose levels in the blood exceed the renal threshold for reabsorption of the glucose from the urine, so blood glucose levels rise in the urine. This creates an osmotic imbalance, which forces more water into the urine, leading to polyuria (frequent urination). This is not due to urea production (and, since a type 1 diabetic does not produce insulin, insulin cannot be stimulating urea production). It is not due to an increase of ketones in the blood. And, since insulin is not present, it cannot be due to insulin stimulation of glucose resorption in the kidney.

18 **The answer is B: Cortisol stimulation of amino acid release from the muscle.** The weight loss seen in type 1 diabetics (untreated) results from the need of the liver for gluconeogenic precursors, many of which are derived from amino acids obtained from muscle protein breakdown. Cortisol release will signal the muscle to release amino acids for use by the liver. Glucagon signals triglyceride degradation, not production. Insulin does signal an inhibition of fatty acid oxidation, but that is not occurring in an individual who does not make insulin (type 1 diabetic). Since the muscle is

oxidizing fatty acids for energy, there is no activation of the AMP-activated protein kinase, as the energy levels are not low. Muscle acetyl-CoA carboxylase 2 (which produces malonyl-CoA, which would inhibit fatty acid oxidation via inhibiting carnitine palmitoyl transferase 1) is not activated under these conditions, due to the lack of insulin.

19 **The answer is B: The anabolic effects of insulin.** In pregnancy, the placenta preferentially shunts glucose to the developing fetus. This, along with placental hormones, causes a functional "insulin resistance" in the mother. Because of the higher glucose level in the fetus, the fetal pancreas produces more insulin. Insulin is the major anabolic hormone of the body stimulating glucose uptake into the cells and stimulating extra growth. Glucagon, growth hormone, epinephrine, corticosteroids, and thyroid hormone are all catabolic hormones that counter insulin and stimulate glucose release from the cells to increase blood glucose. Glucose itself is neither anabolic nor catabolic. Large for gestational age babies, dehydrated babies (from the osmotic diuresis of hyperglycemia), and a fivefold increase in stillborn rates are all complications of uncontrolled gestational diabetes.

20 **The answer is B: The baby's relative hyperinsulinemia.** During pregnancy, the fetus is oversupplied with glucose from the mother causing the fetal pancreas to overproduce insulin. At delivery, the glucose supply from the mother is suddenly terminated and the relative hyperinsulinemia of the baby causes hypoglycemia until the baby's body can adjust to this new environment by decreasing insulin release and increasing glucose release. Hypoglycemia in the first few hours of the newborn's life is a common complication of gestational diabetes. Newborn hyperglycemia would not give a heel stick of 30 mg/dL of glucose. The placenta does not make insulin and the insulin molecule cannot cross the placenta, so the mother's relative hyperinsulinemia is not the cause of this problem. While the mother's hyperglycemia has led to the baby's relative hyperinsulinemia, the mother's blood glucose levels do not cause the drop in the baby's blood glucose levels after birth.

Chapter 20

Nutrition and Vitamins

This chapter covers cofactors derived from vitamins, as well as the basic concepts of biochemical nutrition.

QUESTIONS

Select the single best answer.

1 Consider a 40-year-old man who has just initiated a 24 h fast. Which of the following cofactors are necessary so that his blood glucose levels can be kept constant?
(A) B_6, biotin, and niacin
(B) B_6, niacin, and vitamin D
(C) B_6, biotin, and vitamin D
(D) Biotin, niacin, and B_{12}
(E) Biotin, niacin, and vitamin K

2 In a laboratory study, volunteers were made experimentally vitamin B_6 deficient, and much to the investigator's surprise, a mild hypoglycemia, with ketosis, was noted. The hypoglycemia is a result of which of the following?
(A) Inhibition of phosphoenolpyruvate carboxykinase
(B) Inhibition of pyruvate carboxylase
(C) Reduced activity of glucose-6-phosphatase
(D) Reduced activity of liver glycogen phosphorylase
(E) Reduced insulin secretion

3 An individual who has been on a long-term diet will have reduced the transcription of which of the following enzymes?
(A) Malic enzyme
(B) Carnitine acyltransferase 1
(C) Carnitine acyltransferase 2
(D) Medium chain acyl-CoA dehydrogenase
(E) Fatty acyl-CoA synthetase

4 Which one of the fatty acids listed below can be synthesized by humans?
(A) Cis Δ9, 12 C18:2
(B) Cis Δ9, 12, 15 C18:3
(C) Cis Δ5, 8, 13 C20:3
(D) Cis Δ5, 8, 11, 14 C20:4
(E) Cis Δ10 C16:1

5 A patient has been diagnosed with abetalipoproteinemia. A possible deficiency in which of the following vitamins could occur in this patient?
(A) Vitamin B_1
(B) Vitamin B_2
(C) Vitamin C
(D) Vitamin E
(E) Niacin

6 A deficiency in which of the following vitamins will lead to a functional folate deficiency?
(A) Thiamine
(B) Niacin
(C) Riboflavin
(D) B_{12}
(E) Vitamin C

7 A woman, who eats a standard meat-containing diet, has had one child born with a neural tube defect, and is considering becoming pregnant again. Blood work showed normal levels of B_{12} and total folic acid (specific type of folic acid not specified). One possible explanation for the woman's difficulties in her first pregnancy is a thermolabile variant of which of the following enzymes?
(A) N5, N10-methylenetetrahydrofolate reductase
(B) Serine hydroxymethyl transferase
(C) Ornithine transcarbamoylase
(D) Phenylalanine hydroxylase
(E) Tyrosine aminotransferase

8 Concerning the woman in the previous question, alteration of her diet in which of the following ways would be beneficial for her future pregnancies?
(A) B_{12} supplementation
(B) Folate supplementation
(C) Iron supplementation
(D) A meat-free diet
(E) Homocysteine supplementation

9 A high-protein low-carbohydrate diet has, as its biochemical basis, the potential to lead to weight loss due to which of the following?

(A) Allosteric inhibition of fatty acid synthesis
(B) Increased glucagon release
(C) Minimal insulin release
(D) Reduced cortisol release
(E) Increased urea production

10 The neurotransmitters GABA, dopamine, and histamine are all derived from an amino acid precursor. The generation of these neurotransmitters from the appropriate amino acids requires which one of the following cofactors?

(A) NAD^+
(B) B_1
(C) B_2
(D) B_6
(E) B_{12}

11 A patient presents with episodes of flushing, diarrhea, abdominal cramping, and wheezing. His blood pressure and pulse rate are normal during these episodes. Physical exam is normal except for scattered telangiectasias. In order to diagnose this problem, a 24-h urine collection showed elevated levels of 5-HIAA (5-hydroxyindole acetic acid). The chemical responsible for this above syndrome is a derivative of which amino acid?

(A) Alanine
(B) Serine
(C) Tyrosine
(D) Tryptophan
(E) Phenylalanine

12 An individual has developed pancreatitis, and with it, steatorrhea. The patient also reports problems with his night vision, although visual acuity appears normal. Another expected finding in this patient would be which of the following?

(A) Nystagmus
(B) Easy bruising
(C) Dermatitis
(D) Loss of teeth
(E) Orange tonsils

13 You are treating a patient with a fat malabsorption problem, and you suggest that the patient switch his or her diet to one that contains which of the following?

(A) Triglycerides with long-chain fatty acids
(B) Triglycerides with medium-chain fatty acids
(C) Triglycerides with short-chain fatty acids
(D) Triglycerides with a mixture of long-chain and short-chain fatty acids
(E) Triglycerides with a mixture of long-chain and medium-chain fatty acids

14 Considering the patient in the previous question, a food that should be incorporated into the patient's diet is which of the following?

(A) Butter
(B) Margarine
(C) Olive oil
(D) Peanut oil
(E) Coconut oil

15 A 9-month-old child of strict vegan parents is brought to the pediatrician due to perceived muscle weakness. Due to their strict dietary beliefs, the child has not been given vitamin supplements. An image of the anterior of the knee reveals cupped and widened metaphyses. As the child is very fair skinned, the parents always cover up the child when they go outside such that minimal skin is exposed to the sun. In order to correct these problems the physician prescribes treatment with which of the following?

(A) Vitamin D
(B) Vitamin K
(C) Folic acid
(D) Vitamin B_{12}
(E) Vitamin E

16 A patient has had a series of blood clots, and has been placed on warfarin to reduce such incidents. Warfarin exerts its effect by blocking which of the following?

(A) Platelet biogenesis
(B) Phospholipid synthesis
(C) Clotting factor synthesis
(D) Vitamin E activity
(E) Formation of γ-carboxyglutamate

17 Considering the patient in the previous question, which food should be avoided in large quantities while the patient is on warfarin?

(A) Trout
(B) Milk products
(C) Green leafy vegetables
(D) Orange-yellow vegetables
(E) Steak

18 Chronic alcoholics often develop fatty and leaky livers, as the primary site of alcohol detoxification is the liver. Protein and VLDL secretion can be impaired in such patients due to which of the following?

(A) Ethanol inhibition of microtubule formation
(B) Ethanol inhibition of gene transcription
(C) Acetate reduction of intracytoplasmic pH
(D) Formation of acetaldehyde adducts with cytoplasmic proteins
(E) Increased ketone body levels within the cytoplasm

19 A 6-year-old girl has a history of seizures, which are only marginally relieved by standard medications. Switching her diet to which of the following may help her condition?

(A) 80% fat, 20% combined carbohydrate and protein, by weight
(B) 50% fat, 50% combined carbohydrate and protein, by weight
(C) 20% fat, 80% combined carbohydrate and protein, by weight
(D) 75% protein, 25% combined carbohydrate and fat, by weight
(E) 50% protein, 50% combined carbohydrate and fat, by weight

20 A 42-year-old woman presents with tiredness and lethargy. She has tingling in her hands and feet. Blood work shows a macrocytic anemia, along with elevated homocysteine levels. One would also expect to see elevated levels of which metabolite?

(A) Acetic acid
(B) Ketone bodies
(C) Methylmalonic acid
(D) Propionic acid
(E) Succinate

ANSWERS

1 **The answer is A: B_6, biotin, and niacin.** Biotin is required for pyruvate carboxylase (the enzyme that converts pyruvate to oxaloacetate), an enzyme necessary for gluconeogenesis from any TCA cycle precursor (and pyruvate). The B_6 is required for glycogen phosphorylase (the ability to produce glucose from glycogen) and for transamination reactions, which are necessary for amino acids (such as alanine, aspartic acid, and glutamic acid) to provide carbons for gluconeogenesis. The niacin is required to produce NADH, which is needed to reverse the glyceraldehyde-3-phosphate dehydrogenase step during gluconeogenesis. It is also needed for lactate to be converted to pyruvate, and lactate (provided by the red blood cell) is a major gluconeogenic precursor. The lipid-soluble vitamins (D and K) are not required for glucose production and release (vitamin D is needed for calcium metabolism, and vitamin K is required for the carboxylation of glutamic acid side chains of proteins involved in blood clotting). Vitamin B_{12} is not required for glucose production directly, and its absence does not lead to hypoglycemia.

2 **The answer is D: Reduced activity of liver glycogen phosphorylase.** Glycogen phosphorylase requires pyridoxal phosphate (derived from vitamin B_6) as an essential cofactor. The role of B_6 in the mechanism of the phosphorolysis reaction is still controversial, but it may play a role in general acid-base catalysis. B_6 is not required for the PEP carboxykinase reaction, the pyruvate carboxylase reaction (which requires biotin), or the glucose-6-phosphatase reaction. B_6 is also not involved in regulating insulin secretion.

3 **The answer is A: malic enzyme.** The transcription of five key enzymes for fatty acid synthesis are regulated by diet; malic enzyme, acetyl-CoA carboxylase, citrate lyase, fatty acid synthase, and glucose-6-phosphate dehydrogenase. The other four enzymes listed in the answer (carnitine acyltransferase I and II, medium-chain acyl-CoA dehydrogenase, and fatty acyl-CoA synthetase) are all involved in fatty acid oxidation, a process which would be increased during fasting, and whose enzyme levels would not be decreased under these conditions.

4 **The answer is C: cis Δ5, 8, 13 C20:3.** Humans can synthesize fatty acids of the ω-7 series or higher, but not of ω-6 or lesser. This is due to the limitation of the desaturase system (see the figure below), which can only introduce double bonds at positions 4, 5, 6 and 9, in a substrate that contains at least 16 carbons. Answer A is an ω-6 fatty acid, as are answers D and E. Answer B is an ω-3 fatty acid. Answer C is an ω-7 fatty acid, and would be synthesized as follows. Start with C16:0 (palmitic acid), and add a double bond at position 9, creating a cis Δ9 C16:1. Elongate that fatty acid by two carbons, creating a cis Δ11 C18:1. Desaturate this 18-carbon fatty acid at position 6, creating a cis Δ6Δ11 C18:2, which is elongated by two carbons, producing a cis Δ8Δ13 C20:2. Desaturate this fatty acid at position 5 and the final product is obtained.

5 **The answer is D: Vitamin E.** Abetalipoproteinemia is a disorder in which neither nascent chylomicrons nor nascent VLDL can be produced due to a defect in the microsomal triglyceride transfer protein. Fat-soluble vitamins are delivered to tissues via chylomicrons; in the absence of chylomicron formation, the fat soluble vitamins will remain in the intestinal epithelial cell, or not even be absorbed from the intestinal tract. Vitamin E is believed to be a major antioxidant factor in cells. All of the other vitamins listed (B_1, B_2, C, and niacin) are water-soluble vitamins, and do not require chylomicron formation for vitamin delivery.

6 **The answer is D: B_{12}.** A B_{12} deficiency will block the methionine synthase reaction, in which homocysteine reacts with N5-methyltetrahydrofolate (THF) to regenerate

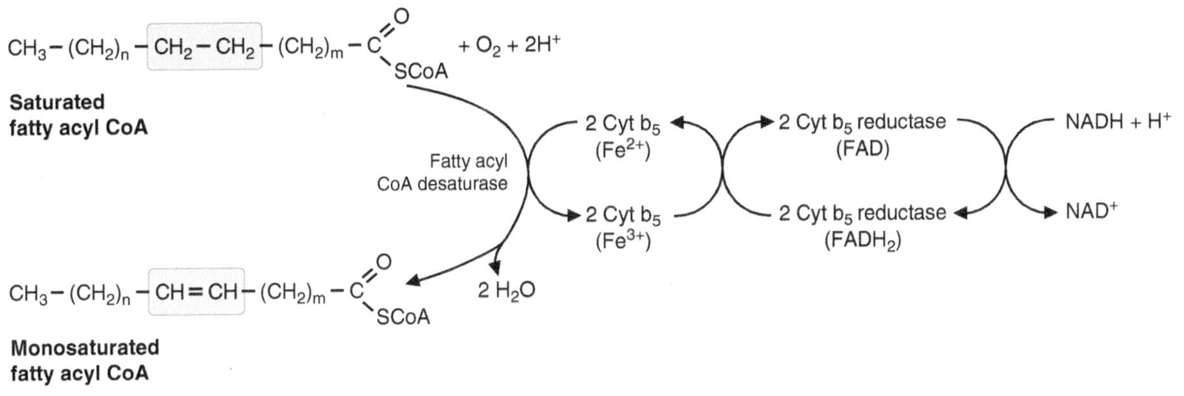

Answer 4: Desaturation of fatty acids in humans. The desaturase system requires a fatty acid which is at least 16 carbons long, and can only insert double bonds between carbons 4–5, 5–6, 6–7, and 9–10.

methionine and free THF. In the absence of such an activity, the N5-methyl THF accumulates, and as that form is the most stable form, eventually all folate will be "trapped" as the N5-methyl derivative. N5-methyl THF cannot go back to N5, N10-methylene THF; once the N5-methyl form is synthesized, the folate is trapped in that form until the methionine synthase reaction occurs. Thus, folate is still available, but in the wrong form; the levels of N5, N10-methylene THF are too low to allow for thymidine synthesis, and the levels of N10-formyl THF are too low to allow for sufficient purine synthesis. Thus, a functional folate deficiency occurs. Deficiencies in the other vitamins listed (thiamine, niacin, riboflavin, and C) will not lead to a functional folate deficiency. The reaction involving folate and vitamin B_{12} is diagrammed below, along with other reactions involved in homocysteine metabolism.

Reaction pathways that involve homocysteine. Defects in numbered enzymes (1, methionine synthase; 2, N5, N10-methylene-THF reductase; 3, cystathionine β-synthase) lead to elevated homocysteine. A B_{12} deficiency will block enzyme 1, leading to a functional folate deficiency as all of the folate will be trapped in the N5-methyl-THF form. This will also lead to an accumulation of homocysteine in the blood.

7 The answer is A: N5, N10-methylenetetrahydrofolate reductase. A thermolabile (temperature-sensitive) N5, N10-methylene-THF reductase would reduce the amount of N5-methyl THF which can be formed (see the figure below; reaction 7 utilizes the N5, N10-methylene-THF reductase), and therefore reduce the amount of homocysteine converted to methionine (reaction 8 of the figure). This would lead to a reduction of S-adenosylmethionine levels, and hypomethylation in the nervous system, which may lead to altered

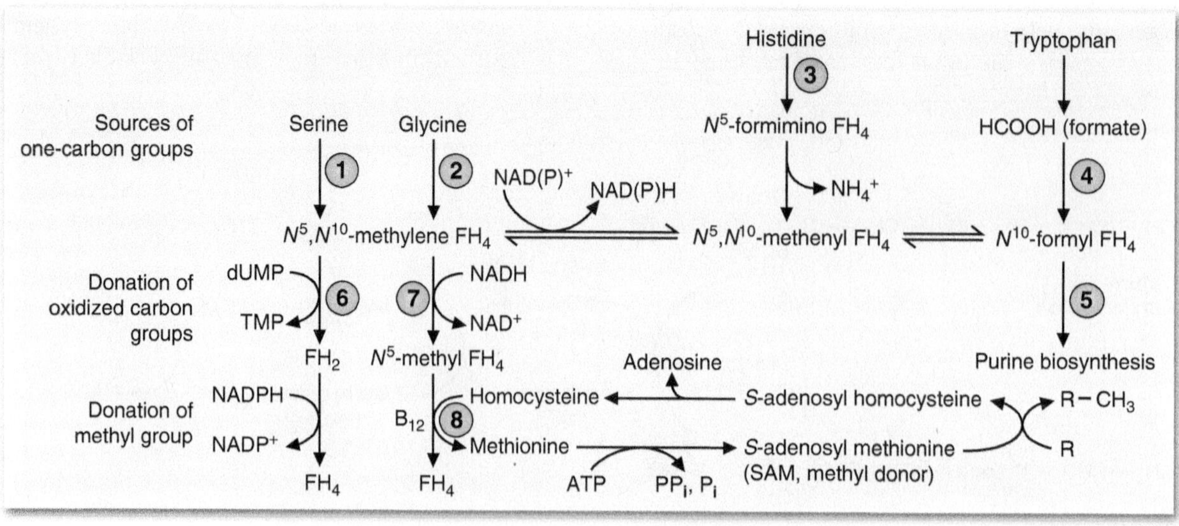

The sources of carbon for the tetrahydrofolate pool are indicated by reactions 1–4. The recipients of carbons from the THF pool are indicated by reactions 5–8. Reaction 7 is catalyzed by the N5, N10-methylenetetrahydrofolate reductase, while reaction 8, which requires vitamin B_{12}, is the methionine synthase reaction. Reaction 1 is catalyzed by the serine hydroxymethyl transferase enzyme.

gene expression and a neural tube defect. Elevated homocysteine would also be evident. This is a common mutation in the general population, and can be overcome by taking folic acid. An inactivating mutation in serine-hydroxymethyl transferase would reduce the major entry point of carbons into the THF pool, but there are other means to do this (reactions 2, 3, and 4 as indicated in the figure on page 180), so a loss of this enzyme would not result in reduced S-adenosylmethionine levels in the nervous system. A defect in ornithine transcarbamoylase (a urea cycle enzyme) would not affect homocysteine and methionine metabolism. Similarly, mutations in phenylalanine hydroxylase, or tyrosine aminotransferase (enzymes involved in phenylalanine and tyrosine metabolism, respectively) would not affect homocysteine and methionine metabolism.

8 **The answer is B: Folate supplementation.** The major problem with the folic acid derivatives which are present in the patient is that almost all of the folate is trapped in the N5, N10-methylene-THF form, leading to reduced levels of N5-methyl THF, and reduced regeneration of methionine from homocysteine. This leads to reduced S-adenosylmethionine levels, and hypomethylation due to a lack of the methylating reagent. Supplementation with N5-methyl THF will overcome this block, and restore methionine levels to normal. Going meat free will not solve the problem, as methionine is found in meat, and is an essential amino acid. B_{12} supplementation also will not help, as the methionine synthase reaction, which requires B_{12}, is not altered; it is just going at a reduced rate due to the lack of one of its substrates (N5-methyl THF). In this condition, homocysteine accumulates due to the reduced effectiveness of the methionine synthase reaction, so supplementation with homocysteine will not help. Iron supplementation will not help in this reaction sequence, as none of the enzymes are iron dependent.

9 **The answer is C: Minimal insulin release.** The biochemical basis of the Atkins diet is to minimize insulin release. Insulin will promote glycogen and fat synthesis, and by minimizing its release (by eating a low carbohydrate, high-protein diet), the ability of the liver to synthesize these energy storage molecules will be greatly reduced. While amino acids can stimulate insulin release (see Table 20-1 and the figure below), the amount released is about 10% that when glucose stimulates insulin release. A high-protein diet will not inhibit, allosterically, fatty acid synthesis. A high-protein diet does not increase glucagon release, nor does it reduce cortisol release. There will be increased urea production on such a diet, due to the increased level of protein degradation, but increasing urea production does not, by itself, lead to weight loss.

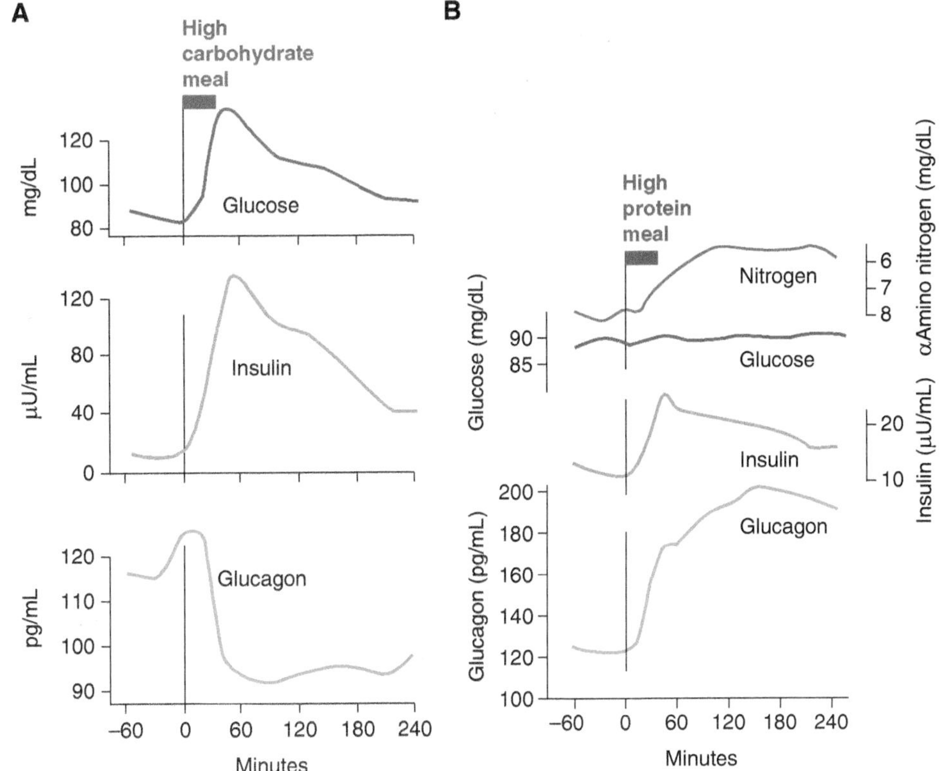

Answer 9: Panel A indicates the increase in blood glucose, insulin, and glucagon levels after a high-carbohydrate meal. Note the scale for the increase in insulin levels. **Panel B** indicates the release of insulin and glucagon in response to a high protein meal (note how little insulin increases under these conditions as compared to that in **panel A**). Also note how glucagon levels increase after the high-protein meal, as compared to the high-carbohydrate meal.

Table 20-1. Regulators of insulin release[a]

	Effect
Major Regulators	
Glucose	+
Minor Regulators	
Amino acids	+
Neural input	+
Gut hormones[b]	+
Epinephrine (adrenergic)	–

[a]+, stimulates

[b]Gut hormones that regulate fuel metabolism include, amongst many others, amylin, galanin, gastric inhibitory peptide, glucagon-like peptide 1 and 2, neuropeptide Y, and somatostatin.

10 **The answer is D: B_6.** All three neurotransmitters (GABA, dopamine, and histamine) are derived via decarboxylation of an amino acid precursor. Such amino acid decarboxylation reactions require pyridoxal phosphate (derived from B_6). GABA is derived from the decarboxylation of glutamate, dopamine from the decarboxylation of dihydroxyphenylalanine, and histamine from the decarboxylation of histidine. NAD, thiamine (B_1), riboflavin (B_2), or cobalamin (B_{12}) are not required for any of these reactions to occur.

11 **The answer is D: Tryptophan.** This patient has the classic presentation of a carcinoid tumor. This type of tumor secretes serotonin which causes these classic symptoms. The breakdown product of serotonin is 5-hydroxyindoleacetic acid (5-HIAA, see the figure below). Elevated

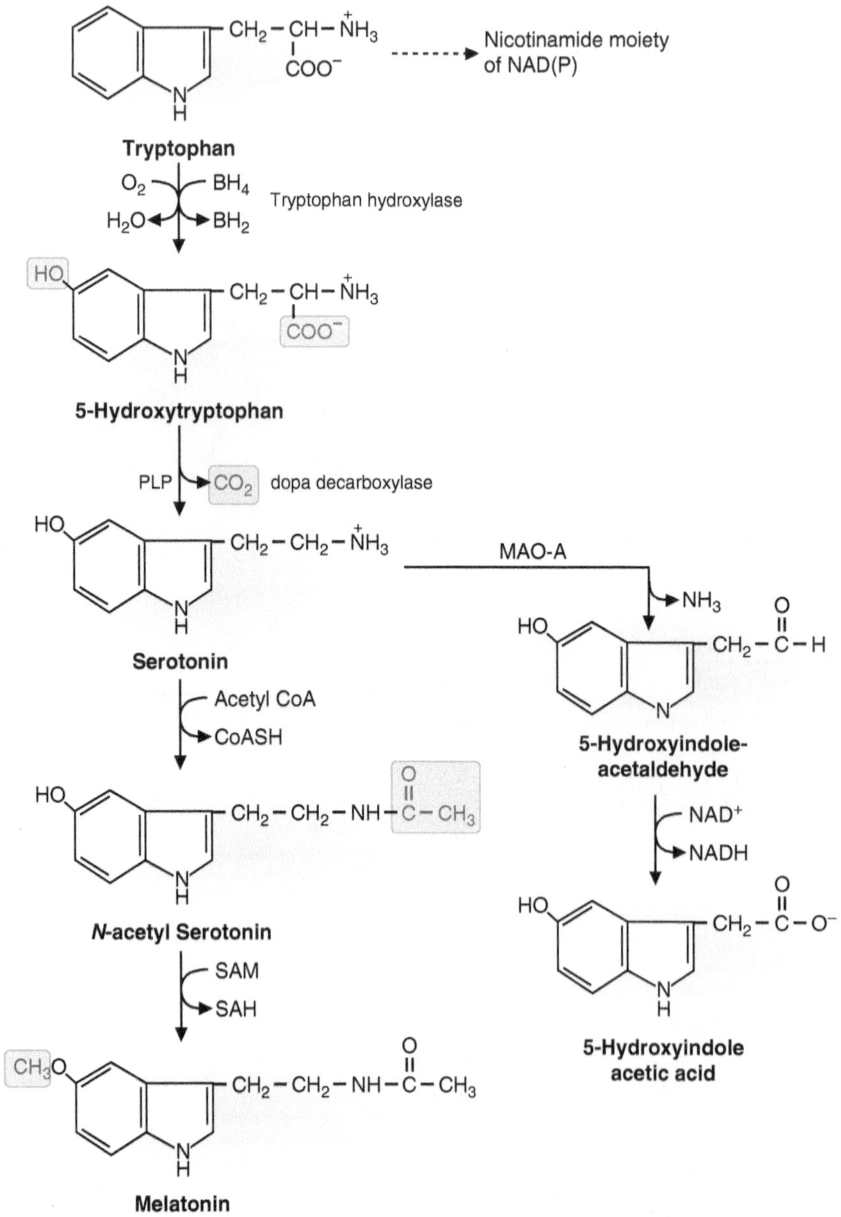

Answer 11: The biosynthesis and degradation of serotonin, leading to 5-HIAA (5-hydroxy indole acetic acid).

levels of 5-HIAA in the urine confirm a high level of serotonin and the diagnosis of a carcinoid. Serotonin is derived from tryptophan, and the patient has a carcinoid tumor secreting serotonin. Elevated levels of alanine, serine, tyrosine, or phenylalanine would not be observed in a patient with a carcinoid tumor.

12 **The answer is B: Easy bruising.** The patient, due to the pancreatitis, is not able to adequately digest triglycerides in the intestinal lumen, which is what leads to the steatorrhea. Fat-soluble vitamin absorption is dependent upon triglyceride digestion and absorption, so under these conditions, the patient can become deficient in fat-soluble vitamins (A, D, E, and K). The loss of night vision is an early warning for lack of vitamin A. If the patient is becoming deficient for vitamin K, bruising would become a problem, due to ineffective clotting with slight internal damage. Nystagmus is a symptom of vitamin B_1 deficiency, a water-soluble vitamin. Dermatitis is a symptom of niacin deficiency (vitamin B_3). Loss of teeth can occur with a vitamin C deficiency, and orange tonsils is not due to a vitamin deficiency, but rather to a lack of ABC-1 activity, and is indicative of Tangier disease.

13 **The answer is B: Triglycerides with medium-chain fatty acids.** Triglycerides containing medium-chain fatty acids are absorbed directly by the intestinal epithelial cells, and sent into the circulation to the liver, bypassing the need to be incorporated into chylomicrons. Thus, conditions which might lead to fat malabsorption, such as pancreatic insufficiency, or decreased bile acid secretion, do not affect the absorption of these triglycerides. Long-chain triglycerides do require the actions of pancreatic lipase and bile salts for absorption. Short-chain fatty acids are not utilized until they reach the large intestine, where colonic bacteria use them primarily for energy. Thus, their nutrient value to humans is very low.

14 **The answer is E: Coconut oil.** Coconut oil contains a high percentage (approximately 65%) of medium-chain triglycerides. Butter also contains some medium-chain fatty acids, but at a lower percentage than coconut oil (about 25%). Margarine is similar to butter in terms of length of fatty acids (although margarine contains more unsaturated fatty acids and no cholesterol, as it is not derived from an animal product). Olive oil is high in unsaturated fatty acids, with about 72% being oleic acid (an 18-carbon fatty acid with one double bond). Peanut oil is also high in unsaturated fatty acids but they are not medium-chain in length.

15 **The answer is A: Vitamin D.** The child has rickets, which is due to a lack of vitamin D. Vitamin D is synthesized via a circuitous route (see the figure below), and due to the parents' (and child's) diet, there is insufficient vitamin D for the child to form healthy bones. UV light is required to form the active form of vitamin D, and the child is also lacking exposure to sunlight. While, due to the diet, the child may become deficient for vitamin B_{12}, lack of B_{12} does not lead to these symptoms. The symptoms are also not consistent with a lack of vitamin K (which would lead to bleeding problems), folic acid (which would lead to anemia), or E (loss of protection against oxidative radicals). The pathway of active vitamin D formation is shown below.

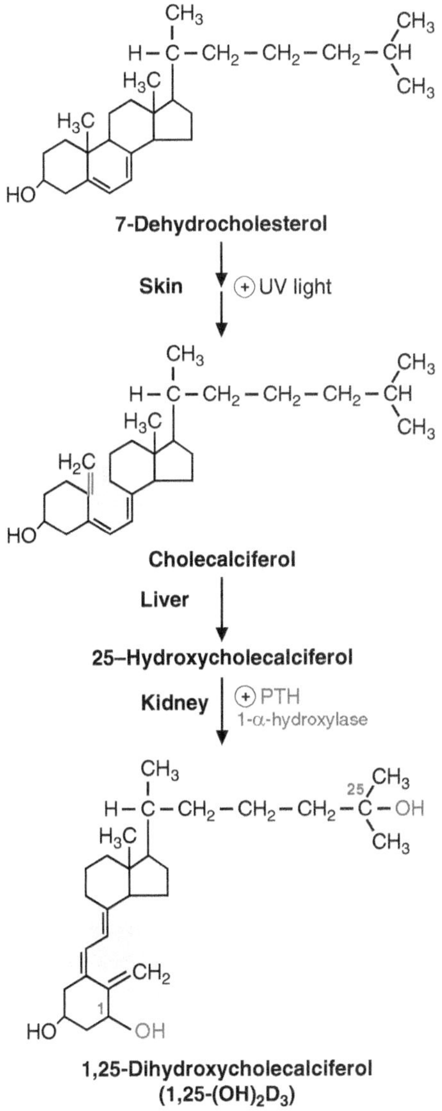

7-Dehydrocholesterol

Skin ⊕ UV light

Cholecalciferol

Liver

25–Hydroxycholecalciferol

Kidney ⊕ PTH, 1-α-hydroxylase

1,25-Dihydroxycholecalciferol ($1,25\text{-}(OH)_2D_3$)

Synthesis of active vitamin D. 1, 25-di (OH)2 D3 is produced from 7-dehydrocholesterol, a precursor of cholesterol. In the skin, ultraviolet (UV) light produces cholecalciferol, which is hydroxylated at the 25th position in the liver and the 1st position in the kidney to form the active hormone.

16 **The answer is E: formation of γ-carboxyglutamate.** Warfarin is a vitamin K antagonist, and blocks the regeneration of active vitamin K after it has participated in its reaction of creating a γ-carboxyglutamate residue (see below). In the absence of this side-chain modification, clotting proteins cannot bind to platelets, and the clotting cascade is inhibited. Warfarin does not interfere with platelet synthesis, nor does it alter phospholipid biosynthesis. Warfarin does not alter the transcription or translation of the clotting factors, and has no relationship with vitamin E, which protects against radical damage within cells and tissues. As seen in the figure below, warfarin blocks the activity of vitamin K epoxide reductase.

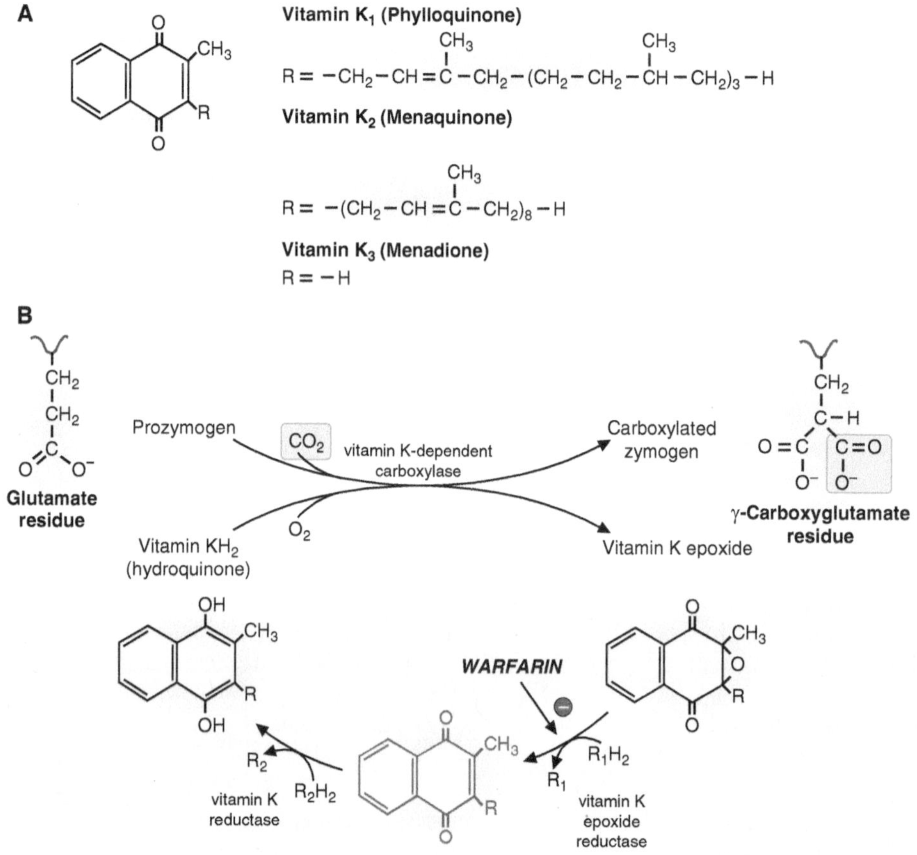

A: Structures of vitamin K derivatives. Phylloquinone is found in green leaves, and intestinal bacteria synthesize menaquinone. Humans convert menaquinone to a vitamin K active form. **B:** Vitamin K-dependent formation of γ-carboxyglutamate residues. The vitamin K-dependent carboxylase uses a reduced form of vitamin K (KH_2) as the electron donor and converts vitamin K to an epoxide. Vitamin K epoxide is reduced, in two steps, back to its active form by the enzymes vitamin K epoxide reductase and vitamin K reductase. As indicated on the figure, warfarin blocks the action of the vitamin K epoxide reductase.

17 **The answer is C: Green leafy vegetables.** Green leafy vegetables contain large amounts of vitamin K, which would overcome the effects of the warfarin. The other foods listed are poor sources of vitamin K (milk is fortified with vitamin D, orange-yellow vegetables are high in vitamin A, trout, and beef are low in fat soluble vitamins, although organs, such as liver, would be high in vitamin K).

18 **The answer is D: Formation of acetaldehyde adducts with cytoplasmic proteins.** As shown on page 185, acetaldehyde, a product of ethanol metabolism, forms covalent adducts with tubulin, which interferes with the movement and secretion of VLDL and other proteins normally secreted from the liver. It is not ethanol that is interfering with microtubule formation, but its metabolite that

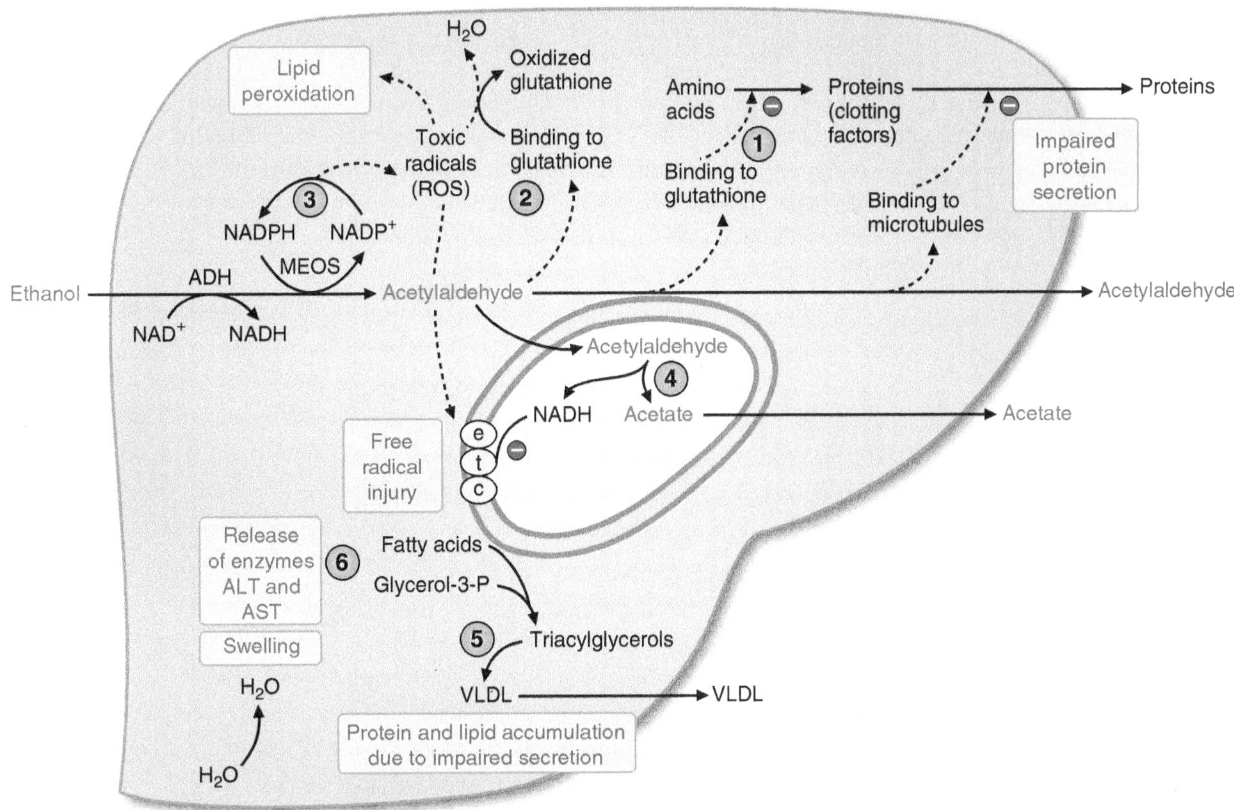

Answer 18: Alcohol-induced damage to microtubules, due to acetaldehyde accumulation. Acetaldehyde-adduct formation decreases protein synthesis and impairs protein secretion, due to microtubule damage. Microtubule damage (via acetaldehdye-adduct formation) also increases the accumulation of VLDL and protein within the liver. Damage to the mitochondria slows the conversion of acetaldehyde to acetate, thereby increasing the availability of acetaldehyde to form adducts with a variety of liver proteins.

interferes with microtubule function. Ethanol does not directly inhibit gene transcription (it actually leads to the transcription of MEOS, the microsomal ethanol oxidizing system). The levels of acetate formed are not sufficient to lower the pH of the liver cytosol. The ethanol carbons can be used for ketone body formation, but the formation of ketones is not related to the impaired secretion of VLDL. The toxic effects of ethanol on the liver are summarized in the figure above.

19 **The answer is A: 80% fat, 20% combined carbohydrate and protein, by weight.** The patient has epilepsy, a disorder of the nervous system which triggers, at times, involuntary muscle movements (seizures). While there are drugs designed to reduce the electrical activity in the nervous system, there is an indication that a strict ketogenic diet can also help to alleviate the frequency of seizures in epileptic patients. The ketogenic diet should be 80%, by weight, fat, with the other 20% split between carbohydrates and protein. If one can use fat containing medium-chain triglycerides, the diet appears to be more effective. The reason for the ketogenic diet having this effect has not yet been elucidated. Of the diets listed as choices, the one with the highest amount of fat would be the most ketogenic.

20 **The answer is C: Methylmalonic acid.** The patient is experiencing the symptoms of vitamin B_{12} deficiency. The macrocytic anemia is due to a lack of precursors for DNA synthesis in the red blood cell precursors due to the B_{12} deficiency. The numbness and tingling is due to hypomethylation in the nervous system, also due to the B_{12} deficiency. Vitamin B_{12} only participates in two reactions in humans. The first is the conversion of homocysteine to methionine, requiring N5-methyl THF. The active form of B_{12} in that reaction is methyl-cobalamin (see the figure below). The second reaction is the conversion of L-methylmalonyl-CoA to succinyl-CoA. The active form of B_{12} in that reaction is adenosyl-cobalamin.

In a B_{12} deficiency, neither of these reactions would proceed, so one would expect to see both homocysteine and methylmalonic acid accumulate in the circulation. B_{12} is not required for the metabolism of acetic acid, ketone bodies, propionic acid (although propionic acid is converted to methylmalonyl-CoA, so in a B_{12} deficiency there may be a slight rise in propionic acid levels as well), or succinate.

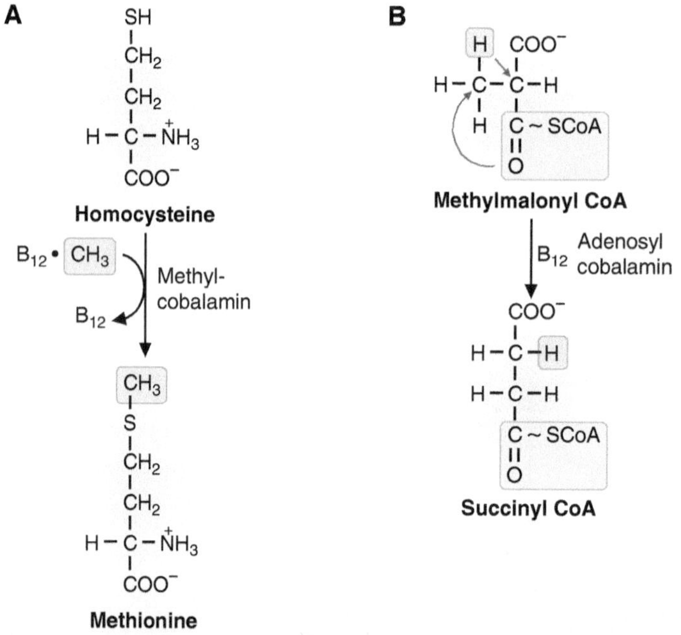

Chapter 21

Human Genetics and Cancer

This chapter will test the reader on basic concepts concerning human genetics, and will also relate to the genetic aspects of cancer and specific signal transduction pathways in certain cancers.

QUESTIONS

Select the single best answer.

1 A couple visits the obstetrician due to a high frequency of miscarriages in the family. Suspecting a chromosomal abnormality, the physician orders karyotype analyses of the couple. For one of the two, the following karyotype was identified; 46, XX, der15 t(9q;15q). The primary reason for the frequency of miscarriages is most likely which one of the following?

(A) Potential regions of trisomy or monosomy in the fertilized egg
(B) Triploidy in the fertilized egg
(C) Chromosomal deletions in the fertilized egg
(D) Abnormal sex chromosomes in the fertilized egg
(E) A Robertsonian translocation in the fertilized egg

2 A 5-year-old boy developed rapidly progressing muscle degeneration resulting in trouble standing with observed quadriceps, hamstring, and gluteal atrophy and hypertrophy of the calves. The chromosomal basis of this disease is most likely which of the following?

(A) A deletion on the X chromosome
(B) A translocation of the X chromosome with chromosome 12
(C) Trisomy X
(D) A microdeletion on the Y chromosome
(E) A pericentric inversion on the X chromosome

3 A woman with $ER^{+}her2^{-}$ breast cancer cells is treated with an agent to block proliferation of such cells. This agent works through which of the following ways?

(A) Inhibiting DNA polymerase
(B) Antagonizing EGF-stimulated cell proliferation
(C) Altering estrogen's induction of new gene transcription
(D) Stimulating the estrogen receptor to leave the nucleus
(E) Blocking the synthesis of the estrogen receptor

4 A boy has a mild case of ornithine transcarbamoylase deficiency, and has volunteered to be part of a study to try and control the disease via genetic engineering. A suitable vector containing a functional ornithine transcarbamoylase deficiency (OTC) gene has been developed, and needs to be targeted to which of the following organs?

(A) Bone marrow
(B) Brain
(C) Kidney
(D) Intestine
(E) Liver

5 A 4-year-old girl was brought to the Emergency Department due to vomiting and lethargy. Blood work showed hyperammonemia and urinalysis demonstrated orotic aciduria. Neither of her parents had ever expressed such symptoms. Genetically, this girl is experiencing these symptoms due to which one of the following?

(A) Inheriting an autosomal recessive disorder
(B) Inheriting an autosomal dominant disorder
(C) Unequal X-inactivation during embryogenesis
(D) Trisomy X gene dosage effects
(E) Monosomy X gene dosage effects

6 A family had an inherited disease that spanned the last three generations. A representation of a Southern blot of the putative disease gene displayed the following:

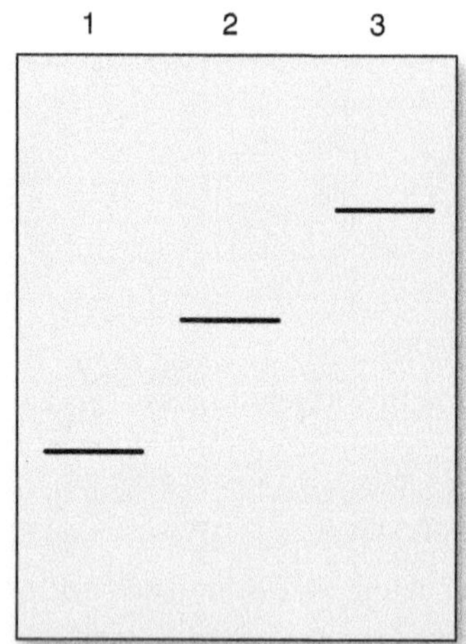

The age of onset of the disease has decreased from the first to the third generation. This disorder may be due to which of the following genetic alterations?

(A) Translocation
(B) Triplet repeat expansion
(C) Trisomy
(D) Deletion
(E) Gene duplication

7 Considering the family in the previous question, which of the following can best describe the finding of earlier age of onset of disease in each succeeding generation?

(A) Uniparental isodisomy
(B) Anticipation
(C) Malformation
(D) Penetrance
(E) Expressivity

8 The disease frequency for an autosomal recessive disorder is one in a million. The carrier frequency for this allele is best estimated as which of the following?

(A) 1 in 500
(B) 1 in 1,000
(C) 1 in 2,000
(D) 1 in 50,000
(E) 1 in 1,000,000

9 A woman has a son with a rare X-linked recessive disease, which has a disease frequency of one in 10,000 in the population. The female carrier frequency in the population is which of the following?

(A) 1 in 5,000
(B) 1 in 10,000
(C) 1 in 20,000
(D) 1 in 50,000
(E) 1 in 100,000

10 The gene frequency for a rare autosomal recessive disease is 1 in 1,000 for the general population. The frequency of affected females is which of the following?

(A) 1 in 1,000,000
(B) 1 in 2,000,000
(C) 1 in 100,000
(D) 1 in 10,000
(E) 1 in 1,000

11 A couple has had a child with a cleft lip and palate. The relative risk of this couple having a second child with this malformation is best described as which of the following?

(A) Same as before their first child was born
(B) Same as the population in general
(C) Greater than before their first child was born
(D) Less than before their first child was born
(E) Less than the population in general

12 Chronic myelogenous leukemia, due to the presence of Philadelphia chromosome, leads to transformation due to the creation of a factor which is nonregulated and aberrant. This factor is best described as which of the following?

(A) Transcription factor
(B) Growth factor receptor
(C) Growth factor
(D) Tyrosine kinase
(E) Ser/thr kinase

13 A patient has been diagnosed with a melanoma, and molecular analysis has indicated that the tumor has sustained a loss of p16(INK4) activity (inhibitor of cyclin-dependent kinase 4). Such a gene would be best classified as which of the following?

(A) A dominant oncogene
(B) A tumor suppressor
(C) A proapoptotic factor
(D) An antiapoptotic factor
(E) A growth factor

14 Considering the pedigree shown below, if I-2 is a carrier of a rare autosomal recessive disease, what is the probability that IV-1 will have the disease?

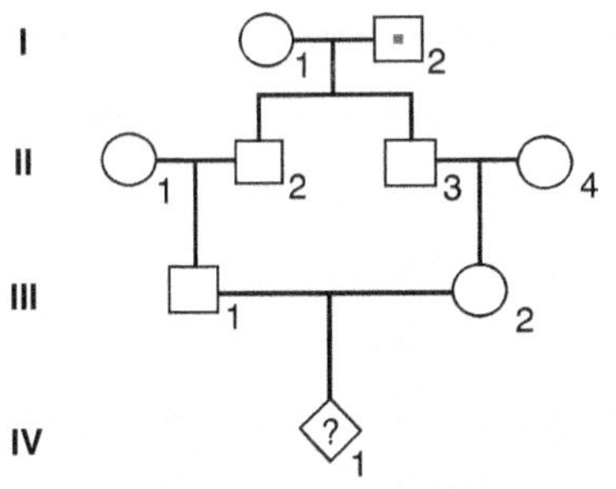

(A) 1 in 4
(B) 1 in 8
(C) 1 in 16
(D) 1 in 32
(E) 1 in 64

15 In the pedigree shown below, assume I-2 is a carrier for sickle cell disease, which occurs in the African American community at a frequency of 1 in 400 live births. Assuming that all of the individuals in the pedigree are members of the African American community, what is the probability that III-2 is a carrier for sickle cell disease?

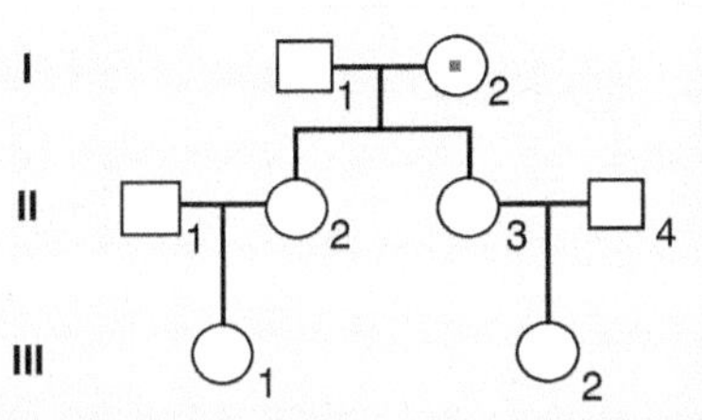

(A) 25%
(B) 32.5%
(C) 37.5%
(D) 50%
(E) 100%

16 Utilizing the same pedigree as indicated in the previous question, what is the probability that III-1 will have sickle cell disease?
(A) 25%
(B) 12.5%
(C) 6.25%
(D) 2.75%
(E) 1.375%

17 A family expresses an X-linked disease, and you have a marker available which can distinguish between 2 polymorphic areas of the X chromosome, designated as A and B. The family pedigree, along with the polymorphic forms of the X chromosome for each family member, is shown below. What is the probability that III-4 is a carrier of this disease?

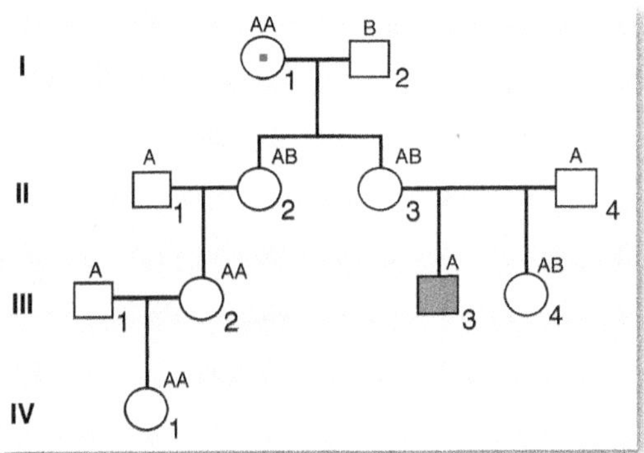

(A) 0%
(B) 12.5%
(C) 25%
(D) 50%
(E) 100%

18 Concerning the pedigree in the previous question, what is the probability that individual IV-1 is a carrier of the mutation?
(A) 0%
(B) 12.5%
(C) 25%
(D) 50%
(E) 100%

19 A 5-year-old presents to the pediatrician due to lethargy and tiredness. The red blood cell count is normal, but molecular analysis indicates that the child is producing 25% of the normal amount of α-globin, compared to 100% of the normal amount of β-globin. Further analysis shows a total deletion of the α-globin genes from one chromosome. What might account for the lower than expected levels of α-globin being produced?
(A) β-globin inhibition of α-globin synthesis
(B) Enhanced expression of γ-globin synthesis
(C) Loss of a β-globin gene
(D) Deletion of a third α-globin gene
(E) Duplication of an α-globin gene

20 A physician in a rural African clinic sees a child with swelling of the jaw, loosening of the teeth, and swollen lymph nodes (see the picture below). Karyotype analysis of blood cells shows a translocation between chromosomes 8 and 14. This rapidly growing tumor is most likely due to which of the following?

(A) EBV activation
(B) Bcr-abl activation
(C) BCl-2 activation
(D) Constitutive myc expression
(E) EGF-receptor activation

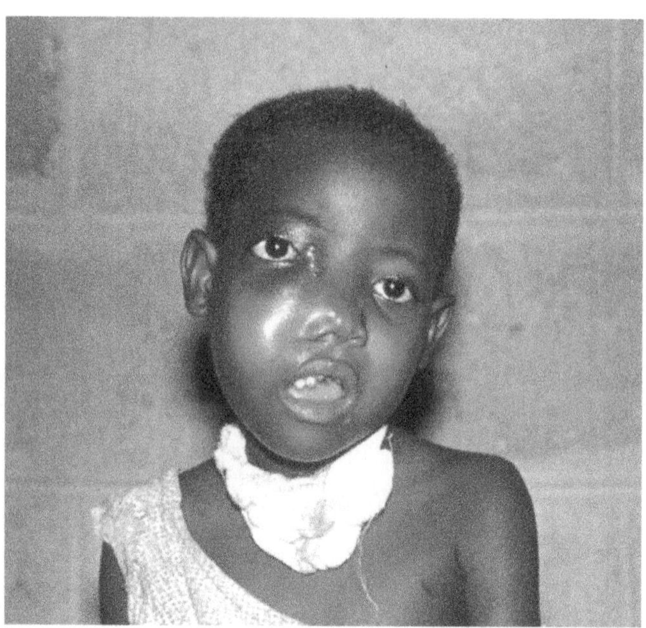

ANSWERS

1 **The answer is A: Potential regions of trisomy or monosomy in the fertilized egg.** The mother carries a translocation (which is not a Robertsonian translocation, as those only occur between acrocentric chromosomes) between chromosomes 9 and 15. A piece of chromosome 9 (from the long arm, 9q) is attached to the long arm of chromosome 15 (the derivative chromosome). As the carrier has all the genes present, she is normal. But when she makes gametes, the following combinations are possible: normal 9 and normal 15; normal 9 and long 15 (carrying a piece of 9q); shorter 9 (missing the 9q area) and normal 15; and shorter 9 and long 15. When each of these four possibilities is fertilized by a sperm carrying a normal 9 and 15, the following four results are possible:

(i) Normal 9 and 15 from mom, normal 9 and 15 from dad—normal pregnancy and birth
(ii) Shorter 9 and long 15 from mom, normal 9 and 15 from dad—normal pregnancy and birth (this child will have the same translocation as the mom, and has all genes represented)
(iii) Normal 9 and long 15 from mom, normal 9 and 15 from dad—abnormal pregnancy, most likely leading to miscarriage. This embryo will have trisomy 9q, and under most conditions, trisomy for a particular region of a chromosome is incompatible with live births.
(iv) Shorter 9 and normal 15 from mom, normal 9 and 15 from dad—abnormal pregnancy, most likely leading to miscarriage. In this case, the embryo is monosomy for the 9q region, expressing too few genes for survival. The only monosomy that leads to a live birth is monosomy X.

These results are also summarized in Table 21-1.

2 **The answer is A: A deletion on the X chromosome.** The boy is showing symptoms of Duchenne muscular dystrophy, which is most often due to a deletion on the X chromosome, removing all or a large part of the gene for dystrophin, an essential component of the muscle cellular membrane. A balanced translocation of the X chromosome with another chromosome would not lead to these symptoms unless the dystrophin gene is split across the two chromosomes (an unlikely event). Trisomy X does not lead to any symptoms. The dystrophin gene is not on the Y chromosome. A pericentric inversion within the X chromosome is also unlikely to lead to disruption of the dystrophin gene.

3 **The answer is C: Altering estrogen's induction of new gene transcription.** The patient is being given tamoxifen, which is a selective estrogen receptor modifier. As the woman's tumor cells are ER^+, the cells are expressing the estrogen receptor, and tamoxifen will be effective in such cells. In breast cells, tamoxifen acts as an antagonist, blocking the actions of estrogen on the cells. In other tissues, however, tamoxifen acts as an agonist, so the other tissues are responding normally to estrogen. Since the breast cancer cells require a supply of estrogen to grow, the use of tamoxifen will reduce the growth rate of tumor cells. Tamoxifen does not stimulate the estrogen receptor to leave the nucleus, nor does it block the synthesis of the estrogen receptor. Rather, the drug binds to the receptor and prevents estrogen from binding to the receptor and altering gene transcription. Tamoxifen does not inhibit DNA polymerase, nor does it antagonize epidermal growth factor (EGF)-stimulated cell proliferation, although in this tumor type ($her2^-$), there are no EGF receptors being expressed such that EGF would not have an effect on these cells.

4 **The answer is E: Liver.** The urea cycle occurs primarily in the liver, so the defective gene only needs to be repaired in the liver for the cycle to become functional again. Targeting the vector to the other tissues listed (bone marrow, brain, kidney, and intestine) will not result in a functional cycle, as those tissues do not express the enzymes at a level sufficient for the cycle to proceed at an adequate rate.

Table 21-1.

Father: 9n and 15n	**Mother: 9n, 9s, 15n, and 15l**		
Father Gametes	**Mother Gametes**	**Genotype**	**Outcome**
9n 15n	9n 15n	9n9n 15n15n	Normal
9n 15n	9n 15l	9n9n 15n15l	Trisomy 9q, lethal event
9n 15n	9s 15n	9n9s 15n15n	Monosomy 9q, lethal event
9n 15n	9s 15l	9n9s 15n15l	Normal, carrier of the translocation (same genotype as the mother)

Note: 9n and 15n represent normal chromosomes 9 and 15. 9s represents the chromosome 9 that has lost a piece of its long arm and that was translocated to chromosome 15. This chromosome 9 is missing a part of 9q. 15l represents the lengthened chromosome 15, which is carrying a piece of 9q at its end.

5 **The answer is C: Unequal X-inactivation during embryogenesis.** The girl is experiencing the symptoms of ornithine transcarbamoylase deficiency (OTC), which is a gene located on the X chromosome. Under usual conditions, women who are carriers of recessive mutated genes located on the X chromosome do not express symptoms of the disease. However, due to gene dosage effects, during early embryogenesis (the 8 to 16 cell stage of the embryo), one X chromosome is inactivated in each cell (and becomes the Barr body) and remains inactivated in all future daughter cells. What has happened in this child is unequal X-inactivation, in that the X chromosome carrying the nonmutated OTC gene was inactivated in the majority of primordial cells, leading to the development of a liver in which the majority of cells expressed only the mutated form of OTC. This led to a female having the symptoms of OTC deficiency. Trisomy or monosomy X will not lead to an OTC deficiency. As the disease gene is X-linked, autosomal dominant and recessive inheritance patterns are not appropriate answer choices.

6 **The answer is B: Triplet repeat expansion.** Triplet repeat diseases (such as myotonic dystrophy or Fragile X syndrome) are due to triplet repeat expansions in or around a gene. The repeats tend to increase in number from one generation to the next, which is indicated in the Southern blot by larger-sized pieces of DNA hybridizing to the probe as the generations increase. As the triplet repeats increase in size, the disease usually becomes more severe, and the age of onset of symptoms is decreased. In some individuals with many repeats, no symptoms appear, and such individuals are considered "sleepers" and can pass the disorder on to their offspring. Nonaffected individuals also have a small number of repeats, but not enough to bring about disease. Translocations, trisomy, deletions, or gene duplications would not show the pattern of signals seen in the Southern blot.

7 **The answer is B: Anticipation.** Anticipation is the term used to describe a genetic disorder that increases in severity from one generation to the next, as is often observed in triplet repeat disorders. Uniparental isodisomy is when a child inherits two copies of a chromosome from one parent. Malformation is a birth defect due to environmental and genetic factors. Penetrance describes the percentage of people who develop symptoms upon inheriting a genetic disease (for example, inheritance of the BRCA1 gene has a penetrance of 85% as 15% of the women who inherit the gene will not develop breast cancer). Expressivity describes the severity of symptoms an affected individual displays (individuals may show mild or severe symptoms depending on the mutation which is inherited).

8 **The answer is A: 1 in 500.** This question requires an understanding of Hardy–Weinberg equilibrium for population genetics in which $p^2 + 2pq + q^2 = 1$ (p is the probability of having the normal allele, q is the probability of having the mutated allele [thus, $p + q = 1$], q^2 is equal to the probability of having the disease, and $2pq$ represents the probability of being a carrier for the disease in the population). For this example, $q^2 = 10^{-6}$, so $q = 10^{-3}$. $2pq$, then, is 2×10^{-3}, or one in 500 people will be a carrier for the disease.

9 **The answer is A: 1 in 5,000.** In the case of an X-linked disease, the disease frequency (1 in 10,000 in this case) indicates that among 10,000 men, one would have the mutated gene on the X chromosome. Since women contain two X chromosomes, a collection of 5,000 women would represent 10,000 X chromosomes, and one of those X chromosomes would contain the mutation. This indicates that 1 in 5,000 women would be a carrier.

10 **The answer is B: 1 in 2,000,000.** Going back to the Hardy–Weinberg equilibrium, $q = 10^{-3}$ (the gene frequency of the mutated allele), so that $q^2 = 10^{-6}$. Thus, the frequency of affected individuals is one in a million. However, the question asked for the frequency of affected females, which would be approximately one half of the affected patients, leading to a frequency of 1 in 2 million females would have the disorder, as would 1 in 2 million males (which, when summed, gives an overall disease frequency of 2 in 2 million, or 1 in 1 million individuals in the population would express the disorder).

11 **The answer is C: Greater than before their first child was born.** Cleft lip and palate is a multifactorial disorder, requiring a large number of genes to interact in a way to create the condition. Each parent needs to contribute a share of "altered" genes such that the condition is observed, and this share needs to be above a threshold amount of "altered" genes. If the threshold is not realized, the condition is not observed. Thus, there is a certain risk in the overall population for having a child with this condition. Once a couple has had a child with this condition, we have identified two individuals who have a large number of "altered" genes. Thus, their risk, as compared to the risk of the population at large (the relative risk), is now greater due to the fact that the prior pregnancy indicated that this couple has a large number of "altered" genes between them.

12 **The answer is D: Tyrosine kinase.** Philadelphia chromosome (a translocation of chromosomes 9 and 22) produces a new gene product, a fusion protein of bcr and abl (bcr from chromosome 22 and abl from chromosome 9,

with the fusion protein being produced from the shorter chromosome 22). Abl is a tyrosine kinase, and when fused with bcr, it is constitutive and no longer properly regulated. The presence of this unregulated kinase leads to a loss of cellular growth control. The bcr–abl protein is not a transcription factor, growth factor receptor, growth factor, or ser/thr kinase. This translocation is shown in the figure below.

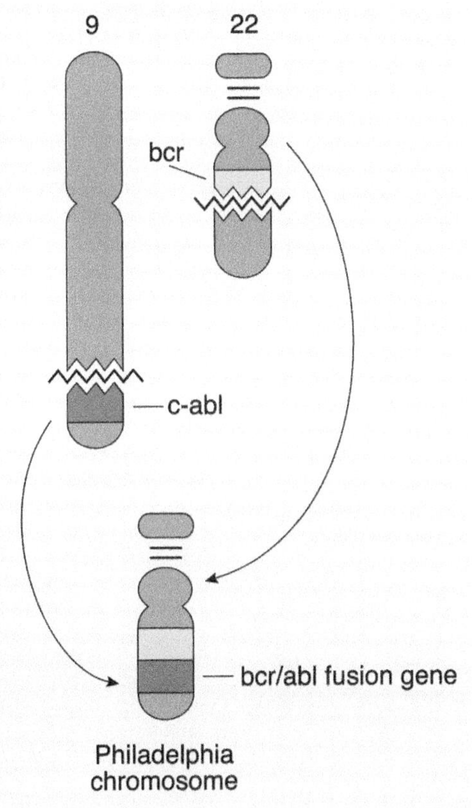

13 **The answer is B: A tumor suppressor.** Cyclin-dependent kinase inhibitors (CKI) act to block the action of kinases that are activated by cyclins (see the figure below). When such an activity is lost (meaning that the gene products from both chromosomes are inactive), uncontrolled cell proliferation can result. Since the activity must be lost, such genes are classified as tumor suppressors, as opposed to the dominant oncogenes, in which an activity is gained via mutation or inappropriate gene regulation. The CKIs are not involved in apoptosis, nor do they act as growth factors.

14 **The answer is E: 1 in 64.** Since this is a rare autosomal recessive disorder, we can assume that the probability of the individuals who married into the family (II-1, II-4) having the altered gene is zero. As such, the probability that II-2 or II-3 has inherited the mutated allele (and will be a carrier) is 50% (a one in two chance of getting the mutated allele from their father, I-2). The probability that III-1 or III-2 would inherit the mutated allele from their fathers is also 50%, such that the overall probability that III-1 and III-2 would carry the mutated allele is 50% times 50%, or 25%. The probability that III-1 would pass the mutated allele to IV-1 is 50%, but since his probability of having the mutated allele in the first place is 25%, the overall probability of passing this gene is 12.5% (1 in 8). This is also true for III-2 passing the mutated allele to IV-1. For IV-1 to have the disease, both mutated alleles would have to be inherited, and the probability of that occurring

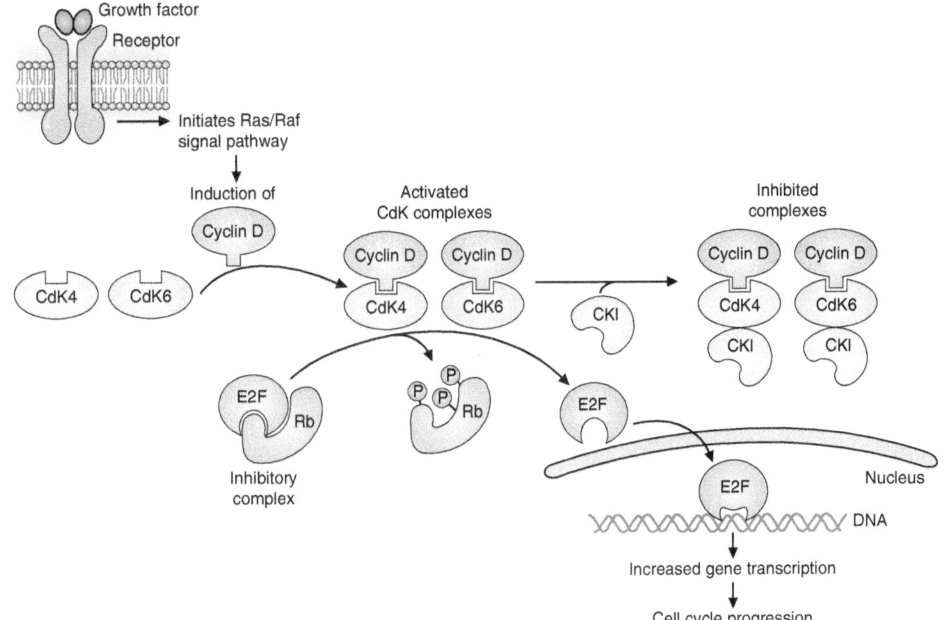

Answer 13: Control of the G1/S transition in the cell cycle. The genes that encode cyclins and CDKs are oncogenes and the gene that encodes the retinoblastoma protein (Rb) is a tumor-suppressor gene, as are the genes that encode CKIs (since the loss of their activity leads to tumor growth). *CDK*, cyclin-dependent kinase; *CKI*, cyclin-dependent kinase inhibitor.

is 12.5% times 12.5%, or 1 in 64. These values are indicated in the pedigree below.

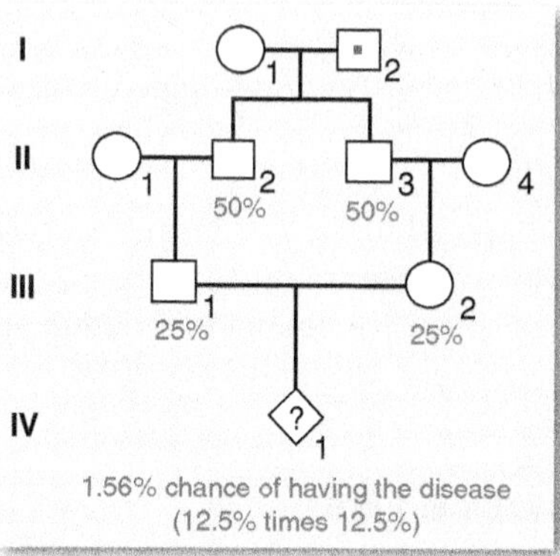

The percentages in red indicate the probability of the individual being a carrier for the disease, until you reach individual IV-1, in which case, the probability is that of the person inheriting the disease.

15 **The answer is B: 32.5%.** For this problem, one cannot assume that the probability of a person marrying into the family has a zero risk of carrying the sickle cell gene. Since the disease frequency is 1 in 400 (q^2), the carrier frequency is $2pq$, or 1 in 10. Thus, the probability that II-3 is a carrier is 55% (a one in two chance of inheriting the gene from her mother, which is 50%, and a 1 in 20 chance of inheriting the gene from her father, which is 5%. Since either event can result in the child being a carrier, the probabilities are added, yielding 55%). The probability that III-2 will be a carrier is the sum of the probabilities of inheriting the mutated gene from either her mother (who has a 55% chance of being a carrier) or her father (who has a 10% chance of being a carrier). This comes out to 32.5% (a 27.5% chance from mom and a 5% chance from dad). These percentages are indicated in the pedigree below.

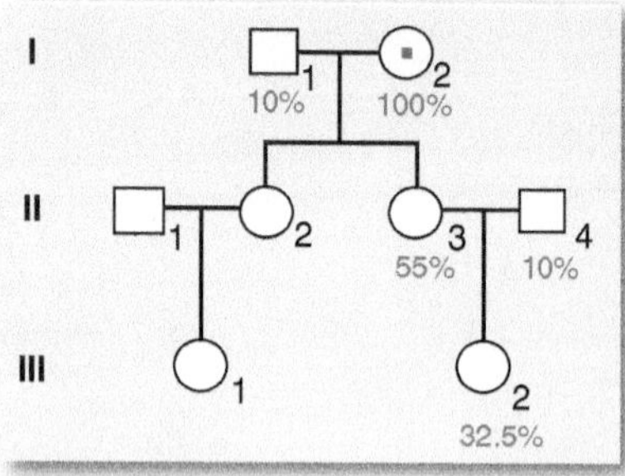

The percentages in red indicate the probability of the individual being a carrier for the disease.

16 **The answer is E: 1.375%.** Based on the answer to the last question, it is known that the probability of II-2 being a carrier is 55% and of II-1 being a carrier is 10%. For III-1 to have the disease, she must inherit the mutated alleles from each parent. There is a 27.5% chance of inheriting the mutated allele from her mother and a 5% chance of inheriting it from her father. For both events to be true (the child to inherit two mutated alleles), the probabilities need to be multiplied, and 0.275 times 0.05 yields 0.01375, or a 1.375% chance.

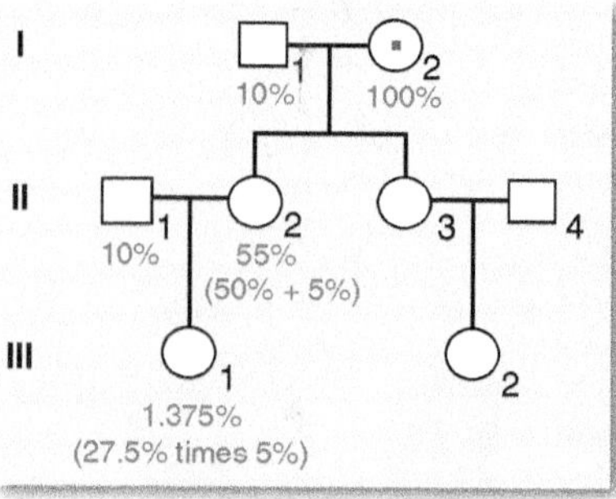

The percentages in red indicate the probability of the individual being a carrier for the disease, except for III-1, in which case, they indicate the probability of that individual having the disease.

17 **The answer is A: 0%.** Individual III-4 has inherited one X chromosome from her father, which contains the A polymorphic marker (indicated by the red A in the figure below). This chromosome does not contain the disease mutation as her father does not express the disease. Her other X chromosome comes from her mother, and contains the B polymorphic marker. III-4's brother has the disease, which came from his mother's X chromosome with the A polymorphic marker (indicated in blue). Since III-4 did not inherit the mother's X chromosome with the A polymorphic marker, she has no risk of being a carrier for the disease. It is important to note in this question that there are two species of X chromosomes with the A polymorphic marker in this family. One carries the disease gene (from II-3), and the other does not (from II-4, and also implied in I-1). This is indicated in the figure below.

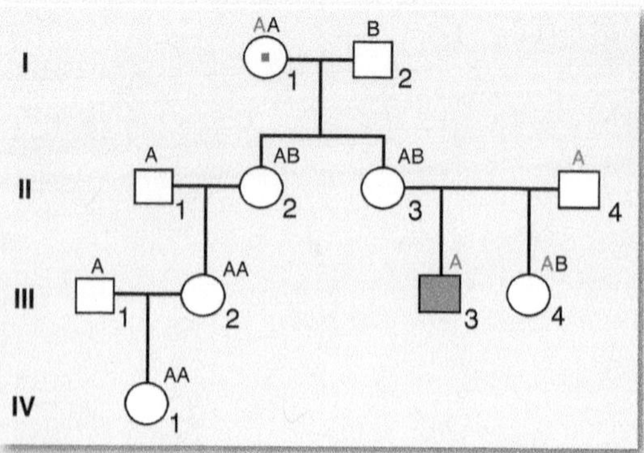

18 **The answer is C: 25%.** I-1 must be a carrier as her daughter (II-3) had a son with the disease. This means that one of the X chromosomes in I-1 carries the disease gene, although both X chromosomes display the A polymorphic marker. Individual II-2 has a 50% chance of inheriting the disease gene with the A polymorphic marker from her mother (the X chromosome with the A polymorphic marker in II-2 had to come from her mother, and there is a one in two chance that it is the one with the disease gene). However, based on the data in the pedigree, individual II-2 passed the X chromosome with the A polymorphic marker (indicated in red in the figure below), and a 50% chance of carrying the disease gene, to her daughter, III-2 (the other A marker X chromosome came from her father). III-2 now has a 50% chance of passing the X chromosome, A polymorphic marker, and disease gene to her daughter IV-1. For IV-1 to be a carrier, all three events must occur, so the overall probability is 50% times 100% times 50%, or 25%.

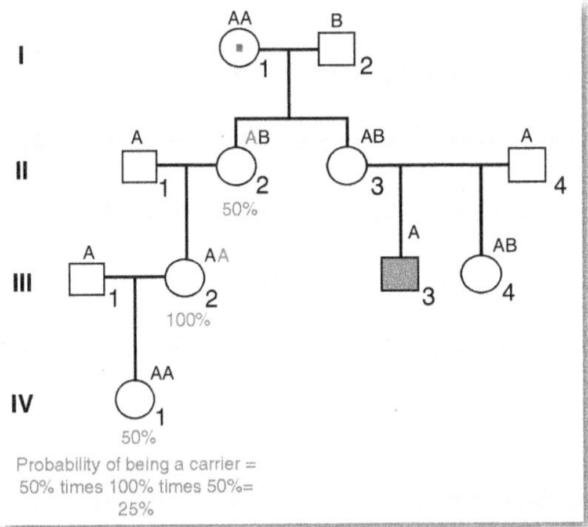

19 **The answer is D: Deletion of a third α-globin gene.** Under normal conditions, a cell expresses 100% α-globin protein. This comes from four α-globin genes, which are transcribed equally (two copies of the α-globin gene on each chromosome 16; see the figure below). Thus, each gene is contributing 25% of the total α-globin protein in the cell. When two of the genes are deleted, one would then expect to see a 50% drop in total α-globin expression. However,

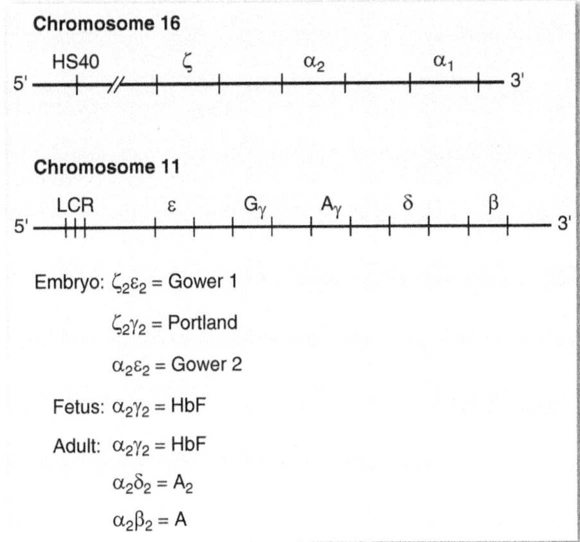

Genomic organization of the globin genes. Note the two active copies of the α-globin gene on chromosome 16.

we are told that the patient is only producing 25% of the normal expected amount of α-globin protein. As there are still two α-globin genes remaining in the patient on chromosome 16, one possibility is to have a deletion of one of the genes on that chromosome, which would reduce overall α-globin gene expression to 25%. β-globin does not inhibit α-globin synthesis, and enhanced expression of γ-globin will not affect α-globin expression. Duplication of an α-globin gene would increase α-globin expression, which would decrease the severity of the disease. Similarly, deletion of a β-globin gene would also alleviate the imbalance in α-globin and β-globin synthesis, and alleviate the severity of the disorder.

20 **The answer is D: Constitutive myc expression.** The patient has Burkitt lymphoma, which in 90% of the cases is due to altered regulation of the myc gene (constitutive activation of transcription), due to a translocation of the myc gene such that it is controlled by an immunoglobulin promoter (which is why this disorder results in abnormal blood cell proliferation, as these are the cells that produce the immunoglobulins). The translocation is shown in the figure below. While Epstein–Barr virus is thought to render individuals susceptible to Burkitt lymphoma, the oncogenic event is the misexpression of the myc gene. Bcr–abl is associated with chronic myelogenous leukemia. Bcl-2 overexpression leads to a loss of apoptotic potential and is not associated with Burkitt lymphoma. EGF-receptor activation (similar to the erbB oncogene) also does not lead to these symptoms.

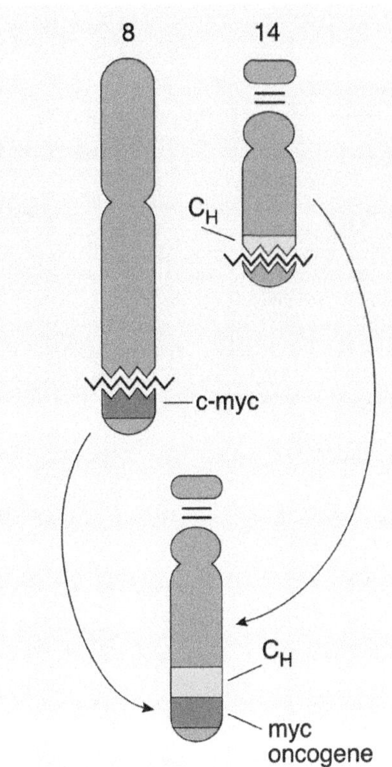

Figure Credits

Chapter 1

A 1-14: From Lieberman M, Marks AD. Marks' Basic Medical Biochemistry: A Clinical Approach. 3rd Ed. Baltimore: Lippincott Williams & Wilkins, 2009, Figure 4-3.

Chapter 2

Q 2-4: Image from Rubin E, Farber JL. Pathology. 3rd Ed. Philadelphia: Lippincott Williams & Wilkins, 1999, Figure 20-26.
Q 2-6: Image from Gold DH, Weingeist TA. Color Atlas of the Eye in Systemic Disease. Baltimore: Lippincott Williams & Wilkins, 2001.
Q 2-7: Image from Rubin E, Farber JL. Pathology. 3rd Ed. Philadelphia: Lippincott Williams & Wilkins, 1999.
Q 2-8: Image from McClatchey KD. Clinical Laboratory Medicine. 2nd Ed. Philadelphia: Lippincott Williams & Wilkins, 2002.
Q 2-18: Image from McClatchey KD, Clinical laboratory Medicine. 2nd Ed. Philadelphia: Lippincott Williams & Wilkins, 2002.
A 2-4: From Lieberman M, Marks AD. Marks' Basic Medical Biochemistry: A Clinical Approach. 3rd Ed. Baltimore: Lippincott Williams & Wilkins, 2009:104.
A 2-5: From Lieberman M, Marks AD. Marks' Basic Medical Biochemistry: A Clinical Approach. 3rd Ed. Baltimore: Lippincott Williams & Wilkins, 2009, Figure 7-19.
A 2-18: From Lieberman M, Marks AD. Marks' Basic Medical Biochemistry: A Clinical Approach. 3rd Ed. Baltimore: Lippincott Williams & Wilkins, 2009, Figure 44-10.

Chapter 3

Q 3-19: Image from Rubin E, Farber JL. Pathology. 3rd Ed. Philadelphia: Lippincott Williams & Wilkins, 1999, Figure 5-25C.
A 3-3: Image from Rubin E, Farber JL. Pathology. 3rd Ed. Philadelphia: Lippincott Williams & Wilkins, 1999, Figure 6-36.
A 3-4: From Lieberman M, Marks AD. Marks' Basic Medical Biochemistry: A Clinical Approach. 3rd Ed. Baltimore: Lippincott Williams & Wilkins, 2009, Figure 13-15.
A 3-6: Image from McClatchey KD. Clinical Laboratory Medicine. 2nd Ed. Philadelphia: Lippincott Williams & Wilkins, 2002.
A 3-8: Image from Anatomical Chart Company. Diseases and Disorders: The World's Best Anatomical Chart. 2nd Ed. Philadelphia: Lippincott Williams & Wilkins, 2005.
A 3-9: From Lieberman M, Marks AD. Marks' Basic Medical Biochemistry: A Clinical Approach. 3rd Ed. Baltimore: Lippincott Williams & Wilkins, 2009, Figure 13-5.

Chapter 4

Q 4-7 & 4-8: Modified from Lieberman M, Marks AD. Marks' Basic Medical Biochemistry: A Clinical Approach. 3rd Ed. Baltimore: Lippincott Williams & Wilkins, 2009, Figure 14-18.
Q 4-9: Image from Fleisher GR, Ludwig S, Baskin MN. Atlas of Pediatric Emergency Medicine. Philadelphia: Lippincott Williams & Wilkins, 2004.
Q 4-12: Image from Anderson, Shauna C. Anderson's Atlas of Hematology. Philadelphia: Lippincott Williams & Wilkins, 2003.
Q 4-16: From Lieberman M, Marks AD. Marks' Basic Medical Biochemistry: A Clinical Approach. 3rd Ed. Baltimore: Lippincott Williams & Wilkins, 2009:220.
A 4-1: From Lieberman M, Marks AD. Marks' Basic Medical Biochemistry: A Clinical Approach. 3rd Ed. Baltimore: Lippincott Williams & Wilkins, 2009, Figure 12-21.
A 4-2: From Lieberman M, Marks AD. Marks' Basic Medical Biochemistry: A Clinical Approach. 3rd Ed. Baltimore: Lippincott Williams & Wilkins, 2009, Figure 14-10.
A 4-3: From Lieberman M, Marks AD. Marks' Basic Medical Biochemistry: A Clinical Approach. 3rd Ed. Baltimore: Lippincott Williams & Wilkins, 2009, Figure 16-19.
A 4-5: From Lieberman M, Marks AD. Marks' Basic Medical Biochemistry: A Clinical Approach. 3rd Ed. Baltimore: Lippincott Williams & Wilkins, 2009, Figure 14-14.
A 4-6: From Lieberman M, Marks AD. Marks' Basic Medical Biochemistry: A Clinical Approach. 3rd Ed. Baltimore: Lippincott Williams & Wilkins, 2009:236.
A 4-10: From Lieberman M, Marks AD. Marks' Basic Medical Biochemistry: A Clinical Approach. 3rd Ed. Baltimore: Lippincott Williams & Wilkins, 2009, Figure 17-12.
A 4-13: From Lieberman M, Marks AD. Marks' Basic Medical Biochemistry: A Clinical Approach. 3rd Ed. Baltimore: Lippincott Williams & Wilkins, 2009, Figure 32-11.

Chapter 5

Q 5-6: From Harnisch JP, Trunca E, Nolan CM. Diphtheria among alcoholic urban adults. Ann Intern Med 1989;111:77, with permission.
A 5-1: From Lieberman M, Marks AD. Marks' Basic Medical Biochemistry: A Clinical Approach. 3rd Ed. Baltimore: Lippincott Williams & Wilkins, 2009, Figure 15-18.
A 5-3: From Lieberman M, Marks AD. Marks' Basic Medical Biochemistry: A Clinical Approach. 3rd Ed. Baltimore: Lippincott Williams & Wilkins, 2009, Figure 30-15.
A 5-6: Adapted from Lieberman M, Marks AD. Marks' Basic Medical Biochemistry: A Clinical Approach. 3rd Ed. Baltimore: Lippincott Williams & Wilkins, 2009, Figure 6-14.
A 5-16: Modified from Lieberman M, Marks AD. Marks' Basic Medical Biochemistry: A Clinical Approach. 3rd Ed. Baltimore: Lippincott Williams & Wilkins, 2009, Figure 15-2.
A 5-18: From Lieberman M, Marks AD. Marks' Basic Medical Biochemistry: A Clinical Approach. 3rd Ed. Baltimore: Lippincott Williams & Wilkins, 2009, Figure 30-13.
A 5-19: From Champe PC, Harvey RA, Ferrier DR. Lippincott's Illustrated Review of Biochemistry. 3rd Ed. Baltimore: Lippincott Williams & Wilkins, 2009, Figure 23-3.
A 5-20: From Lieberman M, Marks AD. Marks' Basic Medical Biochemistry: A Clinical Approach. 3rd Ed. Baltimore: Lippincott Williams & Wilkins, 2009, Figure 30-17.

Chapter 6

Q 6-15: From Lieberman M, Marks AD. Marks' Basic Medical Biochemistry: A Clinical Approach. 3rd Ed. Baltimore: Lippincott Williams & Wilkins, 2009, Figure 44-19.
A 6-1: From Lieberman M, Marks AD. Marks' Basic Medical Biochemistry: A Clinical Approach. 3rd Ed. Baltimore: Lippincott Williams & Wilkins, 2009, Figure 16-4.
A 6-2: From Lieberman M, Marks AD. Marks' Basic Medical Biochemistry: A Clinical Approach. 3rd Ed. Baltimore: Lippincott Williams & Wilkins, 2009, Figure 44-18.
A 6-9: Adapted from Lieberman M, Marks AD. Marks' Basic Medical Biochemistry: A Clinical Approach. 3rd Ed. Baltimore: Lippincott Williams & Wilkins, 2009, Figures 16-21 and 16-22.

Chapter 7

Q 7-11: Image from Goodheart HP. Goodheart's Photoguide of Common Skin Disorders. 2nd Ed. Philadelphia: Lippincott Williams & Wilkins, 2003.
A 7-10: From Lieberman M, Marks AD. Marks' Basic Medical Biochemistry: A Clinical Approach. 3rd Ed. Baltimore: Lippincott Williams & Wilkins, 2009, Figure 17-7.

Chapter 8

Q 8-13 & 8-14: Modified from Lieberman M, Marks AD. Marks' Basic Medical Biochemistry: A Clinical Approach. 3rd Ed. Baltimore: Lippincott Williams & Wilkins, 2009, Figure 8-7.

A 8-1: From Cohen BJ, Taylor JJ. Memmler's The Human Body in Health and Disease. 10th Ed. Baltimore: Lippincott Williams & Wilkins, 2005.

A 8-1: From Lieberman M, Marks AD. Marks' Basic Medical Biochemistry: A Clinical Approach. 3rd Ed. Baltimore: Lippincott Williams & Wilkins, 2009:10.

Chapter 9

Q 9-1: From Goodheart HP. Goodheart's Photoguide of Common Skin Disorders, 2nd Ed. Philadelphia: Lippincott Williams & Wilkins, 2003.

Q 9-12: From McClatchey KD. Clinical Laboratory Medicine. 2nd Ed. Philadelphia: Lippincott Williams & Wilkins, 2002.

Q 9-14: From McClatchey KD. Clinical Laboratory Medicine, 2nd Ed. Philadelphia: Lippincott Williams & Wilkins, 2002.

A 9-2: From Rubin E, Farber JL. Pathology. 3rd Ed. Philadelphia: Lippincott Williams & Wilkins, 1999.

A 9-7: From Lieberman M, Marks AD. Marks' Basic Medical Biochemistry: A Clinical Approach. 3rd Ed. Baltimore: Lippincott Williams & Wilkins, 2009, Figure 11-14.

A 9-8: From Rubin E, Farber JL. Pathology. 3rd Ed. Philadelphia: Lippincott Williams & Wilkins, 1999, Figure 5-30.

A 9-11: Modified from Lieberman M, Marks AD. Marks' Basic Medical Biochemistry: A Clinical Approach. 3rd Ed. Baltimore: Lippincott Williams & Wilkins, 2009, Figure 16-12A.

A 9-13: From Lieberman M, Marks AD. Marks' Basic Medical Biochemistry: A Clinical Approach. 3rd Ed. Baltimore: Lippincott Williams & Wilkins, 2009, Figure 11-16.

A 9-14: From Lieberman M, Marks AD. Marks' Basic Medical Biochemistry: A Clinical Approach. 3rd Ed. Baltimore: Lippincott Williams & Wilkins, 2009, Figure 11-15.

A 9-17: From Lieberman M, Marks AD. Marks' Basic Medical Biochemistry: A Clinical Approach. 3rd Ed. Baltimore: Lippincott Williams & Wilkins, 2009, Figure 18-5.

A 9-19: From Lieberman M, Marks AD. Marks' Basic Medical Biochemistry: A Clinical Approach. 3rd Ed. Baltimore: Lippincott Williams & Wilkins, 2009, Figure 11-4.

Chapter 10

Q 10-3: Image from Gold DH, Weingeist TA. Color Atlas of the Eye in Systemic Disease. Baltimore: Lippincott Williams & Wilkins, 2001. (Courtesy of Thomas D. France, MD.)

A 10-1: Modified from Lieberman M, Marks AD. Marks' Basic Medical Biochemistry: A Clinical Approach. 3rd Ed. Baltimore: Lippincott Williams & Wilkins, 2009, Figure 22.2.

A 10-2: From Lieberman M, Marks AD. Marks' Basic Medical Biochemistry: A Clinical Approach. 3rd Ed. Baltimore: Lippincott Williams & Wilkins, 2009, Figure 29-5.

A 10-6: Modified from Lieberman M, Marks AD. Marks' Basic Medical Biochemistry: A Clinical Approach. 3rd Ed. Baltimore: Lippincott Williams & Wilkins, 2009, Figure 25-2.

A 10-7: From Lieberman M, Marks AD. Marks' Basic Medical Biochemistry: A Clinical Approach. 3rd Ed. Baltimore: Lippincott Williams & Wilkins, 2009, Figure 29-3.

A 10-12: Modified from Lieberman M, Marks AD. Marks' Basic Medical Biochemistry: A Clinical Approach. 3rd Ed. Baltimore: Lippincott Williams & Wilkins, 2009, Figure 31-3.

A 10-17: From Lieberman M, Marks AD. Marks' Basic Medical Biochemistry: A Clinical Approach. 3rd Ed. Baltimore: Lippincott Williams & Wilkins, 2009, Figure 27-12.

Chapter 11

A 11-2: From Lieberman M, Marks AD. Marks' Basic Medical Biochemistry: A Clinical Approach. 3rd Ed. Baltimore: Lippincott Williams & Wilkins, 2009, Figure 20-3.

A 11-3: From Lieberman M, Marks AD. Marks' Basic Medical Biochemistry: A Clinical Approach. 3rd Ed. Baltimore: Lippincott Williams & Wilkins, 2009, Figure 25-2.

A 11-4: From Lieberman M, Marks AD. Marks' Basic Medical Biochemistry: A Clinical Approach. 3rd Ed. Baltimore: Lippincott Williams & Wilkins, 2009, Figure 20-9.

A 11-8: Modified from Lieberman M, Marks AD. Marks' Basic Medical Biochemistry: A Clinical Approach. 3rd Ed. Baltimore: Lippincott Williams & Wilkins, 2009, Figure 21-5.

A 11-13: From Lieberman M, Marks AD. Marks' Basic Medical Biochemistry: A Clinical Approach. 3rd Ed. Baltimore: Lippincott Williams & Wilkins, 2009, Figure 38-3.

A 11-14: From Lieberman M, Marks AD. Marks' Basic Medical Biochemistry: A Clinical Approach. 3rd Ed. Baltimore: Lippincott Williams & Wilkins, 2009, Figure 44-4.

A 11-17: From Lieberman M, Marks AD. Marks' Basic Medical Biochemistry: A Clinical Approach. 3rd Ed. Baltimore: Lippincott Williams & Wilkins, 2009, Figure 22-8.

A 11-20: From Lieberman M, Marks AD. Marks' Basic Medical Biochemistry: A Clinical Approach. 3rd Ed. Baltimore: Lippincott Williams & Wilkins, 2009.

Chapter 12

A 12-1: Image from Rubin E, Farber JL. Pathology. 3rd Ed. Philadelphia: Lippincott Williams & Wilkins, 1999, Figure 6-28.

A 12-4: Image from Becker KL, Bilezikian JP, Brenner WJ, et al. Principles and Practice of Endocrinology and Metabolism. 3rd Ed. Philadelphia: Lippincott Williams & Wilkins, 2001.

A 12-8: Image modified from Lieberman M, Marks AD. Marks' Basic Medical Biochemistry: A Clinical Approach. 3rd Ed. Baltimore: Lippincott Williams & Wilkins, 2009, Figure 28-10.

A 12-10: Image from Rubin E, Farber JL. Pathology. 3rd Ed. Philadelphia: Lippincott Williams & Wilkins, 1999, Figure 27-17B.

A 12-17: Adapted from Lieberman M, Marks AD. Marks' Basic Medical Biochemistry: A Clinical Approach. 3rd Ed. Baltimore: Lippincott Williams & Wilkins, 2009, Figures 30-6 and 10-4.

A 12-19: Modified from Lieberman M and Marks AD. Marks' Basic Medical Biochemistry: A Clinical Approach. 3rd Ed. Baltimore: Lippincott Williams & Wilkins, 2009, Figure 31-3.

Chapter 13

A 13-1: From Lieberman M, Marks AD. Marks' Basic Medical Biochemistry: A Clinical Approach. 3rd Ed. Baltimore: Lippincott Williams & Wilkins, 2009, Figure 35-3.

A 13-4: From Lieberman M, Marks AD. Marks' Basic Medical Biochemistry: A Clinical Approach. 3rd Ed. Baltimore: Lippincott Williams & Wilkins, 2009, Figure 23-8.

A 13-5: From Lieberman M, Marks AD. Marks' Basic Medical Biochemistry: A Clinical Approach. 3rd Ed. Baltimore: Lippincott Williams & Wilkins, 2009, Figure 23-16.

A 13-9: Adapted from Marks 3rd Ed., Figure 23-7 and Lieberman M, Marks AD. Marks' Basic Medical Biochemistry: A Clinical Approach. 3rd Ed. Baltimore: Lippincott Williams & Wilkins, 2009, Figure 23.9.

A 13-10: Modified from Lieberman M, Marks AD. Marks' Basic Medical Biochemistry: A Clinical Approach. 3rd Ed. Baltimore: Lippincott Williams & Wilkins, 2009, Figure 33-8.

A 13-12: From Lieberman M, Marks AD. Marks' Basic Medical Biochemistry: A Clinical Approach. 3rd Ed. Baltimore: Lippincott Williams & Wilkins, 2009, Figure 33-5.

A 13-13: From Lieberman M, Marks AD. Marks' Basic Medical Biochemistry: A Clinical Approach. 3rd Ed. Baltimore: Lippincott Williams & Wilkins, 2009, Figure 23-15.

A 13-15: From Lieberman M, Marks AD. Marks' Basic Medical Biochemistry: A Clinical Approach. 3rd Ed. Baltimore: Lippincott Williams & Wilkins, 2009, Figure 35-3.

A 13-18: From Lieberman M, Marks AD. Marks' Basic Medical Biochemistry: A Clinical Approach. 3rd Ed. Baltimore: Lippincott Williams & Wilkins, 2009. Figure 33-8.

Chapter 14

A 14-1: From Lieberman M, Marks AD. Marks' Basic Medical Biochemistry: A Clinical Approach. 3rd Ed. Baltimore: Lippincott Williams & Wilkins, 2009, Figure 46-5.

A 14-4: From Lieberman M, Marks AD. Marks' Basic Medical Biochemistry: A Clinical Approach. 3rd Ed. Baltimore: Lippincott Williams & Wilkins, 2009, Figure 29-8.

A 14-5: Modified from Lieberman M, Marks AD. Marks' Basic Medical Biochemistry: A Clinical Approach. 3rd Ed. Baltimore: Lippincott Williams & Wilkins, 2009, Figure 29-10.

A 14-6: Modified from Lieberman M, Marks AD. Marks' Basic Medical Biochemistry: A Clinical Approach. 3rd Ed. Baltimore: Lippincott Williams & Wilkins, 2009, Figure 29-10.

A 14-7: Modified from Lieberman M, Marks AD. Marks' Basic Medical Biochemistry: A Clinical Approach. 3rd Ed. Baltimore: Lippincott Williams & Wilkins, 2009, Figure 24-16.
A 14-9: From Lieberman M, Marks AD. Marks' Basic Medical Biochemistry: A Clinical Approach. 3rd Ed. Baltimore: Lippincott Williams & Wilkins, 2009, Figure 24-14A.
A 14-14: Modified from Lieberman M, Marks AD. Marks' Basic Medical Biochemistry: A Clinical Approach. 3rd Ed. Baltimore: Lippincott Williams & Wilkins, 2009, Figure 29-10.
A 14-16: Modified from Lieberman M, Marks AD. Marks' Basic Medical Biochemistry: A Clinical Approach. 3rd Ed. Baltimore: Lippincott Williams & Wilkins, 2009, Figure 29-10.
A 14-20: From Lieberman M, Marks AD. Marks' Basic Medical Biochemistry: A Clinical Approach. 3rd Ed. Baltimore: Lippincott Williams & Wilkins, 2009, Figure 37-6.

Chapter 15

Q 15-2: The image was provided by Steadman's.
A 15-1: From Lieberman M, Marks AD. Marks' Basic Medical Biochemistry: A Clinical Approach. 3rd Ed. Baltimore: Lippincott Williams & Wilkins, 2009, Figure 39-16.
A 15-3: From Lieberman M, Marks AD. Marks' Basic Medical Biochemistry: A Clinical Approach. 3rd Ed. Baltimore: Lippincott Williams & Wilkins, 2009, Figure 38-12.
A 15-4: From Lieberman M, Marks AD. Marks' Basic Medical Biochemistry: A Clinical Approach. 3rd Ed. Baltimore: Lippincott Williams & Wilkins, 2009, Figure 41-14.
A 15-5: From Lieberman M, Marks AD. Marks' Basic Medical Biochemistry: A Clinical Approach. 3rd Ed. Baltimore: Lippincott Williams & Wilkins, 2009, Figure 38-18.
A 15-6: From Lieberman M, Marks AD. Marks' Basic Medical Biochemistry: A Clinical Approach. 3rd Ed. Baltimore: Lippincott Williams & Wilkins, 2009, Figure 44-5.
A 15-8: From Lieberman M, Marks AD. Marks' Basic Medical Biochemistry: A Clinical Approach. 3rd Ed. Baltimore: Lippincott Williams & Wilkins, 2009, Figure 20-9.
A 15-12: From Lieberman M, Marks AD. Marks' Basic Medical Biochemistry: A Clinical Approach. 3rd Ed. Baltimore: Lippincott Williams & Wilkins, 2009, Figure 39-5.
A 15-14: From Lieberman M, Marks AD. Marks' Basic Medical Biochemistry: A Clinical Approach. 3rd Ed. Baltimore: Lippincott Williams & Wilkins, 2009, Figure 40-10.
A 15-15: From Lieberman M, Marks AD. Marks' Basic Medical Biochemistry: A Clinical Approach. 3rd Ed. Baltimore: Lippincott Williams & Wilkins, 2009, Figure 39-15.
A 15-16: Modified from Lieberman M, Marks AD. Marks' Basic Medical Biochemistry: A Clinical Approach. 3rd Ed. Baltimore: Lippincott Williams & Wilkins, 2009, Figure 48-7.
A 15-17: Modified from Lieberman M, Marks AD. Marks' Basic Medical Biochemistry: A Clinical Approach. 3rd Ed. Baltimore: Lippincott Williams & Wilkins, 2009, Figure 48-4.
A 15-18: Modified from Lieberman M, Marks AD. Marks' Basic Medical Biochemistry: A Clinical Approach. 3rd Ed. Baltimore: Lippincott Williams & Wilkins, 2009, Figures 48-6 and 48-7.

Chapter 16

Q 16-9: Image from Rubin E, Farber JL. Pathology. 3rd Ed. Philadelphia: Lippincott Williams & Wilkins, 1999, Figure 26-39.
A 16-1: From Smeltzer SC, Bare BG. Textbook of Medical-Surgical Nursing. 9th Ed. Philadelphia: Lippincott Williams & Wilkins, 2000, Figure 59-6.
A 16-3: From Lieberman M, Marks AD. Marks' Basic Medical Biochemistry: A Clinical Approach. 3rd Ed. Baltimore: Lippincott Williams & Wilkins, 2009:625.
A 16-4: From Lieberman M, Marks AD. Marks' Basic Medical Biochemistry: A Clinical Approach. 3rd Ed. Baltimore: Lippincott Williams & Wilkins, 2009:625.
A 16-6: Image from Rubin E, Farber JL. Pathology. 3rd Ed. Philadelphia: Lippincott Williams & Wilkins, 1999, Figure 6-24.
A 16-7: From Lieberman M, Marks AD. Marks' Basic Medical Biochemistry: A Clinical Approach. 3rd Ed. Baltimore: Lippincott Williams & Wilkins, 2009, Figure 30-18.
A 16-16: From Lieberman M, Marks AD. Marks' Basic Medical Biochemistry: A Clinical Approach. 3rd Ed. Baltimore: Lippincott Williams & Wilkins, 2009, Figure 49-8.
A 16-18: From Bear MF, Connors BW, Paradiso MA. Neuroscience: Exploring the Brain. 3rd Ed. Baltimore: Lippincott Williams & Wilkins, 2007, Figure 2-23.

Chapter 17

A 17-1: From Lieberman M, Marks AD. Marks' Basic Medical Biochemistry: A Clinical Approach. 3rd Ed. Baltimore: Lippincott Williams & Wilkins, 2009, Figure 32-6.
A 17-2: Modified from Lieberman M, Marks AD. Marks' Basic Medical Biochemistry: A Clinical Approach. 3rd Ed. Baltimore: Lippincott Williams & Wilkins, 2009, Figure 34-3.
A 17-3: From Lieberman M, Marks AD. Marks' Basic Medical Biochemistry: A Clinical Approach. 3rd Ed. Baltimore: Lippincott Williams & Wilkins, 2009, Figure 34-11.
A 17-5: From Lieberman M, Marks AD. Marks' Basic Medical Biochemistry: A Clinical Approach. 3rd Ed. Baltimore: Lippincott Williams & Wilkins, 2009, Figure 34-15.
A 17-7: From Lieberman M, Marks AD. Marks' Basic Medical Biochemistry: A Clinical Approach. 3rd Ed. Baltimore: Lippincott Williams & Wilkins, 2009, Figure 34-18.
A 17-8: From Lieberman M, Marks AD. Marks' Basic Medical Biochemistry: A Clinical Approach. 3rd Ed. Baltimore: Lippincott Williams & Wilkins, 2009, Figure 32-14.
A 17-12: Image from Anatomical Chart Company. Diseases and Disorders: The World's Best Anatomical Chart. 2nd Ed. Philadelphia: Lippincott Williams & Wilkins, 2005.

Chapter 18

A 18-1: From Lieberman M, Marks AD. Marks' Basic Medical Biochemistry: A Clinical Approach. 3rd Ed. Baltimore: Lippincott Williams & Wilkins, 2009, Figure 41-19.
A 18-2: Modified from Lieberman M, Marks AD. Marks' Basic Medical Biochemistry: A Clinical Approach. 3rd Ed. Baltimore: Lippincott Williams & Wilkins, 2009, Figure 40-2.
A 18-3: From Lieberman M, Marks AD. Marks' Basic Medical Biochemistry: A Clinical Approach. 3rd Ed. Baltimore: Lippincott Williams & Wilkins, 2009, Figure 41-1.
A 18-4: Modified from Lieberman M, Marks AD. Marks' Basic Medical Biochemistry: A Clinical Approach. 3rd Ed. Baltimore: Lippincott Williams & Wilkins, 2009, Figure 40-5.
A 18-6: From Lieberman M, Marks AD. Marks' Basic Medical Biochemistry: A Clinical Approach. 3rd Ed. Baltimore: Lippincott Williams & Wilkins, 2009, Figure 41-16.
A 18-10: From Lieberman M, Marks AD. Marks' Basic Medical Biochemistry: A Clinical Approach. 3rd Ed. Baltimore: Lippincott Williams & Wilkins, 2009, Figure 41-10.
A 18-12: From Lieberman M, Marks AD. Marks' Basic Medical Biochemistry: A Clinical Approach. 3rd Ed. Baltimore: Lippincott Williams & Wilkins, 2009, Figure 41-19.
A 18-18: Modified from Lieberman M, Marks AD. Marks' Basic Medical Biochemistry: A Clinical Approach. 3rd Ed. Baltimore: Lippincott Williams & Wilkins, 2009, Figure 40-4.

Chapter 19

A 19-3: From Lieberman M, Marks AD. Marks' Basic Medical Biochemistry: A Clinical Approach. 3rd Ed. Baltimore: Lippincott Williams & Wilkins, 2009, Figure 29-4.
A 19-4: From Lieberman M, Marks AD. Marks' Basic Medical Biochemistry: A Clinical Approach. 3rd Ed. Baltimore: Lippincott Williams & Wilkins, 2009, Figure 47-5.
A 19-6: From Champe PC, Harvey RA, Ferrier DR. Lippincott's Illustrated Review of Biochemistry. 3rd Ed. Baltimore: Lippincott Williams & Wilkins, 2009, Figure 23-3.
A 19-10: From Lieberman M, Marks AD. Marks' Basic Medical Biochemistry: A Clinical Approach. 3rd Ed. Baltimore: Lippincott Williams & Wilkins, 2009, Figure 33-35.

Chapter 20

A 20-4: Modified from Lieberman M, Marks AD. Marks' Basic Medical Biochemistry: A Clinical Approach. 3rd Ed. Baltimore: Lippincott Williams & Wilkins, 2009, Figure 33-16.

A 20-6: From Lieberman M, Marks AD. Marks' Basic Medical Biochemistry: A Clinical Approach. 3rd Ed. Baltimore: Lippincott Williams & Wilkins, 2009, Figure 40-10.
A 20-7: From Lieberman M, Marks AD. Marks' Basic Medical Biochemistry: A Clinical Approach. 3rd Ed. Baltimore: Lippincott Williams & Wilkins, 2009, Figure 40-4.
A 20-9: Modified from Lieberman M, Marks AD. Marks' Basic Medical Biochemistry: A Clinical Approach. 3rd Ed. Baltimore: Lippincott Williams & Wilkins, 2009, Figures 26-8 and 26-12.
A 20-11: From Lieberman M, Marks AD. Marks' Basic Medical Biochemistry: A Clinical Approach. 3rd Ed. Baltimore: Lippincott Williams & Wilkins, 2009, Figure 48-7.
A 20-15: From Lieberman M, Marks AD. Marks' Basic Medical Biochemistry: A Clinical Approach. 3rd Ed. Baltimore: Lippincott Williams & Wilkins, 2009, Figure 34-26.
A 20-16: Modified from Lieberman M, Marks AD. Marks' Basic Medical Biochemistry: A Clinical Approach. 3rd Ed. Baltimore: Lippincott Williams & Wilkins, 2009, Figure 45-5.
A 20-18: From Lieberman M, Marks AD. Marks' Basic Medical Biochemistry: A Clinical Approach. 3rd Ed. Baltimore: Lippincott Williams & Wilkins, 2009, Figure 25-7.
A 20-20: From Lieberman M, Marks AD. Marks' Basic Medical Biochemistry: A Clinical Approach. 3rd Ed. Baltimore: Lippincott Williams & Wilkins, 2009, Figure 40-8.

Chapter 21

Q 21-20: Image from Rubin E, Farber JL. Pathology. 3rd Ed. Philadelphia: Lippincott Williams & Wilkins, 1999, Figure 9-9.
A 21-12: Image from Rubin E, Farber JL. Pathology. 3rd Ed. Philadelphia: Lippincott Williams & Wilkins, 1999, Figure 5-25A.
A 21-13: From Lieberman M, Marks AD. Marks' Basic Medical Biochemistry: A Clinical Approach. 3rd Ed. Baltimore: Lippincott Williams & Wilkins, 2009, Figure 18-8.
A 21-19: Modified from Lieberman M, Marks AD. Marks' Basic Medical Biochemistry: A Clinical Approach. 3rd Ed. Baltimore: Lippincott Williams & Wilkins, 2009, Figure 44.18A.
A 21-20: Adapted from Rubin E, Farber JL. Pathology. 3rd Ed. Philadelphia: Lippincott Williams & Wilkins, 1999, Figure 5-25B.

Index

Page numbers in *italics* denote figures; those followed by a t denote tables